Nephrology: A Case Study Approach

Nephrology: A Case Study Approach

Editor: Hudson Palmer

AMERICAN
MEDICAL PUBLISHERS
www.americanmedicalpublishers.com

AMERICAN
MEDICAL PUBLISHERS
www.americanmedicalpublishers.com

Cataloging-in-Publication Data

Nephrology: a case study approach / edited by Hudson Palmer.
p. cm.
Includes bibliographical references and index.
ISBN 979-8-88740-646-6
1. Nephrology. 2. Kidneys--Diseases. 3. Kidneys--Diseases--Treatment. I. Palmer, Hudson.
RC903 .N47 2023
616.61-dc23

American Medical Publishers,
41 Flatbush Avenue,
1st Floor, New York,
NY 11217, USA

ISBN 979-8-88740-646-6 (Hardback)

Contents

Preface

The branch of medicine which deals with the causes, diagnosis and treatment of various kidney diseases and disorders is known as nephrology. Some of the prominent causes of kidney diseases are kidney stones, diabetes, hypertension, glomerulonephritis and polycystic kidney disease. There are various treatment approaches which are used within this field such as medications, dialysis and kidney transplantation. Medications can be used to manage the underlying causes and symptoms of kidney diseases. They are also used to control blood pressure, manage diabetes, reduce inflammation and treat infections. Dialysis is a treatment that performs the functions of the kidneys artificially when they are unable to do so effectively. It involves removing waste products and excess fluids from the blood using a machine. This book provides comprehensive insights into the field of nephrology. It is appropriate for students seeking detailed information in this area of medicine as well as for experts.

This book has been the outcome of endless efforts put in by authors and researchers on various issues and topics within the field. The book is a comprehensive collection of significant researches that are addressed in a variety of chapters. It will surely enhance the knowledge of the field among readers across the globe.

It gives us an immense pleasure to thank our researchers and authors for their efforts to submit their piece of writing before the deadlines. Finally in the end, I would like to thank my family and colleagues who have been a great source of inspiration and support.

Editor

1

Coexistence of Lupus Nephritis, Ulcerative Colitis and Communicating Hydrocephalus: A Report of a 21-Year-Old Male

Bushra Ali Khan, Nida Saleem, Danyal Hassan, Shabaz Kiani, and Muhammad Haneef

Shifa International Hospital, H-8/4, Pitras Bukhari Road, Islamabad, Pakistan

Correspondence should be addressed to Nida Saleem; nidasaa1968@gmail.com

Academic Editor: Sophia Lionaki

Systemic lupus erythematosus (SLE) and ulcerative colitis (UC) are multisystem autoimmune disorders that rarely coexist. We report a case history of a 21-year-old male, presenting with bloody diarrhea and, later, diagnosed to have ulcerative colitis on colonic biopsy. There was clinically silent renal impairment leading to end-stage kidney disease requiring hemodialysis possibly secondary to ongoing lupus nephritis as suggested by positive lupus-specific antibodies' detection. Besides this, the diagnosis of lupus associated with early communicating hydrocephalus was made on CT brain findings which clinically responded well to the initiation of immunosuppressive therapy. It is imperative to keep in mind the remote possibility of ulcerative colitis in an SLE patient with gastrointestinal (GI) manifestations. Communicating hydrocephalus is a rare neurological manifestation of SLE leading to seizures and can respond well to the initiation of steroids and immunosuppressants. Therefore, a trial of immunosuppressant medications must be given even in a patient with end-stage renal disease (ESRD) to halter extra renal rare lupus manifestations.

1. Introduction

Inflammatory bowel disease is a recurrent inflammatory autoimmune disorder involving gastrointestinal mucosa, and it includes Crohn's disease and ulcerative colitis [1]. SLE is an immune complex-mediated disorder common in women of reproductive age group. Although it has been known that many autoimmune disorders coexist, yet, coexistence of SLE and ulcerative colitis has rarely been reported. The reported prevalence of these two disorders is only 0.4% [1, 2]. These two autoimmune disorders share certain common features [3]. In SLE, gastrointestinal manifestations are very common which might be secondary to the disease itself, superimposed infections, or side effects of immunosuppressant medications. SLE can lead to gastrointestinal (GI) vasculitis, peritonitis, pancreatitis, mesenteric ischemia, peptic ulcer disease, acalculous cholecystitis, pseudo-obstruction, and lupus enteritis [4]. Similarly, there are certain manifestations of ulcerative colitis that are similar to SLE. These include oral ulcers and arthritis [3], thus making diagnosis of these coexistent autoimmune disorders extremely difficult.

Although the reported prevalence of neuropsychiatric manifestations of SLE is 50% which include stroke, meningitis, movement disorders, myelopathy, and psychiatric features, the occurrence of communicating hydrocephalus is extremely rare. So far, only a few case series and reports are available [5]. It has been seen that, in patients with coexistent SLE and ulcerative colitis, the overall course of SLE is benign with no marked renal impairment [2] and neurological involvement [3]. However, we report a rare case of coexistent SLE with clinical presentation of ulcerative colitis in a 21-year-old male, requiring permanent hemodialysis secondary to possible lupus nephritis and also who developed lupus-induced nonobstructive hydrocephalus clinically responding well to immunosuppressive therapy.

2. Case

A 21-year-old male, an average student, with no previous comorbidities, was on hearing aid due to hearing impairment noted after several months of a noneventful birth. He was born at 38 weeks of gestation with average birth parameters including weight and height and no immediate developmental abnormality. No family history of hearing loss and chronic kidney disease or ESRD was found among family members. During this admission, he presented with a complaint of bloody diarrhea for one month. Diarrhea was watery in consistency, containing clots of blood, and had a frequency of 7-8 times per day. He initially went to a local hospital, and colonoscopy and colonic biopsy were done, approximately after 20 days of the onset of symptoms. The colonoscopy report showed inflamed and edematous colonic mucosa with multiple bleeding ulcers. The histopathological report showed evidence of focal active colitis with crypt abscess. In order to manage him in lines of inflammatory bowel disease, he was started on tablet mesalazine, loperamide, pantoprazole, rifaximin, and mebeverine. However, he remained noncompliant with medications, and his bloody diarrhea persisted.

Later, he was brought to the Shifa International Hospital emergency department (ER) in a severely dehydrated state with altered mental status. As per the family, there were complaints of generalized weakness, drowsiness, reduced appetite, hiccups, and decrease in the urine output for 1 day. He also had off and on pain in both knee joints for the last 45 days. However, there were no complaints of vomiting, abdominal pain, and fever. He was semioriented and semiresponsive. His vitals at the time of presentation showed a blood pressure of 110/60 mmHg and pulse of 110/min, and he was afebrile. He was clinically pale with sunken eyes and reduced skin turgor. There were no skin rashes, oral ulcers, and enlarged lymph nodes. His systemic examination was unremarkable. He was catheterized immediately, and 500 ml bolus of bicarbonate-based IV fluid was given. His laboratory investigations were sent, which are summarized in Table 1.

Ultrasound of the abdomen was performed in the ER which showed bilateral small echogenic kidneys with grade III renal parenchymal echogenicity as shown in Figure 1.

Given the degree of chronicity and severe metabolic and electrolyte abnormalities, urgent hemodialysis was initiated in the ER via the left femoral temporary dialysis catheter. First session was performed for 2 hours due to marked hyponatremia and uremia with one pack of blood transfusion. He was started on intravenous meropenem and vancomycin given the raised inflammatory and infectious markers.

After a total of 3 sessions of hemodialysis, his conscious level improved. His BUN improved to 77 mg/dL and sodium to 132 mEq/L over 72 hours. Creatinine improved to 4.58 mg/dL and bicarbonate to 22 mEq/L.

In order to identify the exact cause of his renal impairment, his autoimmune workup was sent, which is shown in Table 2.

Table 2 shows low c3 levels and positive ANA, anti-double-stranded (ds) DNA, anti-Golgi apparatus antibodies, and anti-Smith antibodies consistent with the diagnosis of SLE.

Regarding systemic lupus erythematosus (SLE) further management, the rheumatology and gastroenterology departments were taken on board. The patient was initiated on intravenous methylprednisolone pulse therapy which was given at a dose of 500 mg once daily for 5 days, along with mycophenolate mofetil (MMF) at a dose of 1 g twice daily and hydroxychloroquine (HCQ) 200 mg once daily.

A repeat colonoscopy with colonic biopsy was performed. On colonoscopy, multiple ulcers were present throughout the colon, more marked in the terminal ileum leading to narrowing and deformation of the ileocecal valve. Beside pulse methylprednisolone, the patient was prescribed per oral tablet mesalazine 1 g thrice daily.

The histopathology report of the terminal ileum and colonic biopsy showed evidence of moderate chronic active colitis consistent with ulcerative colitis, along with ulceration of colonic mucosa with slough formation and mucin depletion. Besides this, cryptitis and crypt abscesses were also seen. There was evidence of mixed inflammatory infiltrates composed of lymphocytes, plasma cells, neutrophils, and eosinophils in the lamina propria. These findings are shown in Figure 2.

Later on, during the hospital stay, the patient had one episode of generalized tonic clonic seizure associated with frothing from the mouth and uprolling of eyes. While being managed in the Neurology ICU, he suffered two more episodes of seizures, which were settled with intravenous diazepam. Neurology team was taken on board, and levetiracetam was given intravenously at a loading dose and then continued at a maintenance dose. EEG and plain CT scan brain were performed.

CT scan brain without contrast showed evidence of early communicating hydrocephalus. There was dilatation of lateral, third, and fourth ventricles with rounding of frontal horns and empty sella. However, posterior fossa structures including the cerebellum and CP angle cisterns were unremarkable. CT image of the patient is shown in Figure 3.

At that time, his serum sodium was 125 mEq/L, serum magnesium was 1.6 mg/dL, and serum calcium level was also 7.3 mg/dL. Electrolyte imbalance was corrected in the ICU setting, and intravenous mannitol was also given. Lumbar puncture was also advised by the neurological team to rule out the possibility of meningitis. However, the family refused due to financial issues. As the patient's condition stabilized, he was transferred back to the ward after 24–48 hours. His temporary dialysis catheter was then removed, and later on, the right internal jugular tunneled catheter was inserted.

With the initiation of immunosuppressive therapy, antiseizure medications, and correction of electrolyte imbalance and uremia, the patient's level of consciousness improved to his baseline normal. Frequency of diarrhea also reduced, and seizures subsided on per oral levetiracetam; therefore, he got discharged on MMF, hydroxychloroquine (HCQ), levetiracetam, calcium carbonate, calcium acetate, erythropoietin, mesalazine, pantoprazole, and prednisolone.

After two weeks, on follow-up visit, he had gained weight as his appetite improved, and his diarrhea settled, with no

Table 1: Postadmission laboratory investigations.

Hemoglobin (g/dL)	7.1	Serum sodium (mEq/L)	119
Total leucocyte count (cells/cmm)	9490	Serum bicarbonate (mEq/L)	9
Platelet count (cells/uL)	201000	Serum potassium (mEq/L)	5.2
Folic acid	3.1	Serum chloride (mEq/L)	97
Vitamin B12 levels	189	Serum creatinine (mg/dL)	17.2
TSAT	32.5%	BUN (mg/dL)	140
Coagulation profile	Negative	Serum calcium (mg/dL)	7.3
ESR (mm/hour)	140	Serum phosphorous (mg/dL)	4.2
CRP (mg/L)	95.38	Serum albumin (mg/dL)	1.7
Procalcitonin	19.22	Urine R/E	Protein: +, blood: +++, RBCs: 20–25/HPF, WBCs: 1-2/HPF
Stool R/E	No cyst, ovum, or worm	Spot urine protein-to-creatinine ratio	2.2 g/g
Stool for CMV	Negative	Blood C/S	Negative
QuantiFERON-TB	Negative	Urine C/S	Negative
Serum chloride (mEq/L)	97		

ESR: erythrocyte sedimentation rate; R/E: routine examination; RBCs: red blood cells; WBCs: white blood cells; CMV: cytomegalovirus; BUN: blood urea nitrogen.

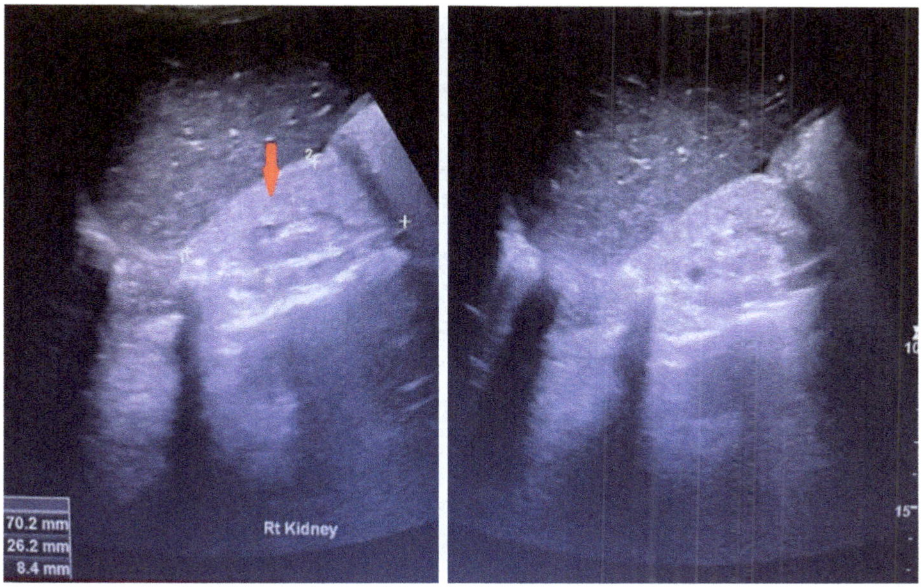

Figure 1: Grade III echogenic right kidney, 70.2 × 26.2 × 8.4 mm in dimensions (red arrow).

Table 2: Autoimmune workup.

ANA	Positive (1 : 80)	Anti-dsDNA antibodies (IU/mL)	Positive (55)
C3	0.67	Anti-Smith antibodies (U/mL)	Positive (37)
c-ANCA	Negative	Antihistone antibodies	Negative
p-ANCA	Negative	Hepatitis B S Ag	Negative
Anti-GBM	Negative	Hepatitis C antibodies	Negative
Anticardiolipin antibodies	Negative	Antilupus anticoagulant antibodies	Negative
Anti-beta-2 glycoprotein antibodies	Negative	Anti-Golgi apparatus antibodies	Positive (1 : 160)

c3: complement-3; p-ANCA: perinuclear antineutrophilic cytoplasmic antibodies; c-ANCA: circulating antineutrophilic cytoplasmic antibodies; ANA: antinuclear antibody; S Ag: surface antigen; ds: double-stranded; anti-GBM: antiglomerular basement membrane antibodies.

seizure activity reported with baseline normal mental status. All his laboratory parameters including CRP and procalcitonin improved. The patient was continued on the tapering dose of steroids, MMF, HCQ, levetiracetam, and erythropoietin and was instructed to continue regular hemodialysis sessions.

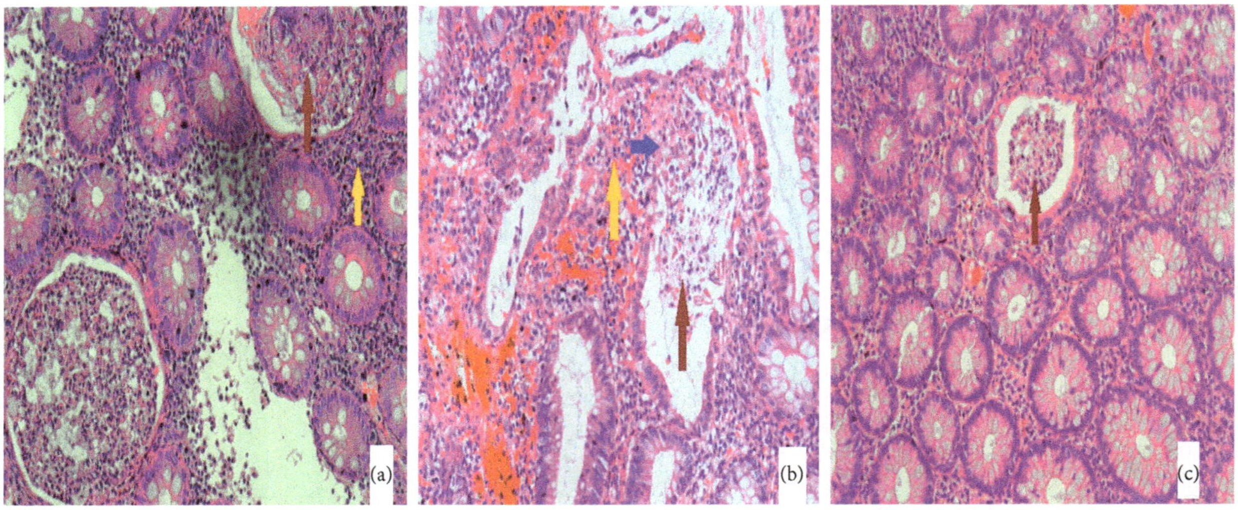

FIGURE 2: (40x): hematoxylin-and-eosin-stained light microscopic images (a–c). Evidence of crypt abscesses (maroon arrow), marked lymphocytic infiltration of the lamina propria (yellow arrow), and colonic mucosal ulceration with mucin depletion.

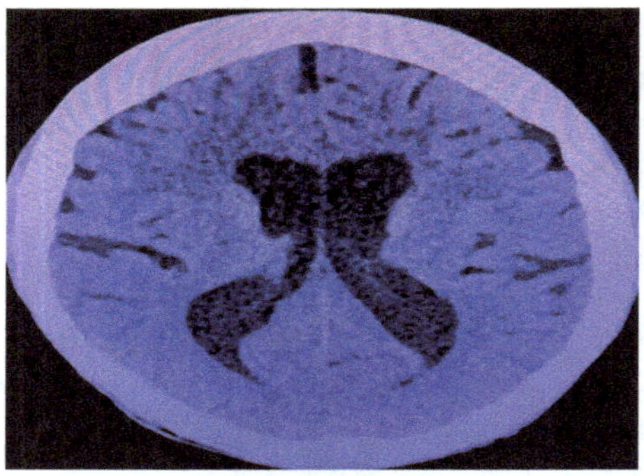

FIGURE 3: Dilated lateral ventricle consistent with hydrocephalus.

Unfortunately, a repeat CT brain was not done due to noncompliance and reluctance on part of the family due to financial strains.

3. Discussion

In summary, we report the first case of lupus nephritis leading to ESRD and communicating hydrocephalus with coexistent ulcerative colitis that has responded well to initiation of steroids and immunosuppressive medications.

It has been suggested as per findings of previously reported cases that SLE precedes ulcerative colitis by several years and usually remains clinically silent with less frequent arthritis, serositis, and other systemic manifestations [2]. Our case history supports this preposition as our patient has clinically silent SLE leading to possible lupus-induced renal impairment, which, later, was diagnosed on a detailed autoimmune workup suggestive of SLE. However, biopsy-proven confirmation of lupus nephritis was not possible due to bilateral shrunken grade-3 echogenic kidneys.

As per previously studied data, it has been suggested that SLE usually runs an indolent course if it coexists with ulcerative colitis; so far, no reported data of severe renal and neurological involvement were obtained [2]. In one systemic review of 9 diagnosed cases of coexistent UC and SLE, not even a single neurological manifestation and dialysis-dependent marked renal impairment was reported [3]. However, as seen from our patient, we can suggest that coexistent UC and SLE can lead to marked renal impairment and even neurological involvement.

Regarding the autoimmune profile, it has been suggested that anti-dsDNA antibodies are positive in 100% of previously reported cases [2, 3], and anti-LA antibodies [6] are also positive in the majority of cases. The finding of anti-dsDNA positivity seen in our patient is consistent with this preposition.

It is well known that the use of certain drugs for the treatment of ulcerative colitis such as sulfasalazine can lead to drug-induced lupus [1, 7]. Furthermore, the use of infliximab for ulcerative colitis has also been associated with the development of hydrocephalus [8]. However, our patient has already developed ESRD prior to mesalazine use, and infliximab has not been prescribed to our patient, thus ruling out these two possibilities.

In SLE, the possible causes of hydrocephalus include superimposed intracranial opportunistic infection, cerebral phlebitis, antiphospholipid antibody (APLA) [9] mediated cerebral venous thrombosis, aseptic meningitis, SLE-induced vasculitis with subarachnoid hemorrhage [5], and postinflammatory aqueductal stenosis [10]. Moreover, the pathological mechanism of SLE-induced hydrocephalus can either be due to direct neuronal and vascular damage or immune complex-mediated and hypercoagulability-induced damage to arachnoid villi, leading to the obstruction of CSF outflow. In our case, the second mechanism is likely a contributing factor in the development of communicating hydrocephalus. However, due to refusal of lumbar puncture and CSF analysis, the possibility of infection-induced nonobstructive hydrocephalus cannot be ruled out. In our patient, the negative APLA antibody workup and coagulation profile are suggestive of non-APLA-associated communicating hydrocephalus.

Regarding the treatment of autoimmune disorder-induced hydrocephalus, several options have been proposed. These include medical management with or without ventriculoperitoneal (VP) shunting [5]. Steroids have been considered as the cornerstone of medical management in autoimmune disorder-induced hydrocephalus. However, the reported outcome has been much better with VP shunting as compared to medical management [5]. As our patient had early-onset communicating hydrocephalus and seizures with coexistent electrolyte abnormalities, therefore, we had given a trial of medical management with simultaneous correction of electrolyte imbalances. Unfortunately, a repeat CT brain was not done due to noncompliance and reluctance on part of the family due to financial strains. Hence, we cannot for sure report an improvement in hydrocephalus, though the patient's clinical improvement may suggest an improvement in the neurological involvement of SLE and hydrocephalus.

The major limitation of this case report is the lack of histopathological confirmation of lupus nephritis due to evidence of bilateral grade-3 echogenic, shrunken kidneys which can predispose to postprocedure complications. However, the presence of positivity of ANA, anti-dsDNA, anti-Smith, and anti-Golgi apparatus antibodies along with hypocomplementemia, proteinuria, and hematuria is highly suggestive of the likely diagnosis of lupus nephritis.

4. Conclusion

From this case description, it can be concluded that SLE and ulcerative colitis can coexist, though rarely as suggested by the previous case reports. Therefore, in an SLE patient with GI manifestation, the remote possibility of UC must be kept in mind. As reported previously, SLE usually runs an indolent course, though, in our case, we have shown that SLE can present with severe symptoms including renal insufficiency and ESRD. Although hydrocephalus is a rare manifestation of SLE, depending on the patient's symptoms and severity of ventricular dilatation, decision must be made promptly whether to manage it medically alone or with surgical intervention. However, in less severe cases, a trial of steroids and immunosuppressant medications can be considered alone.

References

[1] K. H. Katsanos, P. V. Voulgari, and E. V. Tsianos, "Inflammatory bowel disease and lupus a systematic review of the literature," *Journal of Crohn's and Colitis*, vol. 6, no. 7, pp. 735–742, 2012.

[2] D. Medeiros and D. Isenberg, "Systemic lupus erythematosus and ulcerative colitis," *Lupus*, vol. 18, no. 8, pp. 762-763, 2009.

[3] O. Nitzan, M. Elias, and W. R. Saliba, "Systemic lupus erythematosus and inflammatory bowel disease," *European Journal of Internal Medicine*, vol. 17, no. 5, pp. 313–318, 2006.

[4] M. C. Abdulla and M. EJIJoS, "Lupus enteritis—an unusual cause for acute abdominal pain," pp. 1–3, 2020.

[5] B. Ma, H. Wu, H. Yin et al., "Management of hydrocephalus associated with autoimmune diseases: a series of 19 cases," *Autoimmunity*, vol. 50, no. 7, pp. 422–427, 2017.

[6] H. E. Mansour, S. G. Arafa, and W. A. Shehata, "Systemic lupus erythematosus with inflammatory bowel disease-ulcerative colitis: case report," *Lupus*, vol. 27, no. 7, pp. 1198–1201, 2018.

[7] I. D. Griffiths and S. P. Kane, "Sulphasalazine-induced lupus syndrome in ulcerative colitis," *BMJ*, vol. 2, no. 6096, pp. 1188-1189, 1977.

[8] A. Maclennan, M. D. Long, and H. H. Herfarth, "Development of communicating hydrocephalus after infliximab infusion," *Inflammatory Bowel Diseases*, vol. 17, no. 2, pp. E2–E3, 2011.

[9] P. R. Mortifee, R. A. Bebb, and H. Stein, "Communicating hydrocephalus in systemic lupus erythematosus with antiphospholipid antibody syndrome," *Journal of Rheumatology*, vol. 19, no. 8, pp. 1299–1302, 1992.

[10] R. Nayak, J. N. Behera, A. Mallick, and S. Mohapatra, "Communicating hydrocephalus in systemic lupus erythematosus," *Indian Pediatrics*, vol. 51, no. 7, pp. 577-578, 2014.

2

Two Cases of Strictures after Percutaneous CT-Guided Radiofrequency Ablation for Renal Cell Carcinoma

Ortwin Heißler, [1] **Stephan Seklehner**, [1,2] **Maximilian Fingernagel**, [1] **Paul F. Engelhardt**, [1,2] **and Claus Riedl** [1]

[1] *Department of Urology, Landesklinikum Baden-Mödling, Baden, Austria*
[2] *Paracelsus Medical University, Salzburg, Austria*

Correspondence should be addressed to Ortwin Heißler; ortwin@heissler.at

Academic Editor: Fumitaka Koga

Percutaneous radiofrequency ablation is a safe and effective minimally invasive treatment option in selected patients with T1a tumors of the kidney with a low complication rate. We describe two cases that developed the rare but severe complication of thermal injury-induced strictures of the upper urinary tract and its consecutive management.

1. Introduction

Percutaneous radiofrequency ablation (RFA) has proven to be a safe and effective treatment option for small renal masses (T1a) in selected patients [1]. The European Association of Urology (EAU) 2018 guidelines list RFA as an alternative treatment option to nephron-sparing surgery [2].

RFA induces thermal destruction of tumor cells at temperatures of approximately 100°C. Tumors are ablated by convective heat in concentric spheric zones around the RFA needle, so the risk of nontarget thermal damage of adjacent organs, e.g., bowel and ureter, needs to be taken into consideration. Pyelocalyceal injuries leading to stricture formation or ureteric strictures that require surgical, endoscopic, or radiological intervention are rare with a percentage of up to 4% [3].

We report the cases of two patients who developed asymptomatic hydronephrosis and kidney function deterioration as a result of stricture formation induced by nontarget thermal injury and its management.

2. Case Report One

A 70-year-old man underwent percutaneous RFA of an 18 mm renal tumor (Figure 1), after detailed explanation about risks, benefits, and the possibility of active surveillance, which he refused. The tumor was located medially in a duplex kidney with a ureter fissus to the level of lumbar vertebral body III. Biopsy was taken prior to RFA, showing a papillary renal cell carcinoma (RCC), Type 1, Fuhrman nuclear grade 1.

Since the patient wanted active treatment, percutaneous RFA was suggested because of significant comorbidities (coronary heart disease with a history of myocardial infarction and implantation of two coronary stents, arterial hypertension, and an increased body mass index) classified as ASA III.

In December 2016, a percutaneous CT-guided RFA (Modell 1500 RF Generator, 25 cm StarBurst XL Semi-Flex RFA Device, AngioDynamics, Queensbury, NY, USA) with two overlapping ablation zones, each 4 cm in diameter, with an average ablation temperature of 105°C and an ablation duration of eight and ten minutes was performed (Figures 1(b) and 1(c)). A final CT scan, excluding postinterventional urinoma, perirenal bleeding, hydronephrosis, and pneumothorax, was performed, and the patient was discharged on the first postinterventional day.

After four months, he was referred by his urologist because of an asymptomatic de novo hydronephrosis of the upper as well as the lower part of the duplex kidney and elevated serum creatinine that had increased from 1.3 mg/dl before RFA to 2.1 mg/dl.

A retrograde pyelography was performed, showing hydronephrosis of the upper part of the kidney and a jet

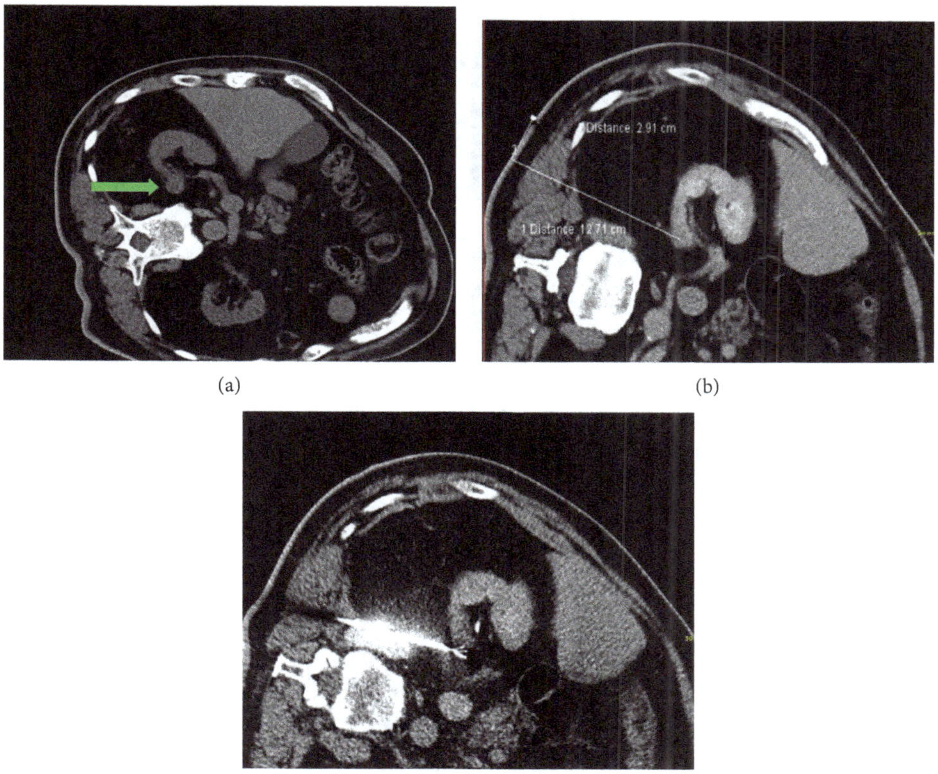

(a) (b) (c)

Figure 1: (a) 18 mm medially located tumor of the right kidney. (b) Planning the optimal ablation needle insertion path. (c) Placing the needle electrode into the tumor under image guidance.

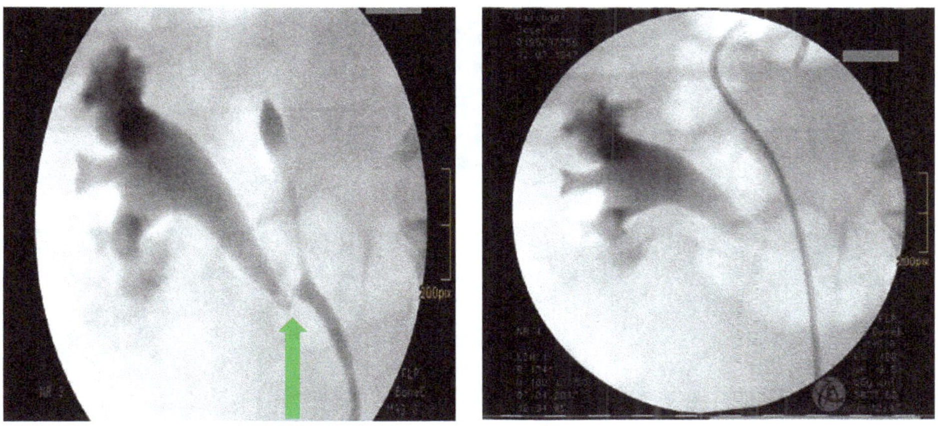

(a) (b)

Figure 2: (a) Ureteral stricture on retrograde pyelogram. (b) Insertion of a double-J stent in the upper part of the duplex kidney.

phenomenon into the lower part, which was also dilated (Figure 2(a)). Semirigid ureteroscopy, using a 8/9.8-French ureteroscope (Wolf, Germany), failed due to a stenosis caused by scar tissue, but a guidewire could be placed in the upper part of the duplex kidney, and consecutively, a 7-French ureteral stent was placed via this guidewire (Figure 2(b)).

As the placement of the ureteral stent did not result in a decline of serum creatinine, a 10-French nephrostomy tube was additionally placed under ultrasound guidance in the dilated lower part of the duplex kidney.

After drainage of both collecting systems of the duplex kidney, serum creatinine levels decreased to 1.9 mg/dl and remained stable during follow-up.

One week after the second procedure, an antegrade nephrostogram was performed, which showed an undisturbed contrast agent discharge into the urinary bladder (with the double-J stent still in place) (Figure 3). Consequently, the

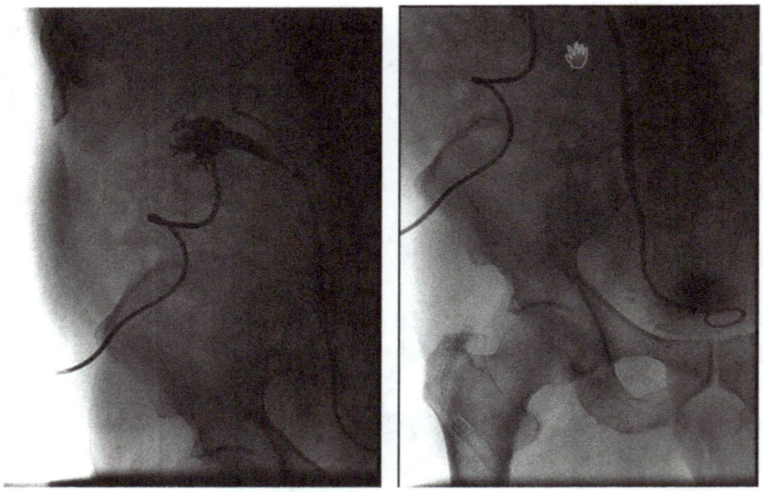

Figure 3: Antegrade nephrostogram with undisturbed contrast medium outflow through the lower kidney cavity system with the double-J stent still in situ.

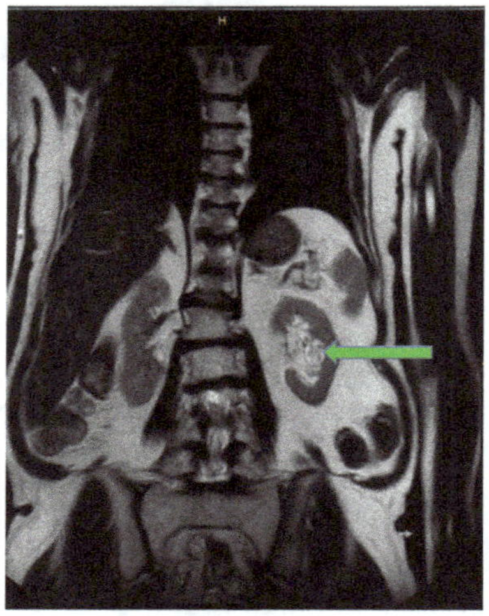

(a)

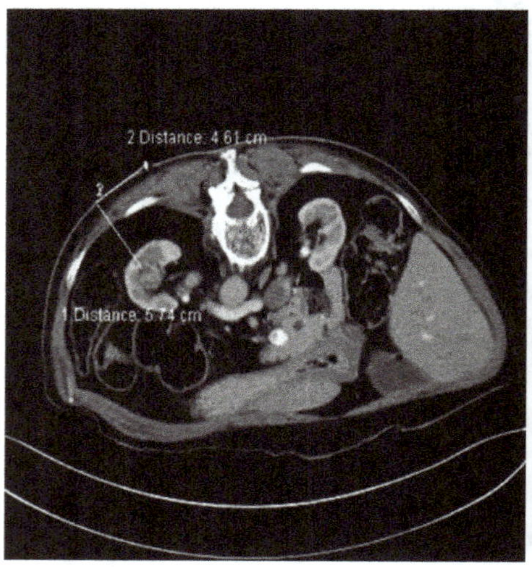

(b)

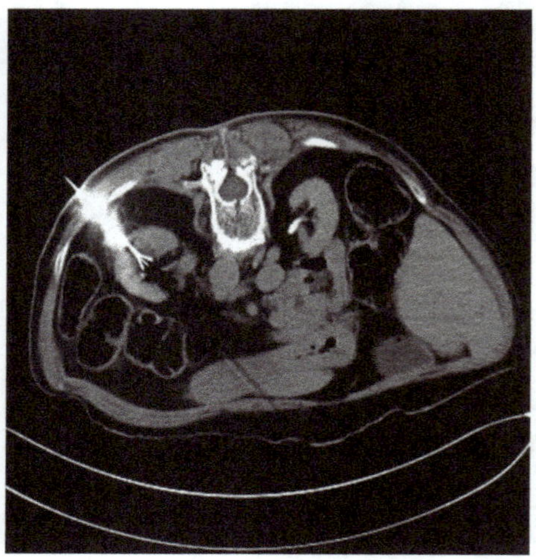

(c)

Figure 4: (a) 2 cm centrally located tumor of the left kidney before percutaneous RFA. (b) Planning the optimal ablation needle insertion path. (c) Needle with fully extended tine electrodes placed in the tumor.

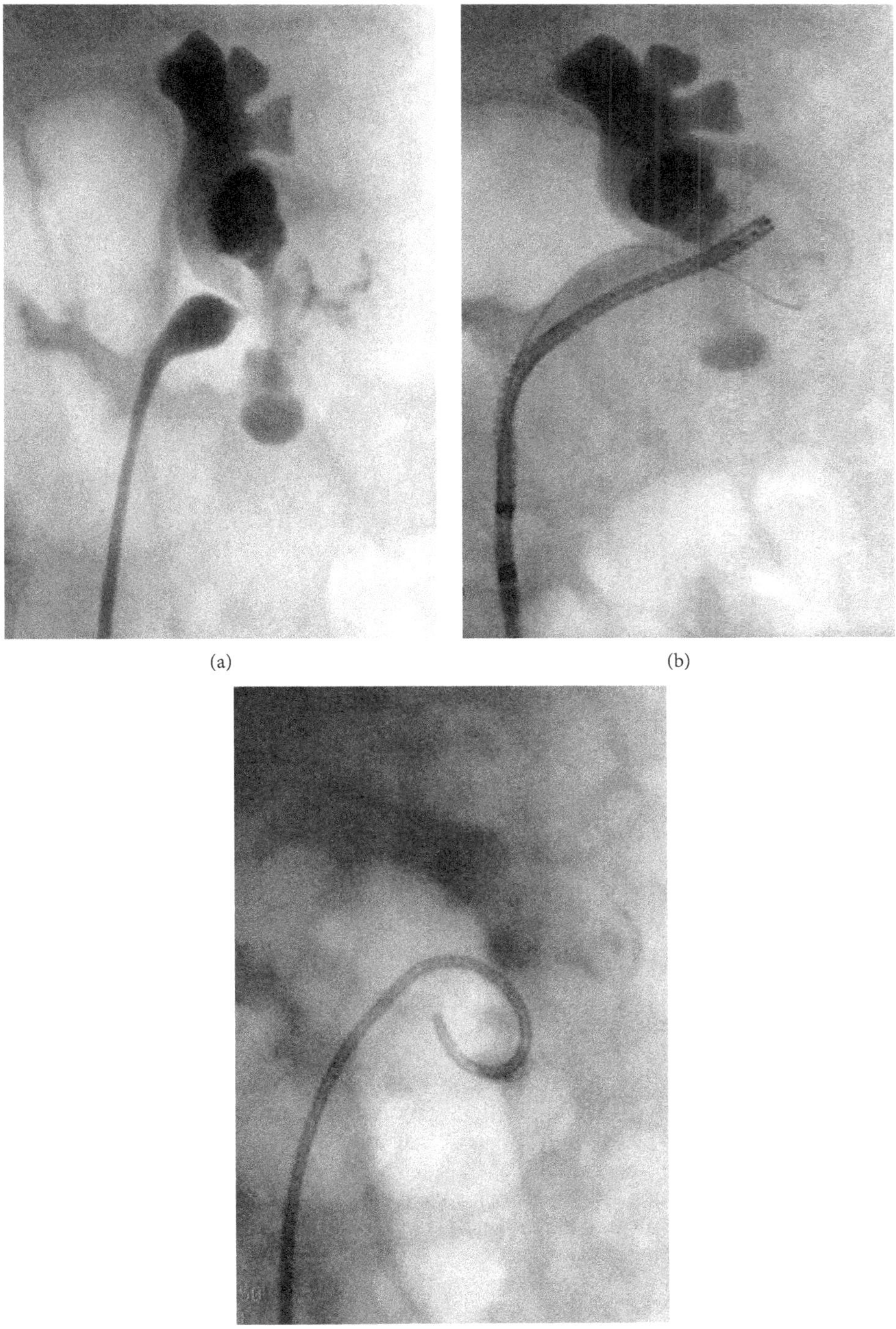

(a) (b) (c)

FIGURE 5: (a) Filiform stenosis at the pyeloureteral junction on retrograde pyelogram. (b) Approach of the middle calyx with flexible ureterorenoscope. (c) Insertion of a double-J stent in the lower calyx.

nephrostomy tube was removed. The double-J stent was removed one month later.

Follow-up magnetic resonance imaging showed no RCC recurrence two years after RFA, the upper part of the duplex kidney was still dilated, the lower part showed no hydronephrosis with stable creatinine level at 1.9 mg/dl, and the patient remained asymptomatic.

3. Case Report Two

Four months after an uncomplicated percutaneous CT-guided RFA (at the request of the patient and performed in the same fashion as described in case 1) of a two-centimeter, biopsy-proven centrally located papillary RCC in the middle third of the left kidney (Figures 4(a)–4(c)), a 78-year-old

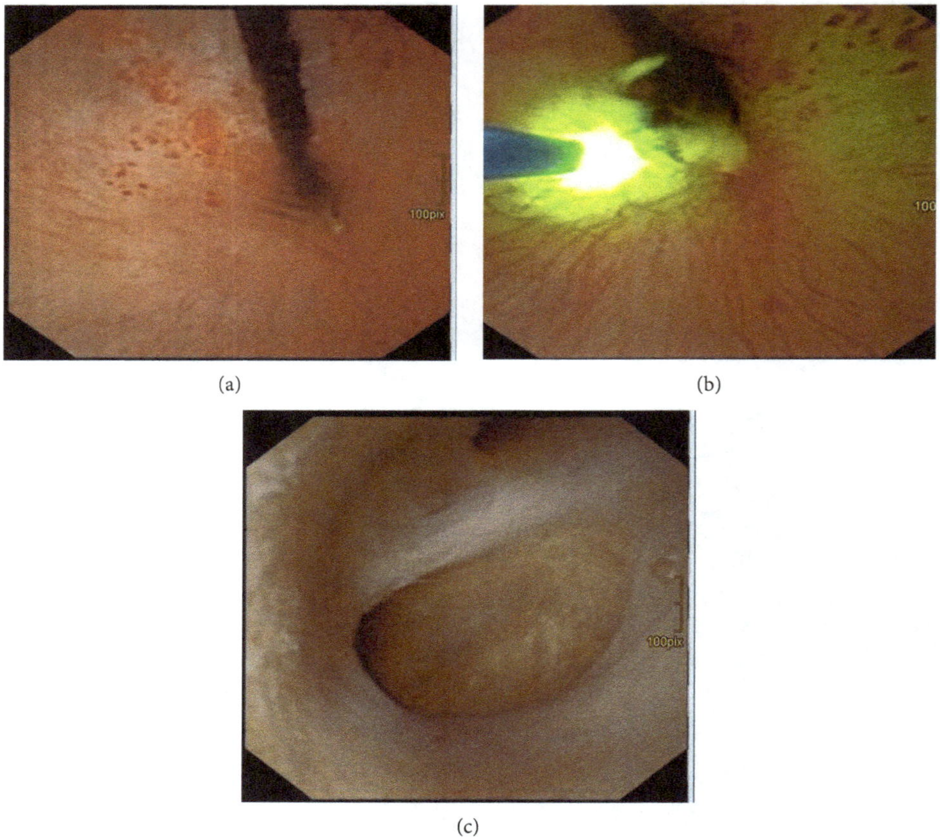

Figure 6: (a) Filiform stenosis at the pyeloureteral junction on flexible ureterorenoscopy. (b) Working up the stricture with a Vela XL Thulium-YAG Laser using a 230-micrometer laserfibre. (c) Access to the middle calyces with the flexible ureterorenoscope.

female patient was sent to our hospital by her urologist because of a grade II hydronephrosis of the upper calyces of the left kidney. She was asymptomatic, but creatinine had increased from 1.2 mg/dl before RFA to 1.9 mg/dl. CT scan showed neither signs of tumor recurrence nor urolithiasis.

A filiform stenosis at the pyeloureteral junction was visible on retrograde pyelography (Figures 5(a) and 6(a)), which could be passed with a 0.035-inch guidewire. Under visual control using a flexible 9.9 F video ureterorenoscope (Olympus, Tokyo, Japan), the stricture was partially vaporized with a Vela XL Thulium-YAG Laser (Boston Scientific, Massachusetts, USA), using a 230-micrometer laserfibre at 25 watts (Figure 6(b)). The lower and middle calyces could be accessed (Figures 5(b) and 6(c)), and an ureteral stent was placed in the lower calyx (Figure 5(c)). The postinterventional creatinine decreased to 1.7 mg/dl, and getting access to the upper calyces is planned in a subsequent procedure, utilizing the same approach and technique.

4. Discussion

Renal cell carcinoma (RCC) is the most common cancer of the kidney and represents 2-3% of all cancers [4]. Small renal masses (SRM) < 4 cm (T1a) are increasingly found incidentally because of the widespread use of diagnostic abdominal imaging, such as ultrasonography, computed tomography, or magnetic resonance tomography for evaluation of other abdominal conditions, and now account for the majority of renal tumors [5, 6]. Surgery is the method of choice for localized RCC; however, there is a significant number of patients who are not ideal candidates for surgery because of comorbidities, chronic kidney diseases, multiple tumors, and anatomical or functional solitary kidney. RFA is emerging as a safe and effective alternative for these patients [1].

Minor complication are observed in 15-20%, e.g., postinterventional pain, fever, or hemorrhage, which resolve with conservative management [7]. Major complications that require interventions, including pneumothorax, injury to the bowel and the renal pelvis, or ureteral strictures, are rare. In a retrospective analysis of 98 percutaneous RFA performed at our institution from 2006 to 2016, no postinterventional stricture was observed [8]. To date, a total of 135 percutaneous RFA have been carried out at our institution, and the two described strictures result in a stricture rate of 1.5%.

Noncentral, posterior, and posterolateral tumors are easier to access and treat with low complication rates, whereas inferior, anterior, and medially located tumors bear higher chance of adjacent organ damage [9].

The "ABLATE algorithm" advocates placement of ureteral stent before ablation to avoid thermal-induced damage to the ureter, collecting system, or bowel. Thus, retrograde pyeloperfusion during the ablation may result

Table 1: "ABLATE" algorithm [10].

ABLATE teaching points
A (axial tumor diameter)
Local treatment failures increase with increasing tumor size.
Ablation-related bleeding complications increase with increasing tumor size
If the tumor is ≥3 cm in diameter, consider cryoablation.
If the tumor is ≥5 cm in diameter, consider preablation tumor embolization.
B (bowel proximity)
Ablation-related bowel injury may result in long-term catheter drainage or surgery.
If the tumor is ≤1 cm from the colon or small bowel, patient repositioning or bowel displacement maneuvers will likely be necessary.
L (location within kidney)
Ablation can be performed safely and effectively in locations other than just the posterior and lateral kidney.
If the tumor is in the anterior kidney, hydrodisplacement will likely be necessary to protect adjacent bowel.
If the tumor is in the anterolateral upper pole of the right kidney, a transhepatic approach may be necessary.
If the tumor is in the anteromedial upper pole of the kidney near the adrenal gland, close blood pressure monitoring and even preablation α-receptor blockade may be necessary.
If the tumor is in the medial lower pole of the kidney, displacement techniques may be required to protect the nerves that run along the anterior surface of the psoas muscle.
A (adjacency to ureter)
Ablation-related ureteral injuries may require long-term stenting or surgery.
If the tumor is ≤1 cm from the ureter, retrograde pyeloperfusion via an externalized ureteral stent or ureteral displacement maneuvers will likely be necessary.
T (touching renal sinus fat)
Local treatment failures are more common with treatment of central tumors (those that touch renal sinus fat).
Ablation-related renal collecting system injuries and major bleeding complications are more frequent with treatment of tumors that touch renal sinus fat.
If the tumor touches renal sinus fat, consider cryoablation.
E (endo/exophytic)
Local treatment failures are more common with treatment of endophytic tumors (those that are completely contained within the renal capsule)
If the tumor is completely endophytic, consider ultrasound guidance, fusion guidance, or IV administration of contrast agent immediately before ablation for better lesion localization.

in a conductive thermal "sink," thereby protecting the ureter. If a renal tumor is 1 cm or less from the proximal ureter, an externalized 5- to 7-French ureteral stent is placed before the procedure and irrigated with sterile fluid during the ablation. The infusate flows retrograde through the stent into the renal pelvis and then returns antegrade within the ureter along the outside of the stent. The bladder is drained via a conventional bladder catheter. An additional advantage of having a ureteral stent in place is that it provides confident visualization of the ureter throughout the ablation procedure. If the tumor is 1 cm or less from the colon or small bowel, maneuvers to minimize the risk of bowel injury include simple changes in patient position (e.g., rolling the patient) and injection of either gas (pneumodisplacement using carbon dioxide) or fluid (hydrodisplacement with 5% dextrose in water) between the tumor and bowel for mechanical displacement [10] (Table 1).

Strictures of the collecting system and the ureter often develop over time and may not be present on the first postinterventional imaging; therefore, in the course of follow-up, special attention should be paid even in asymptomatic patients.

It has to be taken into account that patients who undergo RFA are not the best candidates for major open reconstructive surgery, so if strictures occur, they might be best managed by balloon dilation, endoureterotomy, and/or ureteral stenting, respectively.

5. Conclusion

Thermal injury-induced ureteral strictures may occur after RFA treatment if the ablated lesion is in close proximity to the ureter. The "ABLATE algorithm" may be helpful in reducing complication rates. Endoscopic management of ureteral strictures may be successful and necessary to preserve renal function in the affected kidney.

Abbreviations

RCC: Renal cell carcinoma
CT: Computed tomography
RFA: Radiofrequency ablation
fURS: Flexible ureterorenoscopy.

References

[1] R. J. Zagoria, J. A. Pettus, M. Rogers, D. M. Werle, D. Childs, and J. R. Leyendecker, "Long-term outcomes after percutaneous radiofrequency ablation for renal cell carcinoma," *Urology*, vol. 77, no. 6, pp. 1393–1397, 2011.

[2] https://uroweb.org/guideline/renal-cell-carcinoma/.

[3] D. A. Gervais, R. S. Arellano, F. J. McGovern, W. S. McDougal, and P. R. Mueller, "Radiofrequency ablation of renal cell carcinoma: part 2, Lessons learned with ablation of 100 tumors," *American Journal of Roentgenology*, vol. 185, no. 1, pp. 72–80, 2005.

[4] European Network of Cancer Registries, *Eurocim version 4.0.2010*, Lyon, France, https://ec.europa.eu/jrc/en/network-bureau/european-network-cancer-registries.

[5] B. Escudier, T. Eisen, C. Porta et al., "Renal cell carcinoma: ESMO clinical practice guidelines for diagnosis, treatment and follow-up," *Annals of Oncology*, vol. 23, Supplement 7, pp. vii65–vii71, 2012.

[6] K. Katsanos, L. Mailli, M. Krokidis, A. McGrath, T. Sabharwal, and A. Adam, "Systematic review and meta-analysis of thermal ablation versus surgical nephrectomy for small renal tumours," *Cardiovascular and Interventional Radiology*, vol. 37, no. 2, pp. 427–437, 2014.

[7] J. Rehman, J. Landman, D. Lee et al., "Needle-based ablation of renal parenchyma using microwave, cryoablation, impedance- and temperature-based monopolar and bipolar radiofrequency, and liquid and gel chemoablation: laboratory studies and review of the literature," *Journal of Endourology*, vol. 18, no. 1, pp. 83–104, 2004.

[8] O. Heißler, S. Seklehner, H. Fellner, P. F. Engelhardt, A. Chemelli, and C. Riedl, "Perkutane computertomographie-gezielte Radiofrequenzablation bei kleinen Nierentumoren," *Urologe*, vol. 57, no. 7, pp. 828–835, 2018.

[9] A. Rane, R. Stein, and J. Cadeddu, "Focal therapy for renal mass lesions: where do we stand in 2012?," *BJU International*, vol. 109, no. 4, pp. 491-492, 2012.

[10] G. D. Schmit, A. N. Kurup, A. J. Weisbrod et al., "ABLATE: a renal ablation planning algorithm," *American Journal of Roentgenology*, vol. 202, no. 4, pp. 894–903, 2014.

3

Ketogenic Diet-Induced Severe Ketoacidosis in a Lactating Woman: A Case Report and Review of the Literature

Benedicta Nneoma Nnodum, Eziafa Oduah, David Albert, and Mark Pettus

Berkshire Medical Center, Pittsfield, MA 01201, USA

Correspondence should be addressed to Benedicta Nneoma Nnodum; bnnodum@bhs1.org

Academic Editor: Rumeyza Kazancioglu

The ketogenic diet (KD) is a high-fat, adequate-protein, and low-carbohydrate diet that leads to nutritional ketosis and weight loss. It is known to induce ketosis but is not an established cause of clinically significant ketoacidosis. Lactation ketoacidosis is well established in bovine literature but remains a rare phenomenon in humans. Here we present a life-threatening case of severe ketoacidosis in a nondiabetic lactating mother on a strict ketogenic diet. We review the available case reports of lactation ketoacidosis in humans and the mechanisms thereof. Although ketogenic diet has been shown to be safe in nonpregnant individuals, the safety of this diet in lactating mothers is not known. Health professionals and mothers should be made aware of the potential risk associated with a strict ketogenic diet when combined with lactation. Prompt diagnosis and immediate treatment cannot be overemphasized. To our knowledge, this is the first reported case of life-threatening lactation ketoacidosis associated with ketogenic diet while consuming an adequate number of calories per day.

1. Introduction

Ketogenic diet is a high-fat, adequate-protein, and low-carbohydrate diet that leads to nutritional ketosis and weight loss. Although ketogenic diet is safe in nonpregnant individuals, its safety in lactating mothers is unknown. This case report aims to increase the awareness to healthcare professionals, mothers, and dietitians on the potential risk associated with a strict ketogenic diet when combined with lactation.

2. Case Presentation

A healthy nondiabetic 24-year-old 18 weeks postpartum woman presented to the emergency department with severe nausea, vomiting, and several episodes of diarrhea of 9-hour duration. While in the emergency department, she developed abdominal pain, low back cramps, and malaise. The patient reported adhering to a strict ketogenic diet as a health-conscious life style modification since the recent birth of her 18-week-old son. She had continued to provide her son an exclusively breastfed diet since birth. She reported an intentional 25-pound weight loss in the 18-week postpartum period. She had an unremarkable prenatal care and delivered a healthy baby boy at 40 weeks of gestation by spontaneous vaginal delivery. Her puerperium was otherwise uneventful. She denied smoking and use of alcohol. Dietary review revealed a typical breakfast consisting of egg and bacon; lunch usually consisted of some variation of vegetable salad with cheese, and a dinner consisted of vegetables and meat. Typical food items include vegetables such as peppers, spinach, broccoli, cheese, and carrot soups. For protein, she consumed mostly chicken, salmon, and other white fish. She avoided nuts or shellfish but would have 1-2 tablespoons of peanut butter per day. She eliminated all other forms of carbohydrate including wheat, pasta, bread, or any grain products. She denied any restriction in her daily caloric intake, stating that she consistently tracked her macronutrients at an average of 2200 Kcals per day.

On presentation to the emergency department, her blood pressure was 117/82 mmHg, heart rate of 103 beats/min, respiratory rate of 18 cycles/min, a temperature of 98.1°C, and oxygen saturation 98% on room air. Physical examination was remarkable for dry mucous membranes, comfortable

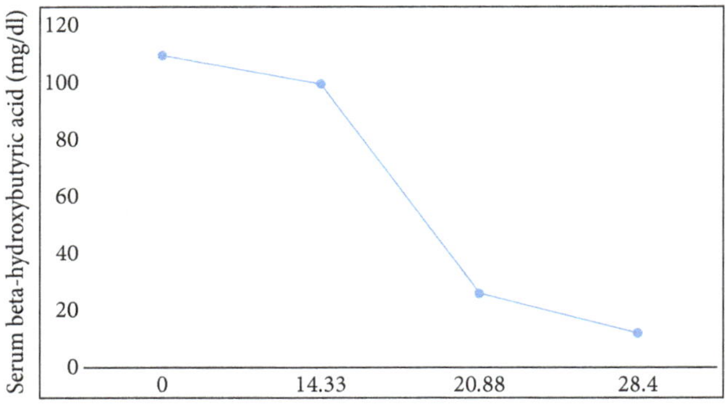

FIGURE 1: Trend of serum beta-hydroxybutyric acid level during hospitalization.

resting tachypnea though she was breathing more deeply, mild epigastric/right upper quadrant tenderness, but was otherwise unremarkable.

Laboratory studies revealed a chemistry panel with sodium of 138 meq/L; potassium, 4.3 meq/L; chloride, 109 meq/L; urea, 10 mg/dl; creatinine, 0.84 mg/dl; bicarbonate, 6 meq/L; glucose 68mg/dl; calculated anion gap of 27.3 meq/L; phosphorus of 2.3meq/L; calcium of 9.7mg/dl; and venous lactate of 1.3 mmol/L. Hematologic indices were grossly unremarkable with hemoglobin of 14.4 g/dl; white blood cells at 9.4; and neutrophils, 7.8. Her beta-hydroxybutyric acid level was initially markedly elevated at 109.5mg/dl (Figure 1). Urinalysis revealed trace protein, ketones 4+, and hemoglobin A1c, 4.8%. Osmolar gap was normal. An arterial blood gas evaluation showed a compensated AG metabolic acidosis acidaemia with pH- 7.11; partial pressure of carbon dioxide, 17 mmHg; bicarbonate (HCO_3), 5.3 mmol/L; base excess, -22.2 mmol/L. Electrocardiogram revealed normal sinus rhythm with a rate of 87 and prolonged QTc interval of 506. Ultrasound of the abdomen was unremarkable. Toxicology screen was negative except for cannabinoids.

She was initially managed with a combination of IV fluids including NS, Isotonic Bicarbonate, and D5W. A repeat arterial blood gas in six hours showed improved pH- 7.28; partial pressure of carbon dioxide, 15.8 mmHg; bicarbonate (HCO_3), 7.8 mmol/L; base excess, -16.9 mmol/L. She was immediately restarted on oral carbohydrate diet. She was allowed to continue to breastfeed her infant as she preferred. She received insulin with glucose supplementation as part of the treatment of nondiabetic ketoacidosis. Insulin levels measured at different times during hospitalization showed appropriate response to blood glucose levels ruling out euglycemic diabetic ketoacidosis. During her treatment, she developed significant metabolic derangements including worsening hypophosphatemia down to 1.0, hypokalemia to a nadir of 2.6, and hypocalcemia down to 7.3. These were closely monitored and were repleted accordingly. She experienced associated symptoms of digital tingling, perioral anesthesia, and trousseau syndrome which gradually improved with therapy. Interestingly, she did not develop respiratory failure associated with severe hypophosphatemia.

With the initiation of carbohydrates and dextrose her blood B-hydroxybutyric acid normalized and her anion gap closed in less than 24 hours of hospitalization. She was successfully discharged on day 4 of hospitalization (Table 2) with close nephrology and primary care follow-up and symptom resolution. Follow-up labs after discharge remained normal (Table 2).

3. Discussion

There are several established causes of ketoacidosis including diabetic ketoacidosis, starvation ketoacidosis, alcoholic ketoacidosis, and some inborn errors of metabolism including succinyl CoA:3 ketoacid CoA transferase deficiency, mitochondrial 2-methylacetoacetyl CoA thiolase deficiency, and methylmalonyl-CoA mutase deficiency [1]. Lactation ketoacidosis is well described in postpartum lactating cattle in the veterinary literature [2]. However, only a few case reports of lactation ketoacidosis in human have been reported to date. Most of these cases were precipitated by situations of starvation or infection requiring lactating mothers to be nil per mouth (Table 1). To our knowledge, this is the first case report of this uncommon phenomenon in humans in the setting of a ketogenic diet with adequate number of calories, above 2000 kcal/day.

Ketogenic diet (KD) is described as a high-fat, adequate-protein, and low-carbohydrate diet (<50g/day) [3]. It has been used as an alternative weight loss tool against obesity due to proven results of greater weight loss compared to other balanced diets [4, 5]. The underlying mechanism appears to culminate in nutritional ketosis induced by the low availability of carbohydrate as the body is forced to burn fats instead of carbohydrate for energy metabolism. This process involves the conversion of fats by the liver into fatty acids thus producing ketone bodies. The resultant effect is the accumulation of ketones in blood and urine but to a level not associated with changes in blood pH, which is the hallmark of life-threatening ketoacidosis as seen in such conditions as diabetic ketoacidosis [3]. The importance of the ketogenic diet can be traced back to the 1920s [6]. It is one of the most studied interventions for weight loss as it has a physiological and biochemical basis to induce effective weight loss [7].

We came across few studies that evaluated the acid-base safety of patients on ketogenic diet, one showed that majority had a ketone level less than 54mg/dl and none was greater than 106 mg/dl while the other study reported patients had a mild compensated metabolic acidosis with no significant metabolic derangement [8, 9]. Studies carried out by Mohammed et al. showed that healthy lactating women on low-carbohydrate diet or 42-hour fast had a significantly increased hydroxybutyric acid compared with nonlactating women due to decreased carbohydrate oxidation and increased fat oxidation [10, 11]. This condition commonly referred to as "bovine ketosis" is common in dairy cows when they are unable to compensate for high energy requirements of milk production by sufficient energy intake [12].

Table 1: Literature review of existing case reports and their precipitating factor.

Case Report	Precipitating Factor
A case of lactation "bovine" ketoacidosis [14]	Breastfeeding twins in the setting of a "selected diet"
A severe case of iatrogenic lactation ketoacidosis [15]	Nil per oral for 3 days to treat a bowel obstruction
"Bovine ketosis" in a nondiabetic postpartum woman [16]	Urinary tract infection in the setting of a weight reduction diet
Severe spontaneous "bovine" ketoacidosis in a lactating woman [17]	Urinary tract infection in the setting of a high protein, carbohydrate-free reduction diet
A case of bovine ketoacidosis in a lactating woman [18]	2-day nausea & vomiting in the setting of several small high-protein carbohydrate-free meals
Ketoacidosis associated with low-carbohydrate diet in a non-diabetic lactating woman [19]	Low carbohydrate, high fat diet for 10 days
Starvation ketosis in a breastfeeding woman [20]	Bariatric surgery during lactation
Severe ketoacidosis in breastfeeding woman with low energy and carbohydrate intake [21]	Illness while on a low carbohydrate diet
Ketoacidosis in a non-diabetic woman who was fasting during lactation [22]	Starvation during lactation due to abdominal pain
Lactation ketoacidosis: an unusual entity and a review of the literature [23]	No precipitating factor except for lactation
Life-threatening lactation or Bovine ketoacidosis [24]	Frequent skipping of meals while on a high protein, low carbohydrate diet
A rare cause of metabolic acidosis: ketoacidosis in a non-diabetic lactating woman [25]	Gastroenteritis in the setting of a low carbohydrate diet

Table 2: Table demonstrating serial pertinent laboratory values during hospitalization and after discharge.

	On admission, June 15th	June 16th	June 17th	June 18th	On discharge, June 19th	1 week after discharge, June 26th
Serum bicarbonate (meq/L)	6	10	24	30	29	23
Glucose (mg/dl)	50	124	112	105	99	77
Insulin level (uiu/ml)	3.4	11.1				
Phosphorous (mg/dl)	2.3	1.4	1.0	2.4	3.3	3.9
Potassium (meq/l)	4.2	3.0	2.6	3.1	4.3	4.0
Calcium (mg/dl)	7.3	7.9	8.8	8.6	9.2	8.8
Urine Ketone	4+					
pH ABG	7.11	7.28				
pCO_2 ABG	17.0	15.8				
Bicarbonate ABG	5.3	7.3				

ABG: arterial blood gas.

Postpartum mothers are at an increased pressure to lose weight gained during pregnancy and may resort to this proven efficacious method of rapid weight loss. The increased energy demands of lactation which results in increased glucose utilization may lead to a dysregulation of the compensatory mechanism regulating normal ketone levels in lactating women on ketogenic diet [13]. Lactation ketoacidosis can occur by adhering to a low-carbohydrate diet which leads to depletion of the glycogen stores forcing the body into using gluconeogenesis as an energy substrate for production of breast milk [1].

Existing case reports like ours demonstrated complete resolution of symptoms, ketoacidosis, and laboratory derangements with rehydration and restarting normal diet.

4. Conclusion

Although ketogenic diet is being considered a safe nutritional intervention for weight loss and has grown to be a popular implementation for successful weight loss in the medical literature, social media, and fitness blogs, the index case may provide caution in lactating mothers on/or considering a ketogenic diet. It is important for clinicians to educate lactating mothers interested in weight.

Disclosure

The case submitted in this paper was also accepted as an abstract case at the American Society of Nutrition (ASN) conference on June 10th, 2019. The current manuscript presents novel contributions in the following ways. The manuscript adds distinct information to the medical literature that was not reported in the ASN conference abstract including (a) a detailed diary of our patient's typical diet and average number of calories consumed in a day, (b) more extensive detail surrounding the specific acid-base disturbances the patient experienced, (c) full clinical presentation and day-to-day management of our patient till she was discharged home, (d) specific values regarding remarkable improvement in deranged laboratory values, and (e) an extensive review of published lactation ketoacidosis cases and how ours differs from these.

References

[1] S. Gleeson, E. Mulroy, and D. E. Clarke, "Lactation ketoacidosis: an unusual entity and a review of the literature," *The Permanente Journal*, vol. 20, no. 1, pp. 71–73, 2016.

[2] P. Holtenius and K. Holtenius, "New aspects of ketone bodies in energy metabolism of dairy cows: A review," *Journal of Veterinary Medicine Series A: Physiology Pathology Clinical Medicine*, vol. 43, no. 10, pp. 579–587, 1996.

[3] L. Gupta, D. Khandelwal, S. Kalra et al., "Ketogenic diet in endocrine disorders: Current perspectives," *Journal of Postgraduate Medicine*, vol. 63, no. 4, pp. 242–251, 2017.

[4] A. Paoli, M. Canato, L. Toniolo et al., "The ketogenic diet: an underappreciated therapeutic option?" *Clinical Therapeutics - Journal*, vol. 162, no. 5, pp. 145–153, 2011.

[5] B. J. Brehm, R. J. Seeley, S. R. Daniels, and D. A. D'Alessio, "A randomized trial comparing a very low carbohydrate diet and a calorie-restricted low fat diet on body weight and cardiovascular risk factors in healthy women," *The Journal of Clinical Endocrinology & Metabolism*, vol. 88, no. 4, pp. 1617–1623, 2003.

[6] A. Paoli, A. Rubini, J. S. Volek, and K. A. Grimaldi, "Beyond weight loss: a review of the therapeutic uses of very-low-carbohydrate (ketogenic) diets," *European Journal of Clinical Nutrition*, vol. 67, no. 8, pp. 789–796, 2013.

[7] A. Paoli, "Ketogenic diet for obesity: friend or foe?" *International Journal of Environmental Research and Public Health*, vol. 11, no. 2, pp. 2092–2107, 2014.

[8] D. Gomez-Arbelaez, A. B. Crujeiras, A. I. Castro et al., "Acid–base safety during the course of a very low-calorie-ketogenic diet," *Endocrine Journal*, vol. 58, no. 1, pp. 81–90, 2017.

[9] W. S. Yancy, M. K. Olsen, T. Dudley, and E. C. Westman, "Acid-base analysis of individuals following two weight loss diets," *European Journal of Clinical Nutrition*, vol. 61, no. 12, pp. 1416–1422, 2007.

[10] M. A. Mohammad, A. L. Sunehag, S. K. Chacko, A. S. Pontius, P. D. Maningat, and M. W. Haymond, "Mechanisms to conserve glucose in lactating women during a 42-h fast," *American Journal of Physiology-Endocrinology and Metabolism*, vol. 297, no. 4, pp. E879–E888, 2009.

[11] M. A. Mohammad, A. L. Sunehag, and M. W. Haymond, "Effect of dietary macronutrient composition under moderate hypocaloric intake on maternal adaptation during lactation," *American Journal of Clinical Nutrition*, vol. 89, no. 6, pp. 1821–1827, 2009.

[12] J. Goff, "Major advances in our understanding of nutritional influences on bovine health," *Journal of Dairy Science*, vol. 89, no. 4, pp. 1292–1301, 2006.

[13] G. R. Oetzel, "Herd-level ketosis diagnosis and risk factors," in *Proceedings of Presentation at the 40th annual conference of the American Association of Bovine Practitioners*, 2007.

[14] A. C. Heffner and D. P. Johnson, "A case of lactation "bovine" ketoacidosis," *The Journal of Emergency Medicine*, vol. 35, no. 4, pp. 385–387, 2008.

[15] A. Szulewski, D. Howes, and A. R. Morton, "A severe case of iatrogenic lactation ketoacidosis," *BMJ Case Reports*, 2012.

[16] B. Chernow, C. Finton, T. G. Rainey, and J. T. O'Brian, ""Bovine ketosis" in a nondiabetic postpartum," *Diabetes Care*, vol. 5, no. 1, pp. 47–49, 1982.

[17] P. Altus and J. W. Hickman, "Severe spontaneous 'bovine' ketoacidosis in a lactating woman," *The Journal of the Indiana State Medical Association*, vol. 76, no. 6, pp. 392-393, 1983.

[18] H. S. Sandhu, M. F. Michelis, and M. V. DeVita, "A case of bovine ketoacidosis in a lactating woman," *Clinical Kidney Journal*, vol. 2, no. 4, pp. 278-279, 2009.

[19] L. Von Geijer and M. Ekelund, "Ketoacidosis associated with low-carbohydrate diet in a non-diabetic lactating woman: A case report," *Journal of Medical Case Reports*, vol. 9, no. 1, 2015.

[20] D. Monnier, T. Goulenok, J. Allary, V. Zarrouk, and B. Fantin, "Starvation ketosis in a breastfeeding woman," *Europe PMC*, vol. 36, no. 12, pp. 854–858, 2015.

[21] J. Wuopio, R. Schiborr, and G. Charalampakis, "Severe ketoacidosis in breastfeeding woman with low energy and carbohydrate intake," *Europe PMC*, vol. 112, 2015.

[22] S. K. Hudak, D. Overkamp, R. Wagner, H.-U. Häring, and M. Heni, "Ketoacidosis in a non-diabetic woman who was fasting during lactation," *Nutrition Journal*, vol. 14, no. 117, 2015.

[23] S. Gleeson, E. Mulroy, and D. E. Clarke, "Lactation ketoacidosis: an unusual entity and a review of the literature," *The Permanente Journal*, vol. 20, no. 2, pp. 71–73, 2017.

[24] D. J. Greaney and P. Benson, "Life-Threatening Lactation or "Bovine" Ketoacidosis: A Case Report," *A & A case reports*, vol. 7, no. 4, pp. 81–84, 2016.

[25] G. Sloan, A. Ali, and J. Webster, "A rare cause of metabolic acidosis: ketoacidosis in a non-diabetic lactating woman," *Endocrinology, Diabetes & Metabolism Case Reports*, vol. 2017, 2017.

4

A Case Report of COVID-19 in a Living Kidney Transplant Recipient: A Challenging Case with Complete Rehabilitation

Mahtab Poor Zamany Nejat Kermaney,[1] Mohammad Hamidi Madani,[2] Milad Bonakdar Hashemi,[2] Alireza Zadmehr,[2] Mehdi Dadpour,[3] and Fatemeh Roodneshin[1]

[1]*Department of Anesthesiology, Shahid Beheshti University of Medical Sciences, Tehran, Iran*
[2]*Resident of Urology, Labbafinezhad Hospital, Urology Nephrology Research Center (UNRC), Shahid Beheshti University of Medical Sciences, Tehran, Iran*
[3]*Urology and Nephrology Research Center, Shahid Labbafinezhad Hospital, Shahid Beheshti University of Medical Sciences, Tehran, Iran*

Correspondence should be addressed to Fatemeh Roodneshin; dr_roodneshin_f2007@yahoo.com

Academic Editor: Walid Farhat

Adjustment of immunosuppressive and COVID-19 treatment in terms of drug interactions is still challenging. Herein, we report a 45-year-old woman with end-stage renal disease due to autosomal dominant polycystic diseases (ADPKD) with COVID-19 and pulmonary involvement following kidney transplantation. The patient was properly treated by discontinuation of immunosuppressive drugs, bronchoscopy, and high volume of blood transfusions. The fact that we quickly used early intubation and a new treatment regimen that suppressed immune systems may help physicians develop optimal treatment strategies for similar severe cases. However, this treatment method requires more detailed evaluations due to the contradictory results in reviewing other studies.

1. Introduction

In late December 2019, China officially declared several cases of severe acute respiratory disease in humans, leading to a pandemic by novel coronavirus SARS-CoV-2.1 [1]. The epidemic coronavirus disease rapidly spread worldwide; on 11 March (2020), it was officially stated a pandemic by the World Health Organization (WHO) [2]. By May 1, 2020, around 247,000 people deaths resulting from COVID-19 were recorded worldwide [3]. It is assumed that RNA beta coronavirus enters the cell and impacted the function of angiotensin-converting enzyme 2 (ACE2) receptors present in the lungs, kidneys, heart, and vascular endothelium [4]. The clinical presentations of infected patients vary from mild symptoms, for instance, flu-like symptoms, including fever, cough, and also shortness of breath, to severe and advanced diseases; it was demonstrated that acute respiratory distress syndrome may result in cardiopulmonary collapse [5]. There are several underlying health conditions such as chronic respiratory diseases, chronic immunosuppression, diabetes mellitus, and hypertension that make patients vulnerable to infectious diseases [6]. Immunosuppressive therapy in kidney transplant recipients including antilymphocyte therapy, a calcineurin inhibitor (CNI, e.g., tacrolimus), high-dose corticosteroids, and mycophenolate mofetil (MMF) may have influence on health status making patients more susceptible to COVID-19 [7, 8]. Consequently, adjustment of immunosuppressive and COVID-19 treatment in terms of drug interactions is still challenging. Herein, we report a case of COVID-19 with pulmonary involvement following kidney transplantation, which was properly treated by discontinuation of immunosuppressive drugs, bronchoscopy, and high volume of blood transfusions.

2. Case Presentation

A 45-year-old married woman with end-stage renal disease due to autosomal dominant polycystic diseases (ADPKD) with a history of routine hemodialysis three times a week was a candidate for receiving a donated kidney from his spouse and underwent living-related kidney transplantation on February 18, 2020. The patient's clinical laboratory outcome before her kidney transplantation is revealed in Table 1. Her previous medical history (including hypertension, diabetes mellitus, coagulopathy, and elective surgery) was negative. The donor was the patient's husband. Both the recipient and the organ donor had no previous international travel or exposure to contaminated or suspected patients infected with COVID-19. A preoperative ultrasound and abdominopelvic CT scan of the patients' native kidneys revealed high-volume native kidneys and confirming ADPKD. As a result, it was decided that the patient should undergo simultaneous unilateral nephrectomy and living-related kidney transplantation.

Since then, on February 18, 2020, she successfully underwent living-related kidney transplantation and nephrectomy surgeries. Throughout postoperative monitoring in the recovery ward at the first evaluation, the patient developed an episode of hypotension and tachycardia. The patient was immediately taken back to the operating room for exploratory surgery with the surgery team's opinion. During exploratory surgery, it was revealed that there are multiple areas of bleeding despite adequate blood coagulation. These bleeding areas were treated with packing lap sponges, which remained in the field for two days. After that, the patient was taken to the intensive care unit (ICU), and she remained intubated due to hypoxia. For routine checkups after surgery, in the emergency tests, acidosis was detected (Table 1). The patient was started on an appropriate immunosuppressive regimen, consisting of tacrolimus (1 to 1.5 mg per 12 hours and the concentration remained 4.0 to 5.0 ng/mL), mycophenolate mofetil (250 mg every 12 hours), and prednisolone (50 mg daily). The initial ventilator settings were TV = 500 ml/kg/FIO_2 = 90%/RR = 20 -30, which were adjusted over the following days based on the patient's clinical condition and laboratory tests. Lap sponges were removed two days later, and she was still connected to a ventilator, and O_2 saturations were around 92%. On July 22, a decrease in oxygen saturation was detected. Despite the tracheal tube replacement, the O_2 saturation was still about 83%, blood pressure was 120/80 mmHg, and no other findings like fever were detected (Table 1).

As a consequence, the patient underwent diagnostic and therapeutic bronchoscopy after consulting with a pulmonologist. During the procedure, copious amounts of clotted blood and mucus were removed. A bronchoalveolar lavage (BAL) sample was submitted for further examination; real-time reverse transcriptase-polymerase chain reaction (RT-PCR) of the BAL sample was confirmed positive COVID-19. In addition, the other symptoms, such as fever (37.5 to 38.9°C), frequent cough, breathlessness, diarrhea, and chest computed tomography (CT) (multiple patchy ground-glass opacity and exudative lesion in bilateral lungs), were confirmed. The next day, a second identical bronchoscopy was performed, and the patient's oxygen saturation improved to 90%. Two days later, the patient felt better, with a reduced body temperature (37.1°-36.2°C) and no longer having breathlessness or cough.

Therefore, the patient was extubated. As a result, all immunosuppressive treatments were discontinued, and an infectious disease specialist consultation was conducted to decide the following line of treatment. At the time of the onset of the COVID-19 pandemic, there was no specific protocol for discontinuing immunosuppressive regimen in transplant patients when needed. In this case, we discontinued mycophenolate mofetil, immediately. Tacrolimus was reduced and stopped within 3 days. Prednisolone, which was started at a dose of 50 mg, was reduced to a dose of 5 mg.

The patient received 20 units of packed cell and 25 fresh frozen plasma units (FFP) and 15 units of platelets for four days following surgery.

The patient was dismissed from the hospital on 30 July 2020. From that day forward, she was undergoing regular blood tests. This patient had a routine examination three weeks after being discharged from the hospital, and no fever or other symptoms were reported. The patient lost 8 kg of body weight during hospitalization. It is interesting to note that despite temporary discontinuous of immunosuppressive drugs, the function of the graft kidney is good after one year of follow-up. Serum creatinine is 1.1 mg/dl, and GFR is estimated 63 ml/min/1.73 m^2. The patient's written consent was obtained to report the case descriptions.

3. Discussions

A novel coronavirus (COVID-19) that accompanied significant morbidity and mortality, as newly recognized in late December 2019 in Wuhan, China, is spreading worldwide [9, 10]. In this study, CT chest [11], fever, cough, RT-PCR positive of a sample of the lavage, shortness of breath, and diarrhea are close to the symptoms in the general population of severe COVID-19 pneumonia [12, 13]. Diagnosis mostly depends on radiological findings, laboratory results, and history taking. Initially, symptoms can be subtle, particularly in the early phases consisting of fever and cough with unremarkable lab test results [14]. It is also said to ground pneumonic glass opacities in chest tomography which is highly suggestive [5]. Despite up to 30% of false-negative results stated for the PCR tests from oropharyngeal/nasal swab samples, it is still one of the best methods for detecting suspicious cases [5]. Moreover, we can perform repeated oropharyngeal/nasal swabs or taking bronchoalveolar lavage if the tests are negative. However, clinical indicators like chest tomography scans can illustrate an urgent need for isolation in suspected cases [15].

Recent research suggests that an early intubation strategy is critical for covid19 patients [16, 17]. Thus, the findings of this study are consistent with previous research and confirm it.

In immunocompromised patients, especially in posttransplant patients, COVID-19 pneumonia may not be presented typically. Therefore, the high-risk population requires more careful attention [18]. In addition, clinical manifestations of COVID-19 in posttransplant patients may be uncommon due to prolonged immunosuppression [19].

TABLE 1: Clinical laboratory outcome.

Test	Unit	Reference value	Before the illness	At the admission	At the discharge	3 weeks after discharge
Biochemistry						
Urea	mg/dl	Female (20-50 years): 15-40	76	181	80	61
Sodium	mEq/l	134-148	138	140	139	141
Potassium	mEq/l	3.5-5.3	3.7	4.5	4.0	3.8
LDH	U/I	Adult < 480	410	390	384	407
Albumin	g/dl	3.5-5.2	4.8	5.1	3.5	3.7
Creatinine	mg/dl	Female: 0.6-1.3	6.13	5.31	4.86	4.46
Calcium	mg/dl	Adult: 8.6-10.3	10.1	9.7	9.1	8.8
Phosphorus	mg/dl	Adult: 2.6-4.5	3.1	3.6	4.1	2.9
Magnesium	mg/dl	Female: 1.9-2.5	2.0	2.2	1.9	2.0
Hematology						
WBC	$10^3/\mu l$	4.0-10.1	8.4	8.7	11.5	10.0
RBC	$10^6/\mu l$	Female: 4.2-5.4	4.3	4.26	4.6	4.9
Hb	mg/dl	Female: 12-16	12.4	15.1	13.7	14.9
Hct	%	Female: 32-45	35.6	37	33.1	38.4
MCV	fl	80-96	87.6	87.3	85.6	85.3
MCH	p.g	26-32	29.5	29.1	29.6	29.8
MCHC	gr/dl	30-36	34.1	34.6	33.2	34.2
Platelets	$10^3/\mu l$	150-450	158	149	112	150
Neutrophils	%	47-76	48	47.5	31	46.8
Lymphocytes	%	Adult: 25-45	26.1	25.3	17	25.7
Monocytes	%	—	2	2	1.5	2
Eosinophils	%	—	0.05	0.5	0.00	0.06
PT patient time	Seconds	8.6-12.6	12.1	11.8	12.2	12.6
I.N.R	Seconds	0.9-1.3	1.24	1.14	1.31	1.00
PTT patient time	Seconds	20-35	29.4	23.00	29.8	21.4
Blood gases						
pH	—	—	7.4	7.47	7.43	7.31
$P\ CO_2$	mmHg	—	24	25	35	33
$P\ O_2$	mmHg	—	49	37	35	42
HCO_3	mmol/l	—	17.5	16.6	22.7	16.6
$SO_2\%$	%	—	87	73	69	72

Moreover, we can perform repeated oropharyngeal/nasal swabs or taking bronchoalveolar lavage if the tests are negative. However, clinical indicators like chest tomography scans can illustrate an urgent need for isolation in suspected cases [15].in immunocompromised patients; especially in posttransplant patients, COVID-19 pneumonia may not be presented typically. Therefore, the high-risk population requires more careful attention [18].

Clinical manifestations of COVID-19 in posttransplant patients may be uncommon due to prolonged immunosuppression [19]. However, in this study, CT chest [11], fever, cough, RT-PCR positive of a sample of the lavage, shortness of breath, and diarrhea are close to the symptoms in the general population of severe COVID-19 pneumonia [12, 13].

It is important to note that COVID-19 pneumonia is more severe in immunocompromised individuals than in the general nonsuppressed immune population. Guillen et al. reported kidney transplanted patients with immunocompromised that presented atypical clinical signs and symptoms such as electrolyte disorders (hyponatremia) unilobar pneumonia imaging [20].

The immunosuppressive regimen intake in this study consists of tacrolimus, mycophenolate mofetil, and prednisolone. Zhu et al. [11] describe a kidney transplant and COVID-19 that had decided several therapeutic strategies such as discontinuing all immunosuppressive agents, methylprednisolone (40 mg) daily, intravenous immunoglobulin, biapenem, and interferon α (5 million units) daily. Finally, they successfully recovered their patient because of various novel treatments, but they could not figure out which medical therapy may or may not help [14]. To explain this phenomenon, Zhu et al. hypothesized that long-term suppression of the immune system might delay the clearance of the virus and prolong the course of the disease, as well as prevent the occurrence of fatal critical pneumonia due to an overimmune response [11].

On the other hand, Namazee et al. [21] reported that the discontinued immunosuppressive medications were unsuccessful in a patient with a kidney transplant with COVID-19 pneumonia. They stated that in treating a COVID-19 case with a kidney transplant, drug-drug reactions (DDI) are essential.

Therefore, the fact that we quickly used early intubation and a new treatment regimen that suppressed immune systems may help physicians develop optimal treatment strategies for similar severe cases. However, this treatment 4method requires more detailed evaluations due to the contradictory results in reviewing other studies.

References

[1] D. J. B. Machado and L. E. Ianhez, "COVID-19 pneumonia in kidney transplant recipients-where we are?," *Transplant Infectious Disease*, vol. 22, no. 5, article e13306, 2020.

[2] World Health Organization, *World Health Organization Coronavirus Disease (COVID-19) Dashboard*, World Health Organization, 2020.

[3] J. Hopkins, *COVID-19 Dashboard by the Center for Systems Science and Engineering (CSSE) at Johns Hopkins University (JHU)*, Johns Hopkins University, Baltimore, MD, USA, 2020.

[4] H. K. Siddiqi and M. R. Mehra, "COVID-19 illness in native and immunosuppressed states: a clinical–therapeutic staging proposal," *The Journal of Heart and Lung Transplantation*, vol. 39, no. 5, p. 405, 2020.

[5] W.-J. Guan, Z.-Y. Ni, Y. Hu et al., "Clinical characteristics of coronavirus disease 2019 in China," *New England Journal of Medicine*, vol. 382, no. 18, pp. 1708–1720, 2020.

[6] C.-F. Rate, "Characteristics of patients dying in relation to COVID-19 in Italy Onder G, Rezza G, Brusaferro S," *JAMA*, vol. 23, 2020.

[7] R. San Juan, J. M. Aguado, C. Lumbreras, J. Fortun, P. Muñoz, J. Gavalda et al., "Impact of current transplantation management on the development of cytomegalovirus disease after renal transplantation," *Clinical Infectious Diseases*, vol. 47, no. 7, pp. 875–882, 2008.

[8] D. Bhadauria, A. Goel, A. Kaul et al., "Cryptosporidium infection after renal transplantation in an endemic area," *Transplant Infectious Disease*, vol. 17, no. 1, pp. 48–55, 2015.

[9] P. Sun, X. Lu, C. Xu, W. Sun, and B. Pan, "Understanding of COVID-19 based on current evidence," *Journal of Medical Virology*, vol. 92, no. 6, pp. 548–551, 2020.

[10] S. M. Ghahestani, M. Bonakdar Hashemi, N. Yousefzadeh Kandevani, N. Borumandnia, M. Dadpour, and F. Sharifiaghdas, "Iranian urology association coronavirus disease 2019 (COVID-19) taskforce pamphlet (IUA-CTP) recommended practice based on national epidemiologic analysis," *Urology Journal*, vol. 17, no. 5, pp. 543–547, 2020.

[11] T. Ai, Z. Yang, H. Hou et al., "Correlation of chest CT and RT-PCR testing in coronavirus disease (COVID-19) in China: a report of 1014 cases," *Radiology*, vol. 10, 2019.

[12] C. Hani, N. H. Trieu, I. Saab et al., "COVID-19 pneumonia: a review of typical CT findings and differential diagnosis," *Diagnostic and Interventional Imaging*, vol. 101, no. 5, pp. 263–268, 2020.

[13] L. Zhu, N. Gong, B. Liu et al., "Coronavirus Disease 2019 Pneumonia in Immunosuppressed Renal Transplant Recipients: A Summary of 10 Confirmed Cases in Wuhan, China," *European Urology*, vol. 77, no. 6, pp. 748–754, 2020.

[14] W. Alhazzani, M. Møller, Y. Arabi et al., "Surviving sepsis campaign: guidelines on the management of critically ill adults with coronavirus disease 2019 (COVID-19)," *Intensive Care Medicine*, vol. 46, no. 5, pp. 854–887, 2020.

[15] E. Prompetchara, C. Ketloy, and T. Palaga, "Immune responses in COVID-19 and potential vaccines: lessons learned from SARS and MERS epidemic," *Asian Pacific Journal of Allergy and Immunology*, vol. 38, no. 1, pp. 1–9, 2020.

[16] E. Papoutsi, V. G. Giannakoulis, E. Xourgia, C. Routsi, A. Kotanidou, and I. I. Siempos, "Effect of timing of intubation on clinical outcomes of critically ill patients with COVID-19: a systematic review and meta-analysis of non-randomized cohort studies," *Critical Care*, vol. 25, no. 1, pp. 1–9, 2021.

[17] V. Tsolaki and G. E. Zakynthinos, "Timing of intubation in COVID-19 ARDS: what "time" really matters?," *Critical Care*, vol. 25, no. 1, pp. 1-2, 2021.

[18] E. Akalin, Y. Azzi, R. Bartash et al., "COVID-19 and kidney transplantation," *New England Journal of Medicine*, vol. 382, no. 25, pp. 2475–2477, 2020.

[19] M. G. Michaels, R. M. La Hoz, L. Danziger-Isakov et al., "Coronavirus disease 2019: implications of emerging infections for transplantation," *American Journal of Transplantation*, vol. 20, no. 7, pp. 1768–1772, 2020.

[20] E. Guillen, G. J. Pineiro, I. Revuelta, D. Rodriguez, M. Bodro, A. Moreno et al., "Case report of COVID-19 in a kidney transplant recipient: does immunosuppression alter the clinical presentation?," *American Journal of Transplantation*, vol. 20, no. 7, pp. 1875–1878, 2020.

[21] N. Namazee, H. Mahmoudi, P. Afzal, and S. Ghaffari, "Novel coronavirus 2019 pneumonia in a kidney transplant recipient," *American Journal of Transplantation*, vol. 20, no. 9, pp. 2599–2601, 2020.

5

Complement Factor H Gene Variant in a Patient with Thrombotic Microangiopathy on a Mixed Clinical Background

Yoichi Iwafuchi,[1] Tetsuo Morioka,[2] Yuko Oyama,[1] Shin Goto,[3] and Ichiei Narita[3]

[1]*Department of Internal Medicine, Koseiren Sanjo General Hospital, 5-1-62 Tsukanome, Sanjo 955-0055, Japan*
[2]*Department of Internal Medicine, Kidney Center, Shinrakuen Hospital, 3-3-11 Shindorimınami Nishi-ku, Niigata 950-2087, Japan*
[3]*Division of Clinical Nephrology and Rheumatology, Niigata University Graduate School of Medical and Dental Sciences, 1-754 Asahinachi-Dori, Niigata 951-8510, Japan*

Correspondence should be addressed to Yoichi Iwafuchi; iwafuchiy@hotmail.com

Academic Editor: Rumeyza Kazancioglu

We report the case of a patient with *complement factor H* gene variant, who developed thrombotic microangiopathy on a mixed clinical background. A 79-year-old woman was transferred to Sanjo General Hospital for maintenance hemodialysis. She suffered from gastric non-Hodgkin lymphoma about two years ago and received chemotherapy and radiation therapy, leading to complete remission. About 13 weeks prior to her transfer to our hospital, she was referred to another hospital due to acute kidney injury, hemolytic anemia, and thrombocytopenia. Hemodialysis was immediately initiated, after which intravenous methylprednisolone and oral prednisolone were started; however, she became anuric within approximately week. The possibility of thrombotic microangiopathy was examined. However, she was in poor general condition and did not get the consent of her family, so no invasive searches such as a kidney biopsy were performed. Despite the cause of acute kidney insufficiency being unclear, she was transferred to us for maintenance hemodialysis. Her general condition was stable, and her renal function improved; hence, two months after transfer, a kidney biopsy was performed. Her clinical and typical renal histological findings indicated a diagnosis of thrombotic microangiopathy. There was a possible CFH gene of a very rare variant "c.526 T > C (p.Phe176Leu)" in exon 5. She was able to withdraw from hemodialysis therapy two weeks after the initiation of an angiotensin-converting enzyme inhibitor. Based on her clinical course and kidney biopsy findings, she was diagnosed with thrombotic microangiopathy with a very rare CFH variant. To ensure proper treatment choices such as eculizumab, the presence of complement dysregulation should be considered in cases of secondary thrombotic microangiopathy.

1. Introduction

Thrombotic microangiopathy (TMA) represents a heterogeneous group of syndromes with the same phenotype: a clinical triad of microangiopathic hemolytic anemia, thrombocytopenia, and organ damage [1]. The pathophysiology of TMA is not fully understood. However, it is likely a multifactorial disease in which various genetic and environmental factors overlap. Accurate diagnosis is important because the causes of TMA are diverse, and the treatment and prognosis differ depending on the cause.

The classification of TMA is currently controversial. TMA can be divided into primary (genetic and acquired) and secondary causes [1]. The concept of atypical hemolytic uremic syndrome (aHUS), a type of TMA that has been clarified in recent years, is that it is caused by complement overactivation in the alternative pathway [2]. aHUS, referred to as complement-mediated TMA, is a syndrome that includes congenital caused by multiple complement genes and various acquired causes [2]. aHUS develops when environmental factors are added to genetic factors, but not all can be explained by genetic factors. There are various pathological conditions that cause secondary TMA. In recent years, attention has also been focused on complement gene abnormalities in secondary TMA because these are related to treatment choices, specially to the use of eculizumab (ECZ) [3].

Here, we report the case of a patient with *complement factor H* (CFH) gene variant, who developed TMA on a mixed clinical background, and discuss the possibility of complement dysregulation being present in secondary TMA.

2. Case Presentation

A 79-year-old woman was transferred to Sanjo General Hospital for maintenance hemodialysis and rehabilitation. She had no family history of renal disease. Her medical history was complex. About two years before transfer, she was diagnosed with gastric non-Hodgkin lymphoma (diffuse large B-cell type) in a medical examination at the first hospital. She was treated with six cycles of rituximab, tetrahydropyranyl adriamycin, cyclophosphamide, vincristine, and prednisolone. These drugs, excluding prednisolone, were not used since then. However, two months after her last chemotherapy for lymphoma, a residual tumor was confirmed. Definitive radiotherapy was performed with a curative intent, totaling 40 Gray in 20 fractions. A complete response was confirmed by an upper gastrointestinal endoscopy after radiotherapy, with no progression observed. After 17 months, about 13 weeks prior to her transfer to our hospital, she was noted to have proteinuria, renal dysfunction, hemolytic anemia, and thrombocytopenia for the first time on follow-up medical examinations. She was referred to the second hospital because of acute kidney injury (AKI) with hemolytic anemia and thrombocytopenia (platelet count was 99,000/μL). Her physical examination findings on to the second hospital were as follows: height, 158.0 cm; weight, 53.0 kg; blood pressure, 136/88 mmHg; and body temperature, 36.8°C. On admission, urinalysis revealed microscopic hematuria (urinary sediment, 50–99 erythrocytes/high-power field) and the urine protein/creatinine ratio was 4.7. Her hematocrit was 30.5%, hemoglobin concentration was 9.9 g/dL, platelet count was 178,000/μL, and leukocyte count was 6,690/μL. Red cell fragments were observed on peripheral blood smear. Her serum urea nitrogen level was 36 mg/dL, creatinine (Cre) level was 2.55 mg/dL, and lactate dehydrogenase level was 485 IU/L. The total complement level was 14 (reference range: 30–46) IU/L, complement 3 (C3) level was 41.8 (73–138) mg/dL, and complement 4 (C4) level was <5 (11–31) mg/dL. Additional laboratory data at the second hospital are summarized in Table 1. Abdominal ultrasound revealed mildly atrophic kidneys. Her renal function very rapidly worsened, and she had a severely high blood pressure (200/100 mmHg). Assuming malignant hypertension and a collagen vascular disease-related kidney injury such as lupus nephritis, hemodialysis was immediately initiated; simultaneously, a 3-day course of intravenous methylprednisolone (500 mg/day) followed by oral prednisolone at 45 mg/day was started; however, she became anuric in about a week. The possibility of TMA was investigated. However, she was in poor general condition and did not get the consent of her family, so no invasive searches, such as a kidney biopsy, were performed. Prednisolone was gradually tapered to a dose of 5 mg/day (Figure 1). She was transferred to Sanjo General Hospital for rehabilitation and maintenance hemodialysis.

When we carefully reassessed her, we observed that her urine volume had increased to 700 mL/day. In addition, since her serum Cre level before dialysis was very low (1.59 mg/dL), steroid treatment seemed to be effective to some extent. Kidney atrophy was unnoticeable, so with the consent of her and her family, we performed kidney biopsy to investigate the cause of renal failure.

On performing light microscopy, we observed the following: the biopsied sample contained 43 glomeruli, of which 8 showed global sclerosis, 1 showed segmental sclerosis, and 1 showed a thrombus (Figure 2(a)). Diffuse global or segmental mesangial expansion was seen, which was accompanied by mesangiolysis. Segmental endocapillary hypercellularity, focal double contours without spike formation, and mesangiolysis were observed (Figures 2(b) and 2(c)). Wrinkling of the glomerular basement membrane (GBM) was also observed (Figure 2(d)). A segmental thrombus was observed in one glomerulus (Figure 2(e)). Tubular atrophy and interstitial fibrosis were noticed (Figure 2(a)). Some arterioles revealed thickness of the arterial intima and narrowing or complete obstruction of the vessel lumina (Figures 2(f) and 2(g)). Immunofluorescent examination revealed no significant deposits of immunoglobulins or complement components. Electron microscopy revealed wrinkling of the glomerular basement membrane (GBM), expansion of the subendothelial space, mesangial interposition, and reduplication of the GBM (Figure 3).

Based on her clinical and histological findings, such as double contours and wrinkling of the GBM, mesangiolysis, and thickness of the arterial intima, she was diagnosed with TMA. The course of her disease was variable; hence, we reviewed her past medical history in detail. Gastric non-Hodgkin lymphoma had been in complete remission at the onset of TMA. She presented with severe hypertension; however, she did not meet the criteria for malignant hypertension. Although the disease was pathologically consistent with radiation nephropathy, there was no reliable evidence. Laboratory data revealed normal disintegrin and metalloproteinase with a thrombospondin type 1 motif, member 13 (ADAMTS13) activity (check before the initiation of HD); hence, she was unlikely to have thrombotic thrombocytopenic purpura (TTP). Throughout the course, there was no obvious infection. Due to a complicated medical history and rapid course of AKI, it was difficult to perform a kidney biopsy and identify the definite cause of disease immediately after the onset of AKI. Imidapril, an angiotensin-converting enzyme inhibitor, 5 mg/day was initiated. Her urine volume gradually increased. She was able to withdraw from hemodialysis therapy two weeks after the initiation of imidapril.

To further examine the genetic involvement of the complement system, we performed extensive diagnostic testing to identify the cause of TMA. Samples for the extensive complement analysis were taken. Plasma-soluble

Table 1: Laboratory data upon the first admission of the patient.

Examination	Value	Reference range	Examination	Value	Reference range	Examination	Value	Reference range
(Hematology)			(Coagulation)			(Serology; continued)		
WBC (/μL)	6690	3300–8600	aPTT (second)	23.9	26.9–40.9	ADAMTS13	72.0	70–120
RBC (10^4/μL)	349	386–492	PT (%)	117	70–130	IL-2R (U/ml)	1214	122–496
Hb (g/dL)	9.9	11.6–14.8	Fibrinogen (mg/dl)	438	200–400	Cryoglobulin	—	
Ht (%)	30.5	35.1-44-4	FDP (μg/ml)	25.5	<5	CEA (ng/ml)	2.3	<5.8
Plt ($\times 10^3$/μL)	17.8	15.8–34.8	D-dimer (μg/ml)	7.2	<1.0	CA19-9 (U/ml)	11	<37
						CA125 (U/ml)	112	<35
(Biochemistry)			(Serology)					
Total protein (g/dl)	6.4	6.6–8.1	CRP (mg/dl)	2.47	<0.14	(Infectious marker)		
Albumin (g/dl)	2.8	4.1–5.1	IgG (mg/dl)	1008	861–1747	HBs Ag	—	
Total bilirubin (mg/dl)	0.6	0.4–1.5	IgA (mg/dl)	97	93–393	HBs ab	—	
ALT (U/L)	30	13–30	IgM (mg/dl)	206	50–269	HCV ab	—	
AST (U/L)	11	7–23	C3 (mg/dl)	41.8	73–138	HIV ab	—	
LDH (U/L)	485	124–222	C4 (mg/dl)	<5	11–31	TPHA	—	
ALP (U/L)	427	106–322	CH50 (U/ml)	14	30–46	STS	—	
γGTP (U/L)	94	9–32	IC-1q (μg/ml)	<1.5	<3.0			
BUN (mg/dl)	36	8–20	ANA (INDEX)	72.4	<20	(Urinalysis)		
Cre (mg/dl)	2.55	0.46–0.79	Anti-DNA (RIA)	2.3	<6	Protein	3+	
UA (mg/dl)	7.5	2.6–5.5	Anti-SS-A (INDEX)	149.0	<10	Protein (g/gCr)	4.7	
Na (mEq/l)	140	138–145	Anti-SS-B (INDEX)	<5.0	<15	Glucose	—	
K (mEq/l)	3.1	3.6–4.8	Anti-SM (INDEX)	<5.0	<7	Ketone	—	
Cl (mEq/l)	105	101–108	Anti-Scl-70 (INDEX)	<5.0	<16	Occult blood	3+	
Ca (mg/dl)	7.9	8.8–10.1	Anti-CENPB (INDEX)	<5.0	<10	Sediments		
iP (mg/dl)	3.7	2.7–4.6	Anti-U1 RNP (INDEX)	<5.0	<15	Red blood cells (/hpf)	50–99	
Glucose (mg/dl)	149	73–109	Anti-ARS (INDEX)	<5.0	<25	White blood cells (/hpf)	5–9	
HbA1c (%)	4.8	4.9–6.0	Anti-CLGPI (U/mL)	<1.2	<3.5	Hyaline casts (/hpf)	10–99	
HDL-C (mg/dl)	61	48–103	aPL IgG (U/ml)	<8	<10	B2MG (μg/L)	158	13.0–301.2
LDL-C (mg/dl)	113	65–163	Anti-CCP (U/ml)	<0.5	<4.5			
Triglyceride (mg/dl)	68	30–117	MPO-ANCA (IU/mL)	<1.0	<3.5	(Blood gas analysis)		
			PR3-ANCA (IU/mL)	<1.0	<2.0	pH	7.477	7.35–7.45
			Anti-GBM (IU/mL)	2.0	<3	pCO2 (mmHg)	31.9	32–45
			BNP (pg/dl)	1055	<18.4	pO2 (mmHg)	77.0	83–108
			Ferritin (ng/dl)	210	5–152	HCO_3^- (mmol/L)	21.5	21–28
			Haptoglobin (mg/dl)	<10	19–170	Base excess (mmol/L)	−2.2	

WBC: white blood cell, RBC: red blood cell, Hb: hemoglobin, Ht: hematocrit, Plt: platelet, ALT: alanine aminotransferase, AST: aspartate aminotransferase, LDH: lactate dehydrogenase, ALP: alkaline phosphatase, γ-GTP: γ-glutamyltranspeptidase, BUN: blood urea nitrogen, Cre: creatinine, UA: uric acid, Na: sodium, K: potassium, Cl: chlorine, Ca: calcium, iP: inorganic phosphorus, HbA1c: hemoglobin A1c, HDL-C: high-density lipoprotein cholesterol, LDL-C: low-density lipoprotein cholesterol, aPTT: activated partial thromboplastin time, PT: prothrombin time, FDP: fibrin/fibrinogen degradation products, CRP: C-reactive protein, IgG: immunoglobulin G, IgA: immunoglobulin A, IgM: immunoglobulin M, C3: complement 3, C4: complement 4, CH50: total complement immunoassay, IC-C1q: immune complex C1Q binding assay, ANA: antinuclear antibody, Anti-DNA: anti-DNA antibody, Anti-SS-A: anti-SS-A antibody, Anti-SS-B: anti-SS-B antibody, Anti-SM: anti-Smith antibody, Anti-Scl-70: antitopoisomerase antibody, Anti-CENPB: anticentromere autoantigen B antibody, Anti-U1 RNP: antiribonucleoprotein antibody, Anti-ARS: antiaminoacyl tRNA synthetase antibody, Anti-CLGPI: anticardiolipin antibody, aPL: antiphospholipid antibody, Anti-CCP: anticyclic citrullinated peptide antibody, MPO-ANCA: myeloperoxidase-antineutrophil cytoplasmic antibody, PR3-ANCA: proteinase-3-antineutrophil cytoplasmic antibody, Anti-GBM: antiglomerular basement membrane antibody, BNP: brain natriuretic peptide, ADAMTS13: a disintegrin and metalloproteinase with a thrombospondin type 1 motif, member 13, IL-2R: soluble interleukin-2 receptor, CEA: carcinoembryonic antigen, CA19-9: carbohydrate antigen 19–9, CA125: cancer antigen 125, HBs Ag: hepatitis B surface antigen, HBs Ab: hepatitis B surface antibody, HCV Ab: hepatitis C antibody, HIV Ab: human immunodeficiency virus antibody, TPHA: Treponema pallidum hemagglutination assay, STS: serologic test for syphilis, hpf: high-power field, B2MG β2: microglobulin, pCO2: carbon dioxide partial pressure, pO2: oxygen partial pressure, HCO_3^-: bicarbonate ion.

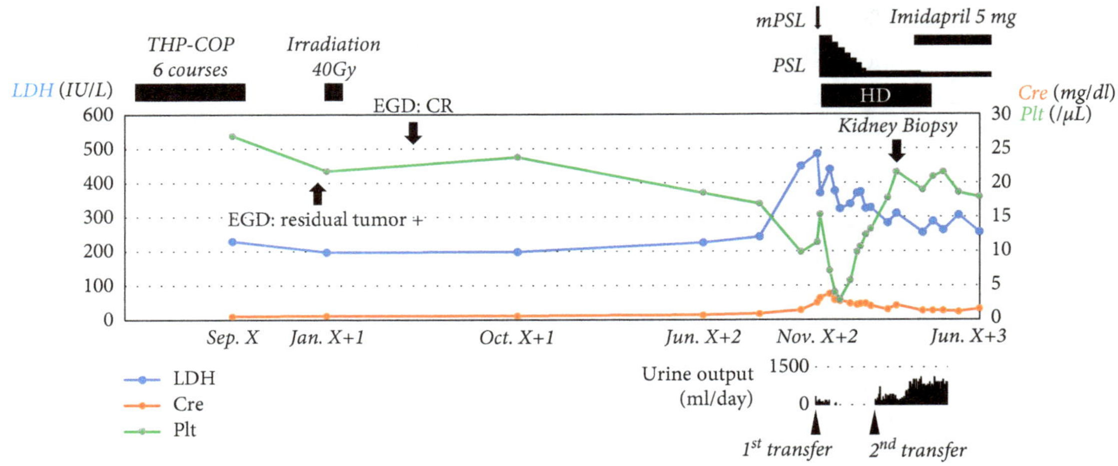

FIGURE 1: Clinical course of the patient. THP-COP: combination of pirarubicin, cyclophosphamide, vincristine, and prednisolone, EGD: esophagogastroduodenoscopy, CR: complete response, mPSL: methyl prednisolone pulse therapy, PSL: prednisolone, HD: hemodialysis, LDH: lactate dehydrogenase, Cre: creatinine, and Plt: platelet.

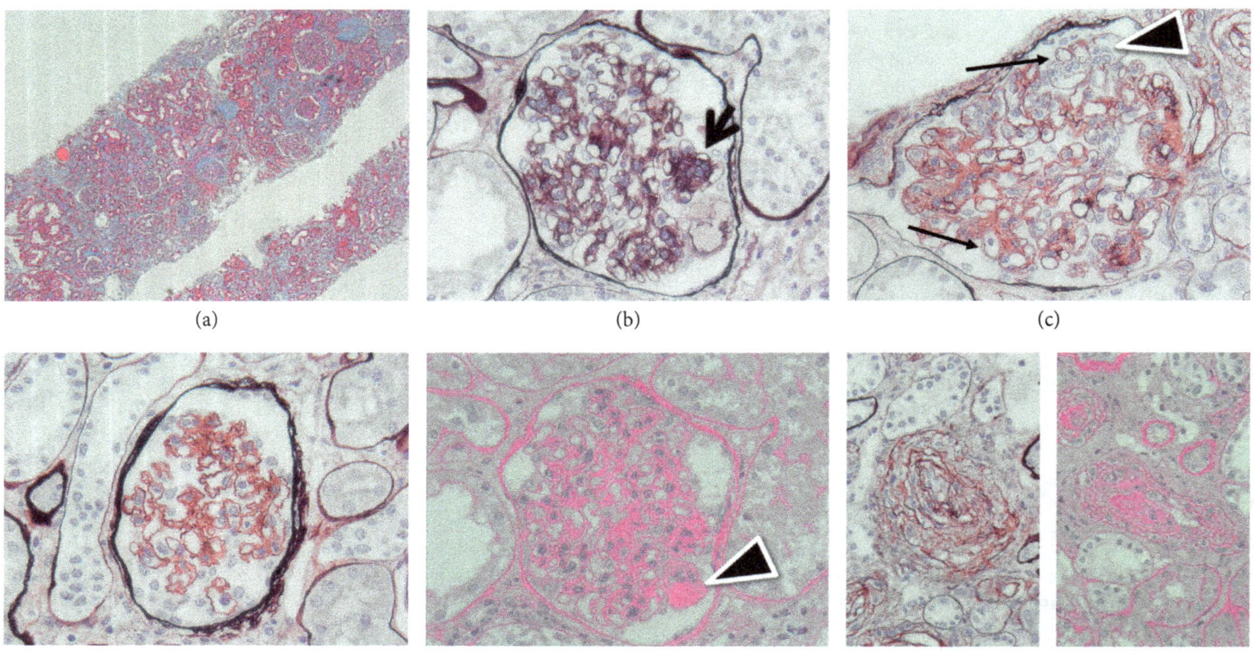

FIGURE 2: (a) Light microscopy of the biopsied sample (Masson's trichrome stain, original magnification ×48). (b) Segmental endocapillary hypercellularity (arrow) (periodic acid-silver methenamine stain, original magnification ×400). (c) Focal double contours without spike formation (arrows) and mesangiolysis (arrowhead) (periodic acid-silver methenamine stain, original magnification ×400). (d) Wrinkling of the glomerular basement membrane (periodic acid-silver methenamine stain, original magnification ×400). (e) Segmental thrombus in one glomerulus (arrowhead) (periodic acid-Schiff stain, original magnification ×400). Some arterioles revealed thickness of the arterial intima and narrowing or complete obstruction of the vessel lumina. (f) Periodic acid-silver methenamine stain, original magnification ×400. (g) Periodic acid-Schiff stain, original magnification ×400.

C5b-9 complement levels were 526.4 (reference range: 37.0–260.6) ng/mL, complement factor Ba levels were 3,970.4 (275.6–685.2) ng/mL, CFH levels were 391.7 (229.8–714.6) μg/mL, and complement 5a levels were 15.84 (0.20–15.62) ng/mL. Enzyme-linked immunosorbent assay for anti-CFH IgG was negative (510.6 (393.9–1069.0) AU/mL). After obtaining informed consent, we collected DNA from the patient. Genomic DNA was extracted from whole blood, and targeted next-generation sequencing of candidate genes for aHUS was performed. Sequencing of the exonic regions of 9 genes (CFH, *CFHR5*, *C3*, *CFI*, *CFB*, *MCP*, *THBD*, *DGKE*, and *PLG*) conducted at the Japanese

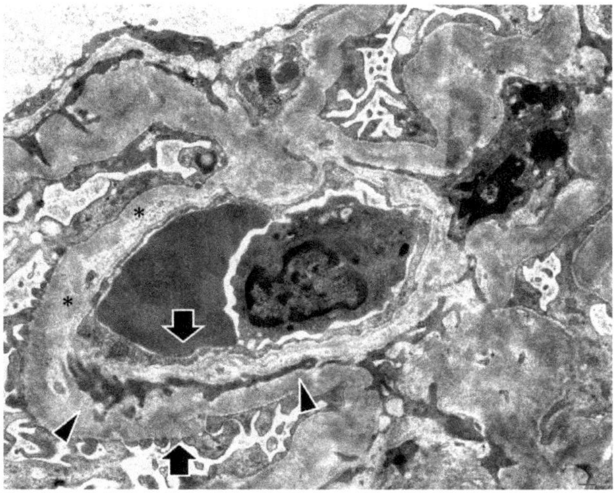

FIGURE 3: Electron microscopy revealed wrinkling of the glomerular basement membrane, expansion of the subendothelial space (asterisks), mesangial interposition (arrowhead), and reduplication of the glomerular basement membrane (arrow) (electron microscopy, original magnification ×3000).

Association for Complement Research revealed a heterogeneous very rare missense variant (exon 5; NM_000186.3: c.526 T > C: p.Phe176Leu) in the CFH gene. Despite the CFH variant, serum and plasma CFH levels were normal. It was not possible to completely deny the possibility that CFH p.Phe176Leu may have some influence as a causative genetic mutation; however, we did not use eculizumab (ECZ). A diagnosis of SLE was considered on account of reduced C3 and C4 counts along with the gradual effect of steroid treatment. However, the hemolytic anemia was attributable to TMA, and there were no other findings to suspect lupus nephritis; hence, a clear diagnosis of SLE could not be made.

The subsequent clinical course was relatively better. Hemodialysis was discontinued. Two years later, her creatinine level stayed at 1.91 mg/dl.

3. Discussion

We reported the case of a patient with the CFH gene variant (p.Phe176Leu in exon 5) who developed TMA on a mixed clinical background. Kidney biopsy findings confirmed that the patient had TMA; however, her medical history was complex. The etiology of TMA is complex, and in some cases, it is difficult to identify the cause. Bayer et al. [4] found that primary TMA accounted for only about 6% of the 564 patients in their study, while the remaining 94% patients had secondary TMA. In addition, they reported that the etiology in 57% of secondary TMA cases was multifactorial. As showed in the case presentation, it must be acknowledged that the diagnosis of background disease was inadequate; however, it was a characteristic finding that the TMA had a CFH variant. Although hypocomplementemia and renal dysfunction are pathological conditions indicating SLE, there were no findings of lupus nephritis, and a clear diagnosis of SLE could not be made.

In aHUS, mutation of CFH is identified in approximately 25% of sporadic cases and in 40% of familial cases [5]. CFH is the most frequent causative gene of aHUS in Europe and the United States (20–30%); however, in Japan, it is <10% [6]. Genetic variations in the CFH gene family are associated with several complex diseases, such as aHUS, C3 glomerulopathy, and age-related macular degeneration (AMD) [7]. In our case, a p.Phe176Leu variant of CFH was revealed. The p.Phe176Leu variant has been reported as a suspected pathological mutation of aHUS [6]. However, that reported case had another aHUS-predisposing variant (p.Arg1215Gln) with known pathogenicity [6]. On the other hand, p.Phe176Leu has recently been reported as a mutation capable of causing AMD [8]. AMD is a disease that is caused by complement dysregulation [9]; hence, it is undeniable that the p.Phe176Leu variant is involved in the amplification of complement activation by the alternative pathway. The p.Phe176Leu variant occurs in the cofactor region of CFH. In our patient, it could not be denied that it solely may lead to a reduction in cofactor activity and may be involved in the amplification of complement activation by the alternative pathway. p.Arg175Trp, an adjacent amino acid of p.Phe176Leu, was reported to be a potentially pathogenic mutation of aHUS [10]. Whether p.Phe176Leu is involved in the pathological condition cannot be determined without a functional analysis; therefore, further studies are required.

Currently, ECZ, a monoclonal antibody that targets complement protein C5, is widely used as a treatment for complement-related HUS [11]. To date, the pathogenesis of secondary HUS has not been fully studied; however, complement dysregulation is involved in some cases of secondary HUS [12]. In general, as shown in our case, the use of ECZ is not required for secondary TMA; however, the use of ECZ for secondary TMA is controversial. Even in some cases of secondary TMA, ECZ is very effective for rapidly resolving TMA and improving renal function [12]. In patients with refractory secondary SLE- and/or antiphospholipid syndrome-related TMA, despite treatment of lupus nephritis, the use of ECZ in 9 patients showed a positive outcome in hematology values, renal function, and other organ functions following treatment with ECZ, suggesting that it involves complement pathways. Unfortunately, a genetic analysis of complement genes was not performed in that study [13]. ECZ is a very effective drug for aHUS; however, ECZ is a very expensive drug. The kind of patient that should be treated and how long treatment should continue are considered important issues. The usefulness of ECZ for secondary TMA should be further investigated in future studies.

We reported the case of a patient with the CFH variant who developed TMA on a mixed clinical background. The pathophysiology of secondary TMA is complex, and it is important to keep in mind that the presence of complement gene abnormalities in secondary TMA should be investigated to help determine whether ECZ should be used.

Consent

Informed consent was obtained from the patient and her family.

Disclosure

The funder was not involved in the manuscript writing, editing, approval, or decision to publish.

Authors' Contributions

Y.I. conceived the article and drafted the manuscript. T.M. contributed to the diagnosis of renal pathology. Y.O., S.G., and I.N. contributed to the review of the literature and provided supervision, assessment, and interpretation of data, along with mentorship. All authors approved the final manuscript.

Acknowledgments

The authors are grateful to Mr. N. Sakamoto, Ms. S. Tsuchida, Ms. M. Yoshinuma, and Ms. M. Igashima (Department of Pathology, Shinrakuen Hospital) for their technical assistance.

References

[1] V. Brocklebank, K. M. Wood, and D. Kavanagh, "Thrombotic microangiopathy and the kidney," *Clinical Journal of the American Society of Nephrology*, vol. 13, no. 2, pp. 300–317, 2018.

[2] T. H. J. Goodship, H. T. Cook, F. Fakhouri et al., "Atypical hemolytic uremic syndrome and C3 glomerulopathy: conclusions from a "kidney disease: improving global outcomes" (KDIGO) controversies conference," *Kidney International*, vol. 91, no. 3, pp. 539–551, 2017.

[3] L. M. P. Palma, M. Sridharan, and S. Sethi, "Complement in secondary thrombotic microangiopathy," *Kidney International Reports*, vol. 6, no. 1, pp. 11–23, 2021.

[4] G. Bayer, F. von Tokarski, B. Thoreau et al., "Etiology and outcomes of thrombotic microangiopathies," *Clinical Journal of the American Society of Nephrology*, vol. 14, no. 4, pp. 557–566, 2019.

[5] C. M. Nester, T. Barbour, S. R. de Cordoba et al., "Atypical aHUS: state of the art," *Molecular Immunology*, vol. 67, no. 1, pp. 31–42, 2015.

[6] M. Fujisawa, H. Kato, Y. Yoshida et al., "Clinical characteristics and genetic backgrounds of Japanese patients with atypical hemolytic uremic syndrome," *Clinical and Experimental Nephrology*, vol. 22, no. 5, pp. 1088–1099, 2018.

[7] R. J. Klein, C. Zeiss, E. Y. Chew, J. Y. Tsai, R. S. Sackler, and C. Haynes, "Complement factor H polymorphism in age-related macular degeneration," *Science*, vol. 308, no. 5720, pp. 385–389, 2005.

[8] S. Cantsilieris, B. J. Nelson, J. Huddleston et al., "Recurrent structural variation, clustered sites of selection, and disease risk for the complement factor H (CFH) gene family," *Proceedings of the National Academy of Sciences*, vol. 115, no. 19, pp. E4433–E4442, 2018.

[9] J. R. W. Yates, T. Sepp, B. K. Matharu et al., "Complement C3 variant and the risk of age-related macular degeneration," *New England Journal of Medicine*, vol. 357, no. 6, pp. 553–561, 2007.

[10] R. W. Thergaonkar, A. Narang, B. S. Gurjar et al., "Targeted exome sequencing in anti-factor H antibody negative HUS reveals multiple variations," *Clinical and Experimental Nephrology*, vol. 22, no. 3, pp. 653–660, 2018.

[11] C. M. Legendre, C. Licht, P. Muus et al., "Terminal complement inhibitor eculizumab in atypical hemolytic-uremic syndrome," *New England Journal of Medicine*, vol. 368, no. 23, pp. 2169–2181, 2013.

[12] T. Cavero, C. Rabasco, A. López et al., "Eculizumab in secondary atypical haemolytic uraemic syndrome," *Nephrology Dialysis Transplantation*, vol. 32, no. 3, pp. 466–474, 2017.

[13] N. Kello, L. E. Khoury, G. Marder, R. Furie, E. Zapantis, and D. L. Horowitz, "Secondary thrombotic microangiopathy in systemic lupus erythematosus and antiphospholipid syndrome, the role of complement and use of eculizumab: case series and review of literature," *Seminars in Arthritis and Rheumatism*, vol. 49, no. 1, pp. 74–83, 2019.

6

Anti-SARS-CoV-2 Antibody Level among Renal Transplant Recipients: A Case Report from Nepal

Kamal Ranabhat,[1,2] Bhuvan Saud,[3] Saroj Adhikari,[4] Suraj Bhattarai,[5] Rojan Adhikari,[6] Bhoj Raj Luitel,[1] and Mahesh Raj Sigdel[1]

[1]*Institue of Medicine, Tribhuvan University, Kathmandu, Nepal*
[2]*Ministry of Health and Population, Kathmandu, Nepal*
[3]*Department of Medical Laboratory Technology, Janamaitri Foundation Institute of Health Sciences, Lalitpur, Nepal*
[4]*National Trauma Center, Ministry of Health and Population Kathmandu, Nepal*
[5]*Global Institute for Interdisciplinary Studies, Kathmandu, Nepal*
[6]*Shahid Dharma Bhakta National Transplant Center, Bhaktapur, Nepal*

Correspondence should be addressed to Bhuvan Saud; link2bhuvan@gmail.com

Academic Editor: Tun-Chieh Chen

Globally, SARS-CoV-2 has caused significant public health burden, mainly in patients with underlying comorbidities including both communicable and noncommunicable diseases. Solid organ transplant recipients under immunesupressive medication are also amongst the high risk group. There is only sparse data on immunity against SARS-CoV-2 infection among renal transplant recipients. In this case report, we present the level of anti-SARS-CoV-2 antibody of three kidney transplant recipients after vaccination against COVID-19 virus. All three cases had received two doses of Oxford-AstraZeneca COVID-19 vaccine AZD1222 (ChAdOx1). Serological analysis showed protective level of circulating antibodies in the blood of all three cases. Although two out of three patients in the study acquired COVID-19 infection after immunization, they recovered with mild clinical course. Hence, we conclude that despite immune-suppressed status of transplant recipients, COVID-19 vaccination could protect them against severe illness.

1. Introduction

Coronavirus disease 2019 (COVID-19) is caused by Severe Acute Respiratory Syndrome Coronavirus-2 (SARS-CoV-2). The virus causes significant morbidity and mortality in individuals with underlying clinical conditions. As of 8th January 2022, more than 302 million positive cases and 5.4 million deaths have been reported globally [1].Generally, pathogenic microorganisms cause pathological manifestations in host system which depends on the host immune response and virulence factors of the infectious agents. Human body activates complex immune mechanism by which it provides protection from the invading foreign substance [2]. In SARS-CoV-2 infection, patients produce virus-specific B and T cells and then initially produce Immunoglobulin M (IgM) and later Immunoglobulin G (IgG) antibodies which are readily detected in serum [3, 4]. Generally, patients with chronic diseases are highly susceptible to the infection. Higher mortality rate in such group may be due to dysregulation of immune system. Studies have suggested that haemodialysis and kidney transplant patients are at high risk of morality from SARS-CoV-2 with 20% mortality rate [5, 6]. Kidney transplant recipients are advised to take immune-suppressive drugs (calcineurin inhibitors, antiproliferative agents, rapamycin inhibitors, and corticosteroids) in order to prevent rejection by the host immune system. Lowered immunity makes such person susceptible to infectious agents [7].

Globally, as of 7th January 2022, 137 different COVID-19 vaccines are in various phases of clinical trials, while

194 are in the preclinical phase; emergency-use approved vaccines are recommended prioritizing people with chronic diseases, with certain clinical conditions and old age [8]. Studies have reported that vaccines show weak immunogenicity among kidney transplant recipients as they do not produce antibodies effectively [9, 10]. Moreover, live or replication component vaccines are contraindicated in transplant recipients [11]. In contrast, some studies have noted that solid organ transplant recipients achieve adaptive immune response similar to immune-competent individuals [12]. A study conducted among kidney transplant recipients in France has revealed that 10.8% of transplant recipients developed antibodies after 28 days of receiving COVID-19 vaccine and that multiple booster doses might be required to reach effective level [13].

In Nepal, immune response to SARS-CoV-2 in immune-compromised individuals, mainly in renal transplant recipients has not been reported till date and very less is known about neutralizing antibody response in them after vaccination. In this study, we estimated circulating anti-SARS-CoV-2 antibody level after vaccination in three renal transplant patients who are concurrently receiving immune-suppressive drugs. It was aimed to understand the humoral immune response in the recipients and the need for additional booster doses of COVID-19 vaccine in such patients.

2. Case Presentation

2.1. Patient 1. A 40-year-old overweight male had kidney transplant in 2008 (13 years ago). He received first dose of ChAdOx1 nCoV-19 vaccine (AZD1222) against SARS-CoV-2 on 16 April 2021 and the second dose on 21 June 2021. A quantitative serological test was performed on 26 June 2021 to detect anti-SARS-CoV-2 antibody level in his blood by Chemiluminescent immunoassay (CLIA) test as per the manufacturer's instructions The test result was 18.15 cutoff index (test positive if value is >1.) Later, on 19 October 2021, the man was admitted to the hospital with mild illness, having fever (101.5°F), body ache and loss of smell. Real-time polymerase chain reaction (RT-PCR) test for COVID-19 was found positive and became negative only after 23 days of first diagnosis. Other clinical laboratory parameter results are shown in Table 1.

2.2. Patient 2. A 38-year-old male had renal transplantation in 2005 (16 years ago). He received the first dose of ChAdOx1 nCoV-19 vaccine (AZD1222) in April 2021 and the second dose in June 2021 (7 weeks later). His anti-SARS-CoV-2 serum antibody level was tested on 25 June 2021 which was 54.5 by enzyme-linked immunosorbent assay (ELISA) where test is positive if value is >11.0. On 24 November 2021, he experienced mild symptoms of COVID-19 such as fever, malaise, sore throat, and loss of smell and taste. He was admitted to the hospital and was found positive for COVID-19 by RT-PCR test. He tested negative for COVID-19 virus gene detection after one month. Before natural infection, the patient's other clinical laboratory reports are listed in Table 1.

2.3. Patient 3. A 41-year-old male had undergone kidney transplantation in 2006 (15 years ago). He took the first dose of ChAdOx1 nCoV-19 vaccine (AZD1222) on 1 June 2021 and the second dose on 8 July 2021. He did not experience COVID-19 infection. His blood was tested for anti-SARS-CoV-2 antibody level on 28 July 2021. Chemiluminescent immunoassay (CLIA) test report showed that anti-SARS-CoV-2 antibody level was 5.91 IU/ml, where test is positive if the value ranged >0.80 IU/ml. Other laboratory parameters are shown in Table 1.

3. Discussion

According to the report published by Shahid Dharma Bhakta National Transplant Center, Bhaktapur, annually, 3000 cases of kidney failure are reported in Nepal and out of them more than 350 kidney transplants are performed [14]. Kidney transplant recipients are at higher risk of microbial infection due to immunosuppressive status. In this case series, we present clinical and laboratory findings of three kidney transplant recipients in Nepal who were vaccinated against SARS-CoV-2 infection. The total leucocyte count and differential leucocyte count of all three cases were normal indicating that the therapeutic indices of the immune-suppressive medications had been maintained. Two recipients got infected by SARS-CoV-2 after completing two doses of vaccine but only presented mild symptomatic illness and successfully recovered without requiring critical care support. Mean age of transplant recipients was 39.6 (range, 38–41 years) and all three were male. Neutralizing antibody was developed in all three cases with significant antibody level. However, since the duration of protection from the vaccine is not clearly known yet, there is need for frequent follow-up for neutralizing antibody levels in such patients which is subjected to drop due to immune-suppressive medication. The result of this study is also different from other studies which reveal that very few individuals who received organ transplant developed anti-SARS-CoV-2 antibody [15, 16]. Kidney transplant recipients are at higher risk of developing COVID-19 severity if the recipients have comorbid diseases (obesity, diabetes, asthma, and chronic pulmonary disease), particularly diabetes and hypertension which are recognized as one of the main factors responsible for severity [16].

In this study, seroconversion occurred in all three transplant patients in an effective level. Studies have suggested that only 4-48% of renal transplant recipients have detectable anti-spike IgGs following two doses of COVID-19 vaccine [17]. In a study conducted among immune-suppressed solid organ transplant recipients from USA, who received Ad26.COV2.S (Janssen COVID-19 vaccine), out of 12 participants, only two (16%) had mounted detectable amount of antibody level [18]. A study from France conducted among kidney transplant recipients after administration of two doses of BNT162b2 mRNA COVID-19 vaccine (Pfizer-BioNTech) found that 5.7% of the patients developed anti-spike antibodies [19]). Furthermore, a case control study conducted in Germany to evaluate the immune response after vaccination in kidney transplant recipients with

Table 1: Different variables of the three renal transplant recipients.

Clinical variables	Patient 1	Patient 2	Patient 3
Age	40	38	41
Gender	Male	Male	Male
Transplant performed	2008	2005	2006
Current medications	Mycophenolate sodium 360 mg and tacrolimus 0.5 mg	Mycophenolate mofetil 500 mg and cyclosporine 25 mg	Mycophenolate mofetil 500 mg and tacrolimus (1 mg* and 0.5 mg**)
Body mass index	Overweight	Normal	Overweight
Comorbidities	No	No	Hypertension
1st dose COVID vaccine	16 April 2021	21 April 2021	01 June 2021
2nd dose COVID vaccine	21 June 2021	08 June 2021	08 July 2021
Serum creatinine (mg/dl)	1.3	1.4	1.2
Serum urea (mg/dl)	41.0	16.96	21.0
Sodium (Na^+) mmol/l	136	139.0	143.0
Potassium (K^+) mmol/l	4.8	3.3	4.0
Hemoglobin (g/dl)	15.8	12.6	12.7
RBC (million/mm^3)	5.48	4.64	4.76
WBC (cells/mm^3)	7900	8400	12500
Differential cell count			
Neutrophil (%)	78	74	77
Lymphocyte (%)	16	21	21
Monocyte (%)	04	4	02
Eosinophil (%)	02	1	0
Basophil (%)	0	0	0
RT-PCR for COVID-19	Positive	Positive	Not tested
COVID-19 sign and symptoms	Fever, body ache, and loss of smell	Fever, malaise, sore throat, and loss of smell and taste	Unknown
Anti-SARS-CoV-2 ab (method)	18.15 COI (ECLIA)	54.5 (ELISA)	5.91 U/ml (ECLIA)
Outcome	Recovered from COVID-19	Recovered from COVID-19	Stable

Note. *Morning dose; **evening dose. NR: normal range; RT-PCR: reverse transcription polymerase chain reaction; ELISA: enzyme-linked immunosorbent assay; ECLIA: electrochemiluminescence immunoassay; ab: antibody; COI: cutoff index.

BNT162b2 mRNA COVID-19 vaccine (Pfizer-BioNTech) found that only 22% of the recipients were positive for anti-SARS-CoV-2 IgG antibodies. The titers were also significantly lower than the control group of heath-care workers. Anti-SARS-CoV-2 IgG antibodies were detected in 100% of the participants in the control group following vaccination [6]. The clinical outcome of the vaccinated renal transplant recipients in our study was favorable. Although two of the three patients got infected with COVID-19, both recovered and are stable. In a study conducted in India among four renal transplant recipients, all of them got infected with COVID-19 despite being vaccinated full doses of ChAdOx1 nCoV-19 vaccine (AZD1222); one of them died, two were admitted on ventilator at the time of the study, and another patient recovered and was stable at home [20].

Tacrolimus induces neutropenia [21] while mycophenolate mofetil leads to reduction of B-lymphocyte count [22]. It is important to maintain the circulating level of these drugs within therapeutic ranges to maintain health and prevent graft rejection. Both renal function tests and complete blood count profile are within normal range and the patients do not present any comorbidity which reflects that the immune-suppressant regimens are maintained within their therapeutic indices. The production of protecting level of humoral immune response against COVID-19 virus after vaccination in the study cases may be attributed to the maintained drug levels.

The limitations of this study are that antibody levels were not estimated periodically nor the antibody level was tested after first dose of vaccine administration. Another limitation is that only ChAdOx1n CoV-19 (AZD1222) vaccinated individuals were enrolled in this study but the immune response to other types of COVID-19 vaccines might be different. Also, periodic reports of serum level of the immune-suppressive drugs could not be obtained which would have better justified the immune status of the participants in the study. For better evidence, similar serological studies should be conducted in large scale to understand the immunogenicity of newer vaccines in the immune-compromised population, the results of which would help the government and concerned authorities to take prompt action.

4. Conclusion

Protective level of humoral immune response against SARS-CoV-2 has been shown after administration of two doses of ChAdOx1 nCoV-19 (AZD1222) vaccine in renal transplant recipients. Routine monitoring of anti-SARS-CoV-2 circulating antibody as well as immune-suppressive drug level is recommended to understand the immune status of transplant recipients and the immunogenicity of newer vaccines in them.

Data Availability

The data used to support the findings of this study are available from the corresponding author upon request. The authors agree that anyone interested can have access to the raw data from the research upon request to the authors. The data will be provided to anyone based on two conditions: upon use of the data, the authors should be acknowledged and also the paper needs to be cited. An agreement in the aforementioned situation will be reached.

Consent

Written informed consent was obtained from the patients for publishing their case details along with their clinical, laboratory, and antibody details.

Disclosure

This research did not receive any specific grant from funding agencies in the public, commercial, or not-for-profit sectors.

Authors' Contributions

Kamal Ranabhat and Bhuvan Saud conceptualized the study. Bhuvan Saud, Saroj Adhikari, and Kamal Ranabhat wrote the first draft and reviewed the literature. Mahesh Raj Sigdel, Suraj Bhattarai, Bhoj Raj Luitel, and Rojan Adhikari provided critical feedback to the draft. All authors read and approved the final version of the manuscript.

Acknowledgments

We thank the patients and their family members for their cooperation and for the written informed consent for the publication of this case report. We acknowledge Mr. Himalaya Tiwari, health staff, Bir Hospital, for his invaluable support and coordination.

References

[1] John Hopkins University and Medicine, *Coronavirus Resource Center*https://coronavirus.jhu.edu/.

[2] C. Wang, X. Zhou, M. Wang, and X. Chen, "The impact of SARS-CoV-2 on the human immune system and microbiome," *Infectious Microbes & Diseases*, vol. 3, no. 1, p. 14, 2021.

[3] P. D. Burbelo, F. X. Riedo, C. Morishima et al., "Sensitivity in detection of antibodies to nucleocapsid and spike proteins of severe acute respiratory syndrome coronavirus 2 in patients with coronavirus disease 2019," *The Journal of infectious diseases*, vol. 222, no. 2, pp. 206–213, 2020.

[4] J. Qu, C. Wu, X. Li et al., "Profile of immunoglobulin G and IgM antibodies against severe acute respiratory syndrome coronavirus 2 (SARS-CoV-2)," *Clinical Infectious Diseases*, vol. 71, no. 16, pp. 2255–2258, 2020.

[5] C. Hugo, M. Stecher, S. Dolff et al., "Solid organ transplantation is not a risk factor for COVID-19 disease outcome," *Transplant international: official journal of the European Society for Organ Transplantation*, vol. 34, no. 2, pp. 378–381, 2021.

[6] J. Korth, M. Jahn, O. Dorsch et al., "Impaired humoral response in renal transplant recipients to SARS-CoV-2 vaccination with BNT162b2 (Pfizer-BioNTech)," *Viruses*, vol. 13, no. 5, p. 756, 2021.

[7] A. Ortiz, M. Cozzolino, R. Duivenvoorden et al., "Chronic kidney disease is a key risk factor for severe COVID-19: a call to action by the ERA-EDTA," *Nephrology Dialysis Transplantation*, vol. 36, no. 1, pp. 87–94, 2021.

[8] WHO, *Draft landscape and tracker of COVID-19 candidate vaccines*, World Health Organization 2021a, 2021, June 2021 https://www.who.int/publications/m/item/draft-landscape-of-covid-19-candidate-vaccineson.

[9] "Immunogenicity of a single dose of SARS-CoV-2 messenger RNA vaccine in solid organ transplant recipients," *Journal of the American Medical Association*, vol. 325, pp. 1784–1786, 2021.

[10] T. Kolb, S. Fischer, L. Müller et al., "Impaired immune response to SARS-CoV-2 vaccination in dialysis patients and in kidney transplant recipients," *Kidney*, vol. 2, no. 9, pp. 1491–1498, 2021.

[11] L. Danziger-Isakov, D. Kumar, and AST ID Community of Practice, "Vaccination of solid organ transplant candidates and recipients: guidelines from the American Society of Transplantation Infectious Diseases Community of Practice," *Clinical Transplantation*, vol. 33, no. 9, p. e13563, 2019.

[12] N. Toapanta, O. Bestard, and M. J. Soler, "SARS-CoV-2 vaccination in patients receiving kidney replacement therapies: where are we now with the protective immune response?,"

Nephrology Dialysis Transplantation, vol. 36, no. 10, pp. 1950–1954, 2021.

[13] I. Benotmane, G. Gautier-Vargas, N. Cognard et al., "Weak anti–SARS-CoV-2 antibody response after the first injection of an mRNA COVID-19 vaccine in kidney transplant recipients," *Kidney international*, vol. 99, no. 6, pp. 1487–1489, 2021.

[14] "Human Organ Transplant Center," https://hotc.org.np/.

[15] M. Elias, D. Pievani, C. Randoux et al., "COVID-19 infection in kidney transplant recipients: disease incidence and clinical outcomes," *Journal of the American Society of Nephrology*, vol. 31, no. 10, pp. 2413–2423, 2020.

[16] D. Banerjee, J. Popoola, S. Shah, I. C. Ster, V. Quan, and M. Phanish, "COVID-19 infection in kidney transplant recipients," *Kidney international*, vol. 97, no. 6, pp. 1076–1082, 2020.

[17] S. Caillard and O. Thaunat, "COVID-19 vaccination in kidney transplant recipients," *Nature Reviews. Nephrology*, vol. 17, pp. 785–787, 2021.

[18] B. J. Boyarsky, T. P. Chiang, M. T. Ou et al., "Antibody response to the Janssen COVID-19 vaccine in solid organ transplant recipients," *Transplantation*, vol. 105, no. 8, pp. e82–e83, 2021.

[19] N. Chavarot, A. Ouedrani, O. Marion et al., "Poor anti-SARS-CoV-2 humoral and T-cell responses after 2 injections of mRNA vaccine in kidney transplant recipients treated with belatacept," *Transplantation*, vol. 105, no. 9, pp. e94–e95, 2021.

[20] H. S. Meshram, V. B. Kute, N. Shah et al., "COVID-19 in kidney transplant recipients vaccinated with Oxford–AstraZeneca COVID-19 vaccine (Covishield): a single-center experience from India," *Transplantation*, vol. 105, no. 9, 2021.

[21] A. De Rycke, D. Dierickx, and D. R. Kuypers, "Tacrolimus-induced neutropenia in renal transplant recipients," *Clinical Journal of the American Society of Nephrology*, vol. 6, no. 3, pp. 690–694, 2011.

[22] G. Weigel, A. Griesmacher, A. Karimi, A. O. Zuckermann, M. Grimm, and M. M. Mueller, "Effect of mycophenolate mofetil therapy on lymphocyte activation in heart transplant recipients," *The Journal of heart and lung transplantation*, vol. 21, pp. 1074–1079, 2002.

7

Donor-Derived Urothelial Carcinoma in Renal Transplant Recipients

Zhiyu Qian,[1] Emily Chou,[2] Jing Yang,[3] Hanwei Zhang,[2] HuiHui Ye,[3] Sandy T. Liu,[4] and Arnold I. Chin[2]

[1]*Division of Urology, Brigham and Women's Hospital, Harvard Medical School, USA*
[2]*Department of Urology, David Geffen School of Medicine at UCLA, USA*
[3]*Department of Pathology, David Geffen School of Medicine at UCLA, USA*
[4]*Department of Medicine, Division of Hematology and Oncology, David Geffen School of Medicine at UCLA, USA*

Correspondence should be addressed to Zhiyu Qian; zhiyu.qian.jason@gmail.com
and Arnold I. Chin; arnoldchin@mednet.ucla.edu

Academic Editor: David Duchene

Cancer is a significant cause of morbidity and mortality in recipients of renal transplantation. The vast majority develop from recipient origins, whereas donor-derived malignancies are exceedingly rare. We report 2 cases of poorly differentiated donor-derived urothelial carcinoma (UC) in renal transplantation recipients. The first patient underwent a living-related-donor renal transplantation 24 years prior and presented with back pain, hematuria, and rising creatinine and was found to have a 14 cm mass in the renal allograft with regional lymphadenopathy and liver metastases. Pathology showed UC with small-cell differentiation. The second patient presented with hematuria and rising creatinine and was initially found to have muscle invasive bladder cancer seven years after a deceased donor renal transplantation. Nine months after radical cystectomy, a large 9 cm mass was found on his allograft, for which radical nephrectomy and excision of prior ileal conduit was performed. Pathology showed UC with sarcomatoid differentiation. Short tandem repeat (STR) genotyping confirmed donor-derived origins. Both patient tumors expressed PD-L1 suggesting an additional therapeutic avenue for these rare tumors.

1. Introduction

Renal transplantation for end-stage renal disease reduces the comorbidity associated with chronic dialysis and can improve patients' quality of life [1]. Among all posttransplantation complications, cancer is a leading cause of morbidity and mortality in recipients of renal transplantation, accounting for up to 56% of deaths in recipients with a functioning renal graft [2, 3]. Cumulative risk for cancer reaches 25% 25 years after transplantation [4]. The majority of these cases arise from recipient origins contributed by the combinatory effects from immunosuppression, infection, and altered cell-specific immunity [2]. In contrast, donor-originated cancers are rare. In a study of the United Kingdom Transplant Registry between 2001 and 2010 with 21,029 cases of renal transplantation, a 10-year incidence of 0.06% was reported [5]. Of these, over 80% were donor-transmitted cancers, where preexisting malignancies within the donor organ were transmitted to graft recipients during transplantation. These cases were typically diagnosed within a year after transplantation in part due to their aggressive biology in the context of immunosuppression accompanying the surgery. The remaining were donor-derived cancers, where malignancies arise *de novo* from donor cells and typically present many years after transplantation.

Literature describing donor-derived urothelial carcinoma (UC) is limited to a series of case reports. The average time of presentation of donor-derived UC is approximately 10 years after renal transplantation [6]. Prior exposure to risk factors for UC could potentially contribute, as well as infection with BK virus and immunosuppression [6, 7]. As such, we felt compelled to contribute to the literature as

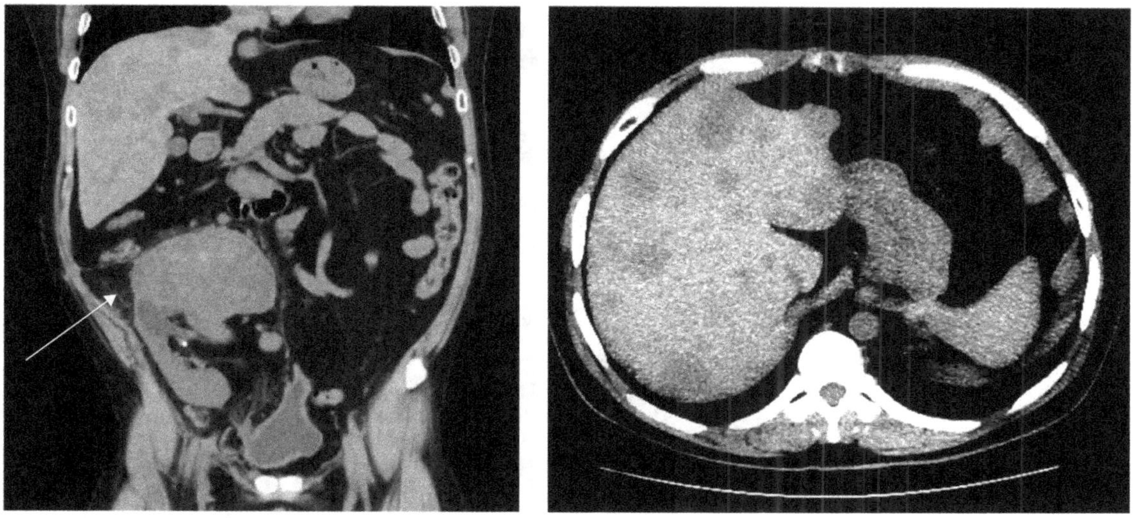

(a) (b)

FIGURE 1: (a) For case 1, coronal view of computer tomographic scan without intravenous contrast visualized 11 cm mass in the renal allograft (arrow). Multiple hypodense masses were vaguely present in the liver. (b) Axial view of the same scan with different brightness and contrast setting visualized numerous hypodense masses in the liver.

screening is not a routine and presentation often insidious. Here, we report 2 cases of poorly differentiated and aggressive donor-derived UC.

2. Case Presentation

2.1. Case 1. The first patient is a 37-year-old male who received a living-donor renal transplantation from his mother at age 13 for end-stage renal disease secondary to obstructive uropathy from posterior urethral valves. The patient developed persistent hydronephrosis after transplantation and received a bladder augmentation and Mitrofanoff procedure four years later. He had a history of recurrent infections involving his bladder and kidney allograft. His right native kidney was resected for a very large staghorn calculi seven years after transplantation. Immunosuppression was maintained on cyclosporin A 100 mg in the am and 75 mg in the pm, mycophenolate mofetil 500 mg daily, and prednisone 4 mg daily.

The patient presented 24 years after his transplantation with worsening lower back pain, hematuria, with a rising creatinine from baseline of 3 to 4.15 milligrams/deciliter (mg/dL). He had a palpable abdominal mass over the allograft. A noncontrast computer tomography (CT) scan showed a 11 cm mass in the renal allograft, multiple hepatic lesions up to 3.2 cm, and marked retroperitoneal lymphadenopathy up to 5 cm (Figure 1). The patient had been followed by routine ultrasound since his transplantation and findings have been unremarkable. His prior imaging study was an ultrasound of the renal graft and native kidneys 10 months prior to his presentation, which showed cortical thinning with unchanged upper pole and interpolar caliectasis. Biopsy of both hepatic and renal masses showed UC with small-cell features. Chromogranin was 5640 nanogram/deciliter (ng/dL) (normal limits (NL) <160 ng/dL), and neuron specific enolase was 361 nanogram/milliliter ng/mL (NL 3.7–8.9 ng/mL).

Immunosuppression was tapered, and the patient was considered for systemic chemotherapy with cisplatin, etoposide, as well as checkpoint immunotherapy in a phase I trial. Prior to initiation of systemic therapy, the patient was admitted for worsening abdominal and back pain and enlarging abdominal mass. After extensive discussion, surgical excision of renal allograft was pursued. Intraoperatively, the tumor was adherent to the colon serosa and anterior and posterior abdominal wall which were partially resected along with regional lymph nodes. Pathology showed a 14 cm mass with majority UC with small-cell differentiation staining diffusely positive for synaptophysin and papillary UC with squamous features in the collecting system (Figure 2). Pathologic stage was pT4N2M1 with 12 of 14 nodes positive and ranging in size of 3.5 to 5 cm. PD-L1 immunohistochemistry (DAKO 22C3) showed 10% tumor expression and <1% tumor infiltrating immune cell expression. TEMPUS 648 gene panel testing showed mutations in TP53, RB1, KDM6A, and KRAS, with a tumor mutational burden of 3.2 m/MB. Microsatellite instability (MSI) based on immunohistochemistry was normal. Short tandem repeat (STR) analysis revealed heterogeneity between tumor and recipient and thus confirmed donor origin (Figure 3). The immediate postoperative course was unremarkable. The patient resumed hemodialysis and was discharged ten days after surgery.

Three weeks later, the patient presented with severe abdominal pain with imaging showing a large pelvic fluid collection. A drain was placed, and its output consisted of feculent material suggesting a perforation of the colon. Despite bowel rest and antibiotic treatment, the patient clinically deteriorated and developed atrial fibrillation with rapid ventricular response leading to hypotension that did

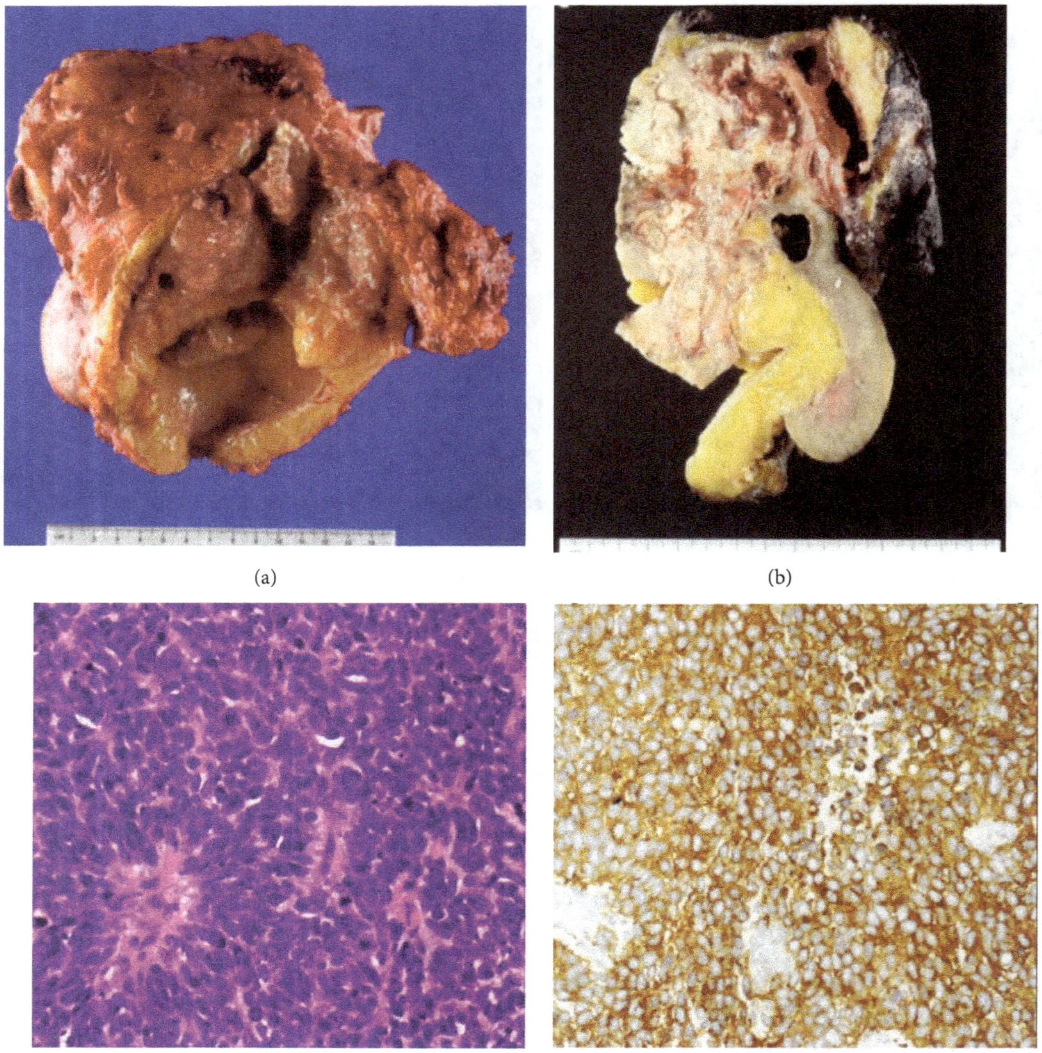

FIGURE 2: (a) For case 1, nephroureterectomy showed the friable tumor in the dilated ureter. (b) The kidney was bivalved to reveal a 17 cm yellow fleshy mass with hemorrhage and focal necrosis. (c) Hematoxylin and eosin stain showed tumor cells consist of diffuse sheets of small round to oval malignant cells with frequent mitotic activity, exhibiting small-cell features (×400). (d) Immunostaining showed tumor cells are strongly positive for synaptophysin (×400).

not improve with therapy. On day 18 of this hospitalization, the family elected to transition the patient to comfort measures, and the patient expired.

2.2. Case 2. The second patient is a 56-year-old-male who received a renal transplantation from a 51-year-old male deceased donor 7 years prior for end-stage renal disease secondary to membranous nephropathy. His posttransplantation course was complicated by BK virus and cytomegalovirus viremia. Allograft biopsy confirmed BK nephropathy, which was treated with intravenous immunoglobulin, ciprofloxacin, and leflunomide. With his elevated creatinine of 1.8 to 2.6 mg/dL, a noncontrast MRI was performed. Only masses within the bladder were detected without lymphadenopathy, allograft hydronephrosis, or allograft masses noted on imaging. Cystoscopy revealed multifocal bladder tumors with transurethral resection confirming the diagnosis of muscle-invasive UC of the bladder. With his creatinine at 2.5 mg/dL and functioning renal allograft, no cisplatin-based neoadjuvant chemotherapy or immunotherapy was given. He underwent radical cystoprostatectomy with ileal conduit and anastomosis of allograft ureter. Pathology showed pT2N0 high-grade urothelial carcinoma with multiple foci involving trigone, anterior and posterior wall, left dome, right distal ureter, and both ureteral orifices, totaling at around 50% bladder surface area (Figure 4). Surgical margins were negative.

The patient underwent surveillance imaging 4 months after surgery. Nine months after cystoprostatectomy, the patient presented with a relapse of gross hematuria. Renal ultrasound showed a hypoechoic area of the renal allograft upper pole with subsequent CT scan confirming a 6.6 cm

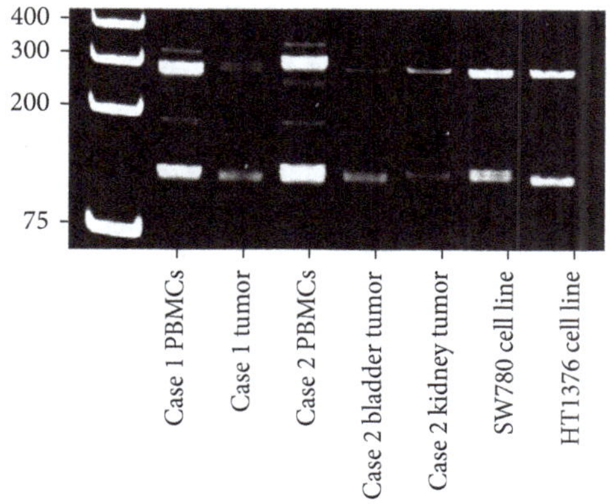

FIGURE 3: Short tandem repeats analysis of loci D18S51 and D3S1358 demonstrated donor-origin. STR analysis of loci D18S51 and D3S1358 of patient purified blood mononuclear cells (PBMC), patient tumors, and two bladder cancer cell lines (SW780 and HT1376) as controls. STR loci and primers were chosen from The National Institute of Standards and Technology.

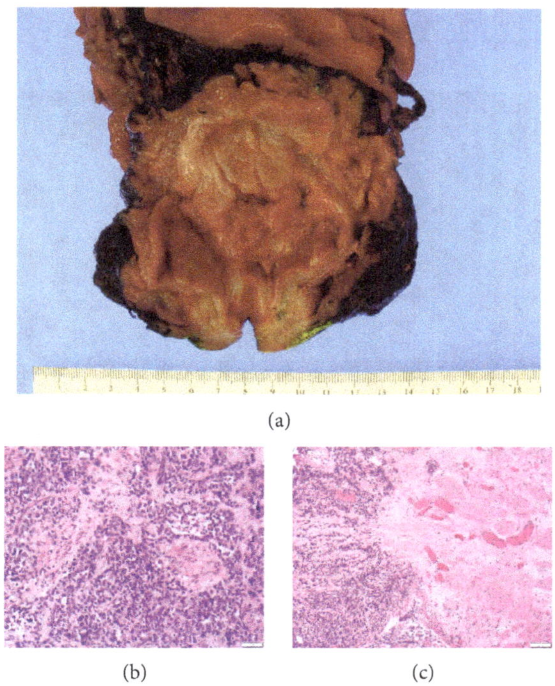

FIGURE 4: (a) For case 2, sectioning of excised bladder revealed a 8.5 cm irregular solid mass grossly invading into the hilar fat and into perinephric fat. (b, c) Hematoxylin and eosin stain showed muscle-invasive urothelial carcinoma on histology of tissue from initial diagnostic transurethral resection of bladder tumor (×200 and ×40 magnification, respectively).

solid renal mass (Figure 5). Biopsy confirmed urothelial carcinoma. CT scan of the chest, abdomen, and pelvis with contrast was negative for metastasis. After discussion with the patient, resection of the renal allograft and ileal conduit was performed. Gross pathology showed a lobulated solid renal mass within the midrenal allograft measuring 6.6 × 4.5 cm with urothelial thickening and nodularity (Figure 6). Tissue pathology confirmed pT4Nx high-grade UC with prominent sarcomatoid features invading through renal parenchyma into perinephric fat, as well as divergent differentiation including clear cell, glandular, plasmacytoid, and signet ring cell differentiation. The tumor also involved the entire length of ureter, invaded through ureteral muscularis propria into periureteric fat, and focally invaded the muscularis propria of the ileal conduit at the anastomosis. Immunohistochemistry (DAKO 22C3) showed 90% tumor tissue expression of PD-L1 and <1% tumor infiltrating immune cells. TEMPUS 648 gene panel revealed TERT and KMT2D mutations and a high tumor mutational burden of 7.8 m/MB with normal MSI status. STR analysis confirmed donor origin of both bladder and allograft tumors, suggesting seeding of the bladder from the transplant allograft (Figure 3). Given high

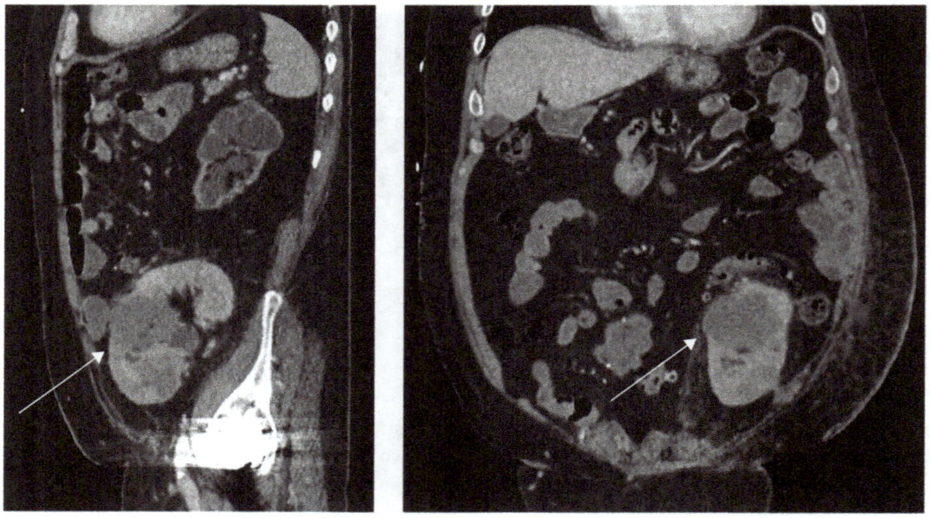

(a) (b)

FIGURE 5: (a) For case 2, sagittal view of computer tomographic scan with intravenous contrast visualized 6.6 cm mass in the renal allograft (arrow). (b) Same mass (arrow) showed in coronal view of the same scan.

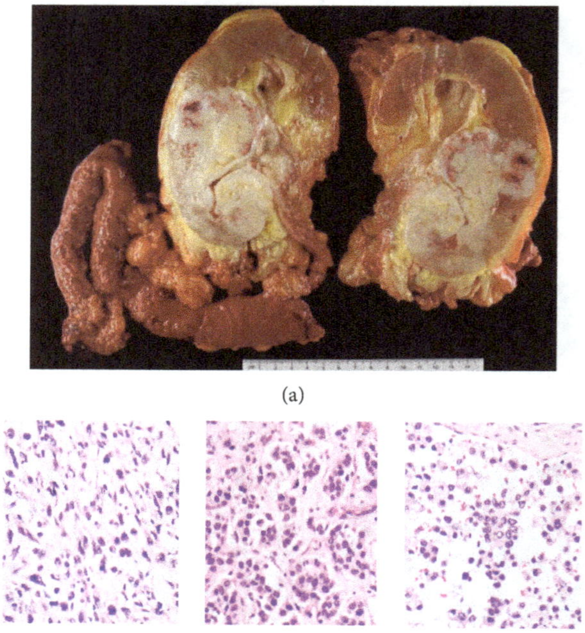

(a)

(b) (c) (d)

FIGURE 6: (a) For case 2, sectioning of the kidney revealed a 9.6 cm irregular solid mass grossly invading into the hilar fat and into perinephric fat. (b–d) Hematoxylin and eosin stain showed invasive high grade urothelial carcinoma with divergent differentiation, including prominent sarcomatoid differentiation (b), glandular (c), plasmacytoid and signet ring cell differentiation (d) (×400 magnification).

PD-L1 expression and mutational burden, the patient was started on 6-week dosing pembrolizumab 400 mg for a planned 2-year maintenance course. One month following surgery, head CT with contrast was performed and showed a 4 mm enhancement in the left parietal lobe with a small amount of perilesional edema, suspicious for metastasis. At 5 months and 10 months following his surgery, additional staging head CT with contrast showed no evidence of disease.

3. Discussion

STRs are short repeating DNA sequences that occupies 3% of human genome that are highly variable among individuals [8]. They are applied in health care and forensic studies for identification purposes [8]. Analyses of STRs confirmed donor origin of our tumors as STRs extracted from tumors are distinct from STRs extracted from patient peripheral blood samples (Figure 3). Regarding the histopathology of our cases, both showed poorly differentiated with variant histologic features. Case 1 demonstrated a rare neuroendocrine differentiation and associated aggressive clinical course, as the patient progressed rapidly within 10 months from his last negative screening ultrasound. Small-cell carcinoma within the urinary tract is a very rare type of UC [9]. Only two prior cases of UC with small-cell differentiation occurring in the bladder of renal transplantation recipients have been reported, and the origin of these tumors were unknown and presumably from the recipient [10]. Our case is the first reported case of donor-derived upper tract small-cell UC.

The clinical course of case 2 mirrored that of the case reported by Ortega et al. in 2016 [11]. Both underwent radical cystectomy initially followed by a metachronous allograft nephrectomy with resection of ileal conduit. The patient reported by Ortega et al. received a final pathological diagnosis of having T3N0 UC of bladder and pT3 UC of graft kidney with positive retroperitoneal node found on image-guided biopsy. On follow-up MRIs, this patient showed no new lesions 12 months after surgical intervention and discontinuation of immunosuppression [11]. These cases should remind us to perform surveillance of the renal allograft following diagnosis of lower urinary tract urothelial carcinoma in renal transplant recipients with routine imaging and urine cytology. Using genotyping techniques such as STR would confirm the donor origin and lead to further scrutiny of the renal allograft. In case 2, this may have prompted an earlier diagnosis.

The optimal method of screening for UC in renal transplantation recipient remains to be elucidated. The rarity of these tumors makes the analysis of the benefits and cost-effectiveness of routine screening challenging [12]. Both cases ultimately presented with gross hematuria and rising creatinine. Case 2 received routine screening with ultrasound imaging every 6 months secondary to his history of hydronephrosis and recurrent infections, but still did not result in early detection of the cancer.

While donor-derived UCs reported in the past often present with extensive involvement and distant, disease-free state of up to 10 years has been achieved from timely surgical intervention alone [13]. This case reported by Olsburgh et al. also received a second kidney transplantation and maintained good renal functions [13]. Research on the optimal timing of redoing allotransplantation after the complete remission of donor-related malignancy is lacking. One center reported 3 patients undergoing retransplant after remission of donor-derived cancer within kidney allografts with one patient remaining healthy and active 20 years after [14].

For muscle-invasive or metastatic urothelial carcinoma, cisplatin-based chemotherapy is first line while checkpoint inhibitor immunotherapy is approved in cisplatin-ineligible or in patients who have progressed following chemotherapy [15]. In transplantation recipients, the decision to use checkpoint inhibitor should be made with caution. In a review containing 29 cases of using checkpoint inhibitors to treat malignancies in kidney transplant recipients, 45% exhibited graft rejection after initiation of checkpoint inhibitor therapy. 1 and 10 out of these 29 patients, respectively, achieved complete and partial response [16]. It is worth noting that only one of these 29 patients had UC, whereas 25 of them had skin cancer with 22 cases of melanoma and 3 cases of squamous cell carcinoma. In addition, a single-institution study reported 39 solid organ transplant recipients diagnosed of malignancies treated with checkpoint inhibitor immunotherapy. While 41% of these patients exhibited various degrees of allograft rejection after the initiation of immunotherapy, a response rate of 47% was reported [17]. 23 out of these 39 patients were renal transplant recipients [17]. However, 79% of all malignancies in this study were skin cancers, and none was from a urothelial origin [17]. Only two prior reported cases have shown benefits of donor-derived renal allograft UC treated checkpoint inhibitors, one showing 15 months of progression-free survival after graft excision and pembrolizumab monotherapy [18]. The other case was locally invasive upon presentation and had partial response to combined treatment with pembrolizumab, bevacizumab, cisplatin, and gemcitabine [19]. Interestingly, no graft rejection was noted in latter case. Here, our two cases both showed elevated tumor mutational burden and PD-L1 CPS score of >10 and 90%, suggesting that checkpoint inhibitor immunotherapy may be a feasible therapeutic modality for these patients.

Abbreviations

UC: Urothelial carcinoma
DDC: Donor-derived cancer
STR: Short tandem repeat
CT: Computer tomography
MRI: Magnetic resonance imaging
mg/dL: Milligrams/deciliter
ng/dL: Nanograms/deciliter
ng/mL: Nanograms/milliliter
NL: Normal limits
MSI: Microsatellite instability
PBMC: Purified blood mononuclear cells.

References

[1] P. Schnuelle, D. Lorenz, M. Trede, and F. J. Van Der Woude, "Impact of renal cadaveric transplantation on survival in end-stage renal failure: evidence for reduced mortality risk compared with hemodialysis during long-term follow-up," *Journal of the American Society of Nephrology*, vol. 9, no. 11, pp. 2135–2141, 1998.

[2] E. Au, G. Wong, and J. R. Chapman, "Cancer in kidney transplant recipients," *Nature Reviews Nephrology*, vol. 14, no. 8, pp. 508–520, 2018.

[3] M. Sarier, O. Yayar, A. Yavuz, H. Turgut, and E. Kukul, "Update on the management of urological problems following kidney transplantation," *Urologia Internationalis*, vol. 105, no. 7-8, pp. 541–547, 2021.

[4] B. Krynitz, G. Edgren, B. Lindelöf et al., "Risk of skin cancer and other malignancies in kidney, liver, heart and lung transplant recipients 1970 to 2008–a Swedish population-based study," *International journal of cancer*, vol. 132, no. 6, pp. 1429–1438, 2013.

[5] R. Desai, D. Collett, C. J. Watson, P. Johnson, T. Evans, and J. Neuberger, "Cancer transmission from organ donors-unavoidable but low risk," *Transplantation*, vol. 94, no. 12, pp. 1200–1207, 2012.

[6] M. I. Bellini, J. P. Gopal, P. Hill, D. Nicol, and N. Gibbons, "Urothelial carcinoma arising from the transplanted kidney: a single-center experience and literature review," *Clinical Transplantation*, vol. 33, no. 6, article e13559, 2019.

[7] L. A. Hickman, D. Sawinski, T. Guzzo, and J. E. Locke, "Urologic malignancies in kidney transplantation," *American Journal of Transplantation*, vol. 18, no. 1, pp. 13–22, 2018.

[8] H. Fan and J.-Y. Chu, "A brief review of short tandem repeat mutation," *Genomics, proteomics & bioinformatics*, vol. 5, no. 1, pp. 7–14, 2007.

[9] L. Wang, B. A. Smith, N. G. Balanis et al., "A genetically defined disease model reveals that urothelial cells can initiate divergent bladder cancer phenotypes," *Proceedings of the National Academy of Sciences*, vol. 117, no. 1, pp. 563–572, 2020.

[10] D. Katkoori, B. L. Cohen, M. S. Soloway, and M. Manoharan, "Small cell carcinoma of the bladder in transplant recipients: a report of 2 cases," *Canadian Urological Association Journal*, vol. 4, no. 1, pp. E4–E6, 2013.

[11] R. M. M. Ortega, D. J. Wolff, C. A. Schandl, and H. A. Drabkin, "Urothelial carcinoma of donor origin in a kidney transplant patient," *Journal for immunotherapy of cancer*, vol. 4, no. 1, pp. 1–4, 2016.

[12] S. A. Acuna, J. W. Huang, A. L. Scott et al., "Cancer screening recommendations for solid organ transplant recipients: a systematic review of clinical practice guidelines," *American Journal of Transplantation*, vol. 17, no. 1, pp. 103–114, 2017.

[13] J. Olsburgh, R. H. Zakri, C. Horsfield et al., "TCC in transplant ureter–when and when not to preserve the transplant kidney," *American Journal of Transplantation*, vol. 16, no. 2, pp. 704–711, 2016.

[14] L. Georgieva, E. Gielis, R. Hellemans et al., "Single-center case series of donor-related malignancies: rare cases with tremendous impact," vol. 48, no. 8, pp. 2669–2677, 2016.

[15] Y. Fradet, J. Bellmunt, D. Vaughn et al., "Randomized phase III KEYNOTE-045 trial of pembrolizumab versus paclitaxel, docetaxel, or vinflunine in recurrent advanced urothelial cancer: results of >2 years of follow-up," *Annals of Oncology*, vol. 30, no. 6, pp. 970–976, 2019.

[16] P. de Bruyn, D. van Gestel, P. Ost et al., "Immune checkpoint blockade for organ transplant patients with advanced cancer: how far can we go?," *Current Opinion in Oncology*, vol. 31, no. 2, pp. 54–64, 2019.

[17] N. Abdel-Wahab, H. Safa, A. Abudayyeh et al., "Checkpoint inhibitor therapy for cancer in solid organ transplantation recipients: an institutional experience and a systematic review of the literature," *Journal for immunotherapy of cancer*, vol. 7, no. 1, p. 106, 2019.

[18] R. S. Chiang, A. A. Connor, B. A. Inman et al., "Metastatic urothelial carcinoma from transplanted kidney with complete response to an immune checkpoint inhibitor," *Case reports in urology*, vol. 2020, 5 pages, 2020.

[19] C.-K. Wu, G.-D. Juang, and H.-C. Lai, "Tumor regression and preservation of graft function after combination with anti-PD-1 immunotherapy without immunosuppressant titration," *Annals of Oncology*, vol. 28, no. 11, pp. 2895-2896, 2017.

8

Acute Interstitial Nephritis in a Patient with Non-Small Cell Lung Cancer under Immunotherapy with Nivolumab

Panagiotis I. Georgianos,[1] Vasilios Vaios,[1] Eleni Leontaridou,[1] Georgia Karayannopoulou,[2] Triantafyllia Koletsa,[2] Athanasios Sioulis,[1] Elias V. Balaskas,[1] and Pantelis E. Zebekakis[1]

[1] *Section of Nephrology and Hypertension, 1st Department of Medicine, AHEPA Hospital, Aristotle University of Thessaloniki, Thessaloniki, Greece*
[2] *Department of Pathology, Aristotle University of Thessaloniki, Thessaloniki, Greece*

Correspondence should be addressed to Panagiotis I. Georgianos; pangeorgi@yahoo.gr

Academic Editor: John A. Sayer

Immune-checkpoint-inhibitors (ICPIs) represent a novel class of immunotherapy against several malignancies. These agents are associated with several "immune-mediated" adverse effects, but the reported renal toxicity of ICPIs is less well defined. We present the case of a 60-year-old man with a history of non-small cell lung cancer, who developed acute kidney injury (AKI) approximately 3.5 months after initiation of immunotherapy with nivolumab. Urinalysis revealed sterile pyuria, without microscopic hematuria or proteinuria. Immunological examination was negative. A renal biopsy showed severe interstitial inflammatory infiltration of T-cells, monocytes, and eosinophils without interstitial granulomas and normal appearance of glomeruli, indicating acute interstitial nephritis (AIN) as the cause of AKI. After a short-term course of corticosteroids and permanent nivolumab discontinuation, partial recovery of renal function was noted. AIN is a rare adverse effect of ICPIs that mandates the close monitoring of renal function in patients under immunotherapy with these agents.

1. Introduction

Immune-checkpoint-inhibitors (ICPIs) are a newly introduced class of immunotherapy against several solid organ and haematological malignancies [1]. These agents are monoclonal antibodies targeting anticytotoxic T-lymphocyte-associated protein 4 (CTLA-4) and antiprogrammed death 1 (PD-1) signalling pathways, which act as negative immunologic regulators on T-cells and other immune cells [1]. Inhibition of these pathways activates tumor-directed immune responses, engaging the patient's own innate and adaptive immune system against tumour cells [1].

ICPIs have been associated with a number of unique "immune-related" adverse reactions, possibly mediated through nonspecific immune activation against self-antigens [2]. The most commonly reported ICPI-related adverse events include skin rash, colitis, hepatitis, hypophysitis, and other endocrinopathies [2]. Although these agents were originally considered as nonnephrotoxic, a growing body of evidence suggests that ICPIs are associated with increased risk for acute kidney injury (AKI), glomerular damage, and electrolyte disturbances [3–6]. However, the clinical spectrum, pathogenesis, and therapeutic approach of ICPI-associated AKI still remain elusive.

Herein, we present the case of a biopsy-proven acute interstitial nephritis (AIN) in a 60-year-old man with a history of non-small cell lung cancer under immunotherapy with the PD-1 inhibitor nivolumab.

2. Case Presentation

A 60-year-old man was admitted to our department due to progressive deterioration of renal function approximately 3.5 months after initiation of immunotherapy with nivolumab. In April 2016, there was a diagnosis of stage IIIa non-small cell lung cancer located in the upper lobe of right lung was made (cT3N2M0). Lung

Table 1: Patient laboratory value after initiation of immunotherapy with nivolumab.

Parameter	Nivolumab therapy			Nivolumab withdrawal				
	Day 0	Day 105	Day 130	Admission	Discharge	Month 1	Month 2	Month 6
Serum creatinine (μmol/L)	79.56	176.8	362.4	433.1	433.2	274.1	194.5	159.1
eGFR* (ml/min/1.73m^2)	92.5	35,2	14,8	11.9	14.8	20.7	31.4	40
Serum sodium (mmol/L)	-	145	-	138	143	137	140	143
Serum potassium (mmol/L)	-	5.3	-	5.8	4.3	5.4	4.5	4.7
Serum calcium (mmol/L)	-	2.45	-	2.2	2.2	2.4	2.2	2.25
Serum phosphate (mmol/L)	-	-	-	1.35	1.32	1.42	0.97	1.23
Eosinophil count (cells/μL, %)	-	-		320 (6.9%)	260 (4.0%)	230 (3.7%)	80 (0.9%)	50, (0.5%)
CRP (nmol/L)	-	-	-	780.0	207.6	138.1	85.7	57.1
UPE (mg/day)	-	-	-	180	-	190	201	266

CRP= C-reactive protein; eGFR= estimated glomerular filtration rate; UPE= urine protein excretion.
*CKD-EPI equation was used to estimate eGFR

cancer was initially treated with combination of radiotherapy and 6 cycles of chemotherapy, including paclitaxel and carboplatin. In March 2017, a positron-emission-tomography/computed-tomography (PET/CT) scan showed malignant extension to tracheobronchial and subcarinal lymph nodes. Immunotherapy with nivolumab was initiated at a dosing regimen of 3 mg/kg every 2 weeks. Immunotherapy started with a normal renal function (serum creatinine: 79.56 μmol/l, estimated-glomerular-filtration-rate (eGFR): 92.5 ml/min/1.73m^2). After the 7th infusion of nivolumab (approximately 105 days after initial exposure), laboratory examinations revealed for first time impaired renal function (serum creatinine: 176.8 μmol/L, eGFR: 35.2 ml/min/1.73m^2). Treating oncologists decided the administration of 2 additional cycles of nivolumab with progressive doubling of serum creatinine and eGFR decline to 14.8 ml/min/1.73m^2 before referral to the renal department (Table 1).

On admission, the patient's medical history revealed that he was a former heavy smoker over the past 35 years (20 cigarettes per day) and had no other comorbidities. He did not receive any medications with the exception of sporadic use of simple analgesics. He denied the use of nonsteroidal anti-inflammatory drugs, proton pump inhibitors, or other nephrotoxic agents, and he reported no drug or food allergies. His family history was unremarkable. The physical examination revealed a normal body temperature (36.7°C), blood pressure 135/70 mmHg, pulse rate 80 bpm, oxygen saturation 98% in the room air, and absence of abnormal clinical signs from the chest auscultation and palpation of the abdomen. Pedal edema, skin rash, joint pain, and swelling were not present. Blood tests revealed mild anemia (hemoglobin: 12.0 g/dl), severely impaired renal function (serum creatinine: 433.1 μmol/L, eGFR: 11.9 ml/min/1.73m^2), and hyperkalemia (serum potassium: 5.8 mmol/L) with no other electrolyte or acid-base disturbances. Urinalysis showed sterile pyuria and absence of both proteinuria and microscopic hematuria. A 24-hour urine collection confirmed the absence of proteinuria. Renal ultrasonography excluded the presence of hydronephrosis and showed kidneys with normal size, contour, and cortical echotexture.

With respect to the diagnostic work-up of AKI, screening for hepatitis B and C viruses and HIV was negative. Immunological tests including antinuclear and anti-DNA antibodies, rheumatoid factor, anti-neutrophil cytoplasmic autoantibodies (ANCA), complement and serum immunoglobin levels were negative or within the normal range. Electrophoresis and immunofixation did not identify the presence of a monoclonal immunoglobin component in the serum. The absence of both proteinuria and microscopic hematuria and the negative immunological examination raised the clinical suspicion of AIN and a renal biopsy was performed to ascertain the cause of AKI. Light microscopy showed severe interstitial nephritis with infiltration of polymorphic inflammatory cells (Figure 1(a)). The interstitial inflammatory infiltrate was predominantly composed of T cells, monocytes, and eosinophils. Inflammatory infiltrates were also present in the tubular basement, and tubular epithelial cells exhibited diffusive degenerative lesions; interstitial granulomas were not present (Figure 1(b)). Glomeruli were normal, except for 2 out of 12, which were fully sclerotic. Immunofluorescence was negative for glomerular or tubular immune deposits.

After the biopsy-proven diagnosis of AIN, the patient received 500 mg/day intravenous methylprednisolone for 3 days, followed by oral prednisolone 1.0 mg/kg/day for the subsequent 2 weeks. Prednisolone dose was progressively tapered and the total duration of corticosteroid therapy was 8 weeks. Immunotherapy with nivolumab was permanently withdrawn. The patient was followed up closely in the Outpatient Nephrology Clinic (Table 1). At month 2 after discharge, renal function was significantly improved (serum creatinine: 194.5 μmol/L, eGFR: 31.4 ml/min/1.73m^2) and then stabilized at 6-month follow-up visit to a slightly higher eGFR level, suggesting a partial, but clinically meaningful, recovery of kidney injury.

3. Discussion

This case report highlights that AIN is a serious ICPI-induced renal adverse event that mandates the close monitoring of renal function in patients receiving immunotherapy with

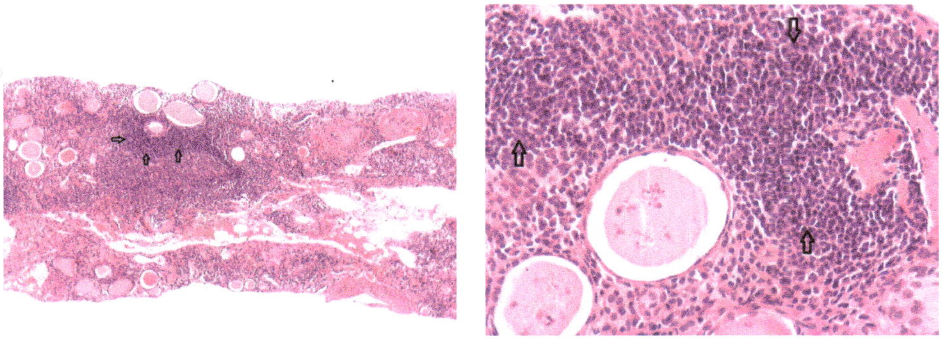

(a) (b)

FIGURE 1: (a) Hematoxylin and eosin stain show typical histopathological appearance of acute interstitial lesions in light microscopy. (b) Hematoxylin and eosin stain shows diffusive interstitial infiltration of polymorphic inflammatory cells, predominantly T-cells, monocytes, and eosinophils.

these agents. Any deterioration in renal function should always raise the suspicion of ICPI-associated nephrotoxicity, particularly in the absence of background therapy with other agents that may induce AIN, as in the patient of our case report. Early recognition of this rare nephrotoxic reaction by treating oncologists may be of major importance for the subsequent clinical course and recovery from AKI.

In a review of renal toxicities reported to the Food and Drug Administration adverse reporting database (FAERS) between the 3rd quarter of 2011 and 1st quarter of 2015, Wanchoo et al. [2] identified 20 cases of renal impairment and another 24 cases of serious electrolyte disturbances attributable to nivolumab use. By analyzing clinical-trial data from 3,695 patients, Cortazar et al. [7] reported an overall incidence of ICPI-associated AKI as high as 2.2%. In a 2018 meta-analysis of 48 randomized trials (incorporating data from 11,845 participants), compared with controls receiving nonnephrotoxic agents, patients treated with PD-1 inhibitors had a 4.2-fold higher risk of AKI [Relative Risk (RR): 4.19; 95% Confidence Interval (CI): 1.57-11.18] [5]. The pooled incidence of AKI among patients treated with PD-1 inhibitors was 2.2% [5]. It has to be noted, however, that these estimates may underestimate or overestimate the true burden of ICPI-inducible nephrotoxicity, given the limitations related to adverse event reporting in clinical trials, the heterogeneity in definitions of AKI across studies, and rarity of biopsy-proven cases that may provide more causal associations. A summary of previously reported cases of nivolumab-associated nephrotoxicity is provided in Table 2 [4, 8–13].

In the patient of our case, the time elapsed from the initial exposure to nivolumab until the onset of AKI was 105 days. This delayed response is in line with the observations of a case-series of 13 patients with ICPI-induced AKI, in which the median time from initiation of an ICPI to AKI was 91 days (range: 21-245 days) [7]. The heterogeneous and delayed onset of AKI is suggestive of a mechanistic pathway distinct from the typical drug-induced hypersensitivity reaction. ICPI-associated AIN is proposed to be mediated through "reprogramming" of the innate and adaptive immune system, a process resulting in loss of immune tolerance against self-antigens at the kidney level [14, 15]. This hypothesis is supported by experimental studies showing that the PD-1 signalling pathway is expressed in tubular epithelial cells and exerts protective actions against T-cell-mediated autoimmunity [14, 15]. Animal studies showed that PD-1 knockout mice were prone to developing AIN and glomerulonephritis [16]. Similarly, administration of anti-PD-1 monoclonal antibody in mice was able to induce interstitial and glomerular damage, possibly mediated through autoimmune overactivity [17]. An alternative mechanistic explanation is that ICPIs may induce suppression of T-cell immunity that results in loss of normal renal tolerance against concomitantly administered drugs known to be associated with AIN [11, 13, 18]. This is a less likely explanation for pathogenesis of AIN in our case presentation, since the patient did not have comorbidities and denied the use of nonsteroidal anti-inflammatory drugs, proton pump inhibitors, or other nephrotoxic agents.

The efficacy of corticosteroids in remission of kidney injury is another area surrounded by controversy in the therapeutic approach of AIN management. A short-term course of corticosteroids is recommended as an approach to hasten the recovery of renal function in biopsy-proven AIN, particularly in patients requiring support with hemodialysis or when withdrawal of the inciting agent is not accompanied by the anticipated improvement in renal function [19, 20]. In the aforementioned case-series of Cortazar et al. [7] complete or partial remission of renal damage was observed in 9 out of 10 patients with AIN who received short-term corticosteroid therapy; in contrast, 2 patients with AIN not given corticosteroids had no improvement in renal function [7]. Undoubtedly, the observational nature of these findings cannot provide cause-and-effect associations, and the efficacy and safety of corticosteroids warrant evaluation in properly designed randomized trials. In addition, duration of AIN and severity of interstitial fibrosis in kidney biopsy are shown to be strong predictors of natural course of AIN [21]. The long duration of AIN, diffusive interstitial inflammatory infiltrate, and severity of tubular lesions that were evident in the kidney

TABLE 2: Case reports associating nivolumab therapy with nephrotoxic reactions.

Author	Patients	Age	Gender	ICPI	Cancer	Renal biopsy	Treatment	Outcome
Hoffman et al. [9]	1	52 yrs	M	Nivolumab	Melanoma	Not available	Steroids	Recovery
Shirali et al. [13]	6	67.5 yrs	3M/3F	Nivolumab/ Pembrolizumab/ Ipilimumab	NSCLC	Tubulointerstitial inflammation with infiltrate of lymphocytes	Steroids in 5 of 6 patients	Recovery
Kishi et al. [10]	1	72 yrs	M	Nivolumab	NSCLC	IgA nephropathy	No steroids	Recovery
Murakami et al. [12]	1	75 yrs	M	Combination of Nivolumab and Ipilimumab	Melanoma	Tubulointerstitial inflammation with infiltrate of lymphocytes	Steroids	Recovery
Koda et al. [11]	1	67 yrs	M	Nivolumab	NSCLC	Acute tubulointerstitial nephritis without granuloma formation	Steroids	Recovery
Bottlaender et al. [8]	1	76 yrs	F	Ipilumumab-Nivolumab	Melanoma	Interstitial edema with dense inflammatory infiltrates	Steroids	Recovery
Jung et al. [4]	1	70 yrs	M	Nivolumab	Kidney cancer	Diffusive tubular injury and complex-mediated glomerulonephritis	Steroids and hemodialysis	Recovery

ICPI= immune checkpoint inhibitor; NSCLC= non-small cell lung cancer; M= male, F= female.

biopsy may be plausible explanations for the only partial recovery of renal function in response to corticosteroid therapy in our case presentation.

Although immune checkpoint inhibitors were originally considered as nonnephrotoxic immunotherapy against solid organ and haematological malignancies, this case-report highlights that acute interstitial nephritis is a rare, but serious, adverse effect of nivolumab. A short course of corticosteroid therapy is a promising therapeutic approach in order to achieve complete or partial remission of nivolumab-induced AIN. Close monitoring of renal function and serum electrolyte balance is required for early recognition of renal toxicities associated with ICPI use in daily clinical practice.

Abbreviations

AIN: Acute interstitial nephritis
AKI: Acute kidney injury
ANCA: Anti-neutrophil cytoplasmic autoantibodies
CI: Confidence interval
CTLA-4: Anticytotoxic T-lymphocyte-associated protein 4
eGFR: Estimated glomerular filtration rate
ICPIs: Immune checkpoint inhibitors
PD-1: Programmed death-1
PET/CT: Positron-emission-tomography/computed-tomography
RR: Relative risk.

Consent

The patient gave written informed consent and waived his rights for the publication of images.

Authors' Contributions

Panagiotis I. Georgianos, Vasilios Vaios, Eleni Leontaridou, Athanasios Sioulis, and Elias V. Balaskas took care of the patient and performed renal biopsy; **Panagiotis I. Georgianos** drafted the paper; **Georgia Karayannopoulou and Triantafyllia Koletsa** performed renal pathology examination; **Elias V. Balaskas and Pantelis E. Zebekakis** critically revised the paper.

References

[1] M. A. Postow, M. K. Callahan, and J. D. Wolchok, "Immune checkpoint blockade in cancer therapy," *Journal of Clinical Oncology*, vol. 33, no. 17, pp. 1974–1982, 2015.

[2] R. Wanchoo, S. Karam, N. N. Uppal et al., "Adverse Renal Effects of Immune Checkpoint Inhibitors: A Narrative Review," *American Journal of Nephrology*, vol. 45, no. 2, pp. 160–169, 2017.

[3] P. Balakrishna and A. Villegas, "Hypokalemic Paralysis Secondary to Immune Checkpoint Inhibitor Therapy," *Case Reports in Oncological Medicine*, vol. 2017, Article ID 5063405, 4 pages, 2017.

[4] K. Jung, X. Zeng, and M. Bilusic, "Nivolumab-associated acute glomerulonephritis: a case report and literature review," *BMC Nephrology*, vol. 17, no. 1, pp. 1–6, 2016.

[5] S. Manohar, P. Kompotiatis, C. Thongprayoon, W. Cheungpasitporn, J. Herrmann, and S. M. Herrmann, "Programmed cell death protein 1 inhibitor treatment is associated with acute kidney injury and hypocalcemia: meta-analysis," *Nephrology Dialysis Transplantation* , 2018.

[6] R. Wanchoo, A. Abudayyeh, M. Doshi et al., "Renal toxicities of novel agents used for treatment of multiple myeloma," *Clinical Journal of the American Society of Nephrology*, vol. 12, no. 1, pp. 176–189, 2017.

[7] F. B. Cortazar, K. A. Marrone, M. L. Troxell et al., "Clinicopathological features of acute kidney injury associated with immune checkpoint inhibitors," *Kidney International*, vol. 90, no. 3, pp. 638–647, 2016.

[8] L. Bottlaender, A.-L. Breton, L. Laforcade, F. Dijoud, L. Thomas, and S. Dalle, "Acute interstitial nephritis after sequential ipilumumab - nivolumab therapy of metastatic melanoma," *Journal for ImmunoTherapy of Cancer*, vol. 5, no. 1, p. 57, 2017.

[9] L. Hofmann, A. Forschner, C. Loquai et al., "Cutaneous, gastrointestinal, hepatic, endocrine, and renal side-effects of anti-PD-1 therapy," *European Journal of Cancer*, vol. 60, pp. 190–199, 2016.

[10] S. Kishi, M. Minato, A. Saijo et al., "IgA Nephropathy after Nivolumab Therapy for Postoperative Recurrence of Lung Squamous Cell Carcinoma," *Internal Medicine*, vol. 57, no. 9, pp. 1259–1263, 2018.

[11] R. Koda, H. Watanabe, M. Tsuchida et al., "Immune checkpoint inhibitor (nivolumab)-associated kidney injury and the importance of recognizing concomitant medications known to cause acute tubulointerstitial nephritis: A case report," *BMC Nephrology*, vol. 19, no. 1, p. 48, 2018.

[12] N. Murakami, T. J. Borges, M. Yamashita, and L. V. Riella, "Severe acute interstitial nephritis after combination immune-checkpoint inhibitor therapy for metastatic melanoma," *Clinical Kidney Journal*, vol. 9, no. 3, pp. 411–417, 2016.

[13] A. C. Shirali, M. A. Perazella, and S. Gettinger, "Association of Acute Interstitial Nephritis With Programmed Cell Death 1 Inhibitor Therapy in Lung Cancer Patients," *American Journal of Kidney Diseases*, vol. 68, no. 2, pp. 287–291, 2016.

[14] E. A. Tivol, F. Borriello, A. N. Schweitzer, W. P. Lynch, J. A. Bluestone, and A. H. Sharpe, "Loss of CTLA-4 leads to massive lymphoproliferation and fatal multiorgan tissue destruction, revealing a critical negative regulatory role of CTLA-4," *Immunity*, vol. 3, no. 5, pp. 541–547, 1995.

[15] Y. Z. Yuan, C. Blank, and T. F. Gajewski, "Negative regulation of T-cell function by PD-1," *Critical Reviews in Immunology*, vol. 24, no. 4, pp. 229–237, 2004.

[16] H. Nishimura, M. Nose, H. Hiai, N. Minato, and T. Honjo, "Development of lupus-like autoimmune diseases by disruption of the PD-1 gene encoding an ITIM motif-carrying immunoreceptor," *Immunity*, vol. 11, no. 2, pp. 141–151, 1999.

[17] G. Zheng, Y. Wang, D. Mahajan, X. Qin, S. I. Alexander, and D. C. H. Harris, "The role of tubulointerstitial inflammation," *Kidney International*, vol. 67, no. 94, pp. S96–S100, 2005.

[18] Z. Spanou, M. Keller, M. Britschgi et al., "Involvement of drug-specific t cells in acute drug-induced interstitial nephritis," *Journal of the American Society of Nephrology*, vol. 17, no. 10, pp. 2919–2927, 2006.

[19] M. R. Clarkson, L. Giblin, F. P. O'Connell et al., "Acute interstitial nephritis: clinical features and response to corticosteroid therapy," *Nephrology Dialysis Transplantation* , vol. 19, no. 11, pp. 2778–2783, 2004.

[20] E. González, E. Gutiérrez, C. Galeano et al., "Early steroid treatment improves the recovery of renal function in patients with drug-induced acute interstitial nephritis," *Kidney International*, vol. 73, no. 8, pp. 940–946, 2008.

[21] M. Praga, A. Sevillano, F. Aunon, and E. Gonzalez, "Changes in the aetiology, clinical presentation and management of acute interstitial nephritis, an increasingly common cause of acute kidney injury," *Nephrology Dialysis Transplantation* , vol. 30, no. 9, pp. 1472–1479, 2015.

9

Intranodal Ultrasound-Guided Percutaneous Methylene Blue Injection for the Identification of Leakage Point during Laparoscopic Repair of Refractory Chylous Ascites after Laparoscopic Lymphadenectomy for Kidney Cancer

Hugo Otaola-Arca,[1,2] Patricio Vargas,[1] Daniel Hasson,[1] Marcelo Orvieto,[1] Carmen Niño-Taravilla,[3] and Hugo Bermúdez[1]

[1]*Clínica Alemana, Santiago, Chile*
[2]*School of Medicine, Clínica Alemana-Universidad del Desarollo, Santiago, Chile*
[3]*Clinica INDISA, Santiago, Chile*

Correspondence should be addressed to Hugo Otaola-Arca; hugotaolarca@hotmail.com

Academic Editor: David Duchene

Chylous ascites is an uncommon complication after surgery that can result in malnutrition and immunodeficiency. Therefore, surgical interventions are reserved for refractory patients, and the primary success factor for these interventions is locating the point of leakage, which is often tricky. We describe a case of a 56-year-old male with chylous ascites after laparoscopic radical nephrectomy and lumbo-aortic lymphadenectomy for kidney cancer. The patient was initially managed with dietary modifications and drainage placement. Afterward, lymphography with Lipiodol, percutaneous embolization of the leakage point, and total parenteral nutrition were established. Finally, the patient underwent laparoscopic repair after identifying the leakage point by injecting methylene blue through an inguinal node. Complete resolution was achieved, and no complications related to the procedure were recorded. Intranodal methylene blue injection can be an invaluable tool to identify the point of leakage in selected patients to improve the outcomes of surgical repair of refractory chylous ascites.

1. Introduction

Chylous ascites (CA) is the accumulation of chyle within the peritoneum secondary to chylous leakage (CL), which can be developed after major abdominal surgery due to an inadvertent iatrogenic injury of cisterna chyle or one of its main tributaries and can be life-threatening as a result of the secondary disorders (electrolyte imbalance, malnutrition, and immunodeficiency).

Nowadays, no standardized treatment guidelines are available, but classifications based on severity have been used to harmonize its management [1]. Dietary modification (high-protein and low-fat diet, medium-chain triglycerides (MCT) supplements) to reduce the intake of long-chain triglycerides (LCT) is accepted as a first-line approach. Absolute fasting with total parenteral nutrition and somatostatin or analogs is often second-line therapy [2]. Paracentesis or drain placement [3], lymphangiography, and embolization are alternatives for non-responders [4]. Surgical interventions are reserved for refractory patients. However, the intraoperative location of the leakage point is the most significant limiting factor in the success of the surgical repair.

This article aims to present a case of refractory CA in a patient with kidney cancer and to describe a successful laparoscopic repair of CL after a percutaneous injection of methylene blue in an inguinal lymph node.

2. Case Presentation

We present a 56-year-old man with hypertension and hypothyroidism under treatment, without known allergies. On

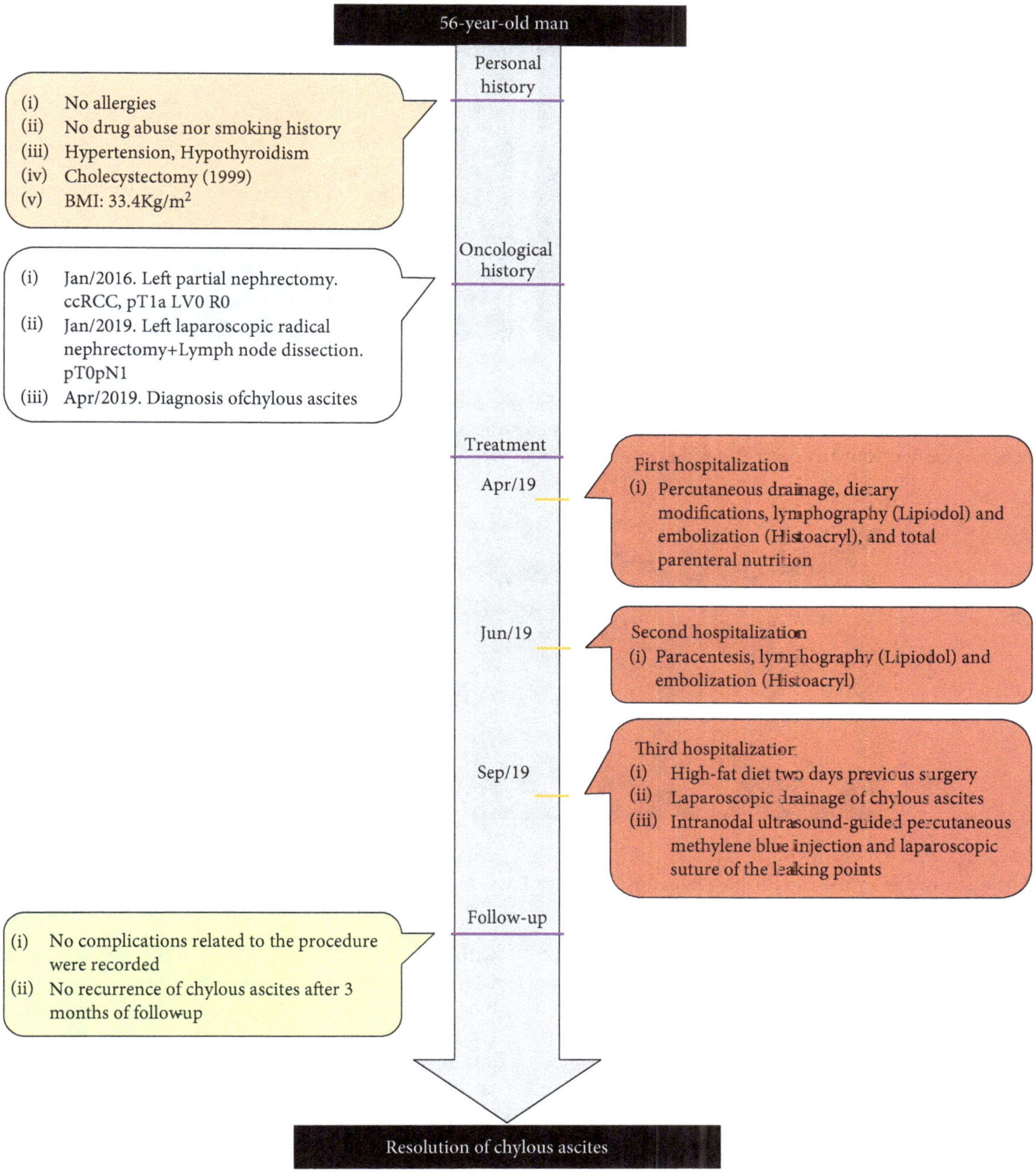

Figure 1: Timeline of interventions and outcomes. BMI = body mass index, ccRCC = clear cell renal cell carcinoma, LV = lymphovascular invasion, R = margin status.

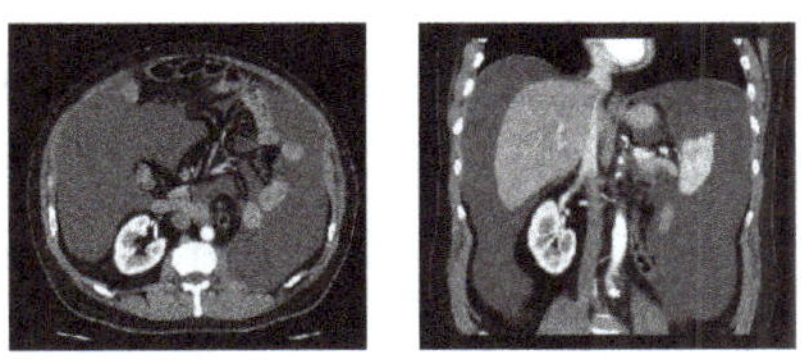

(a) (b)

Figure 2: Computed tomography scan. Massive ascites can be seen in the (a) axial and (b) coronal sections.

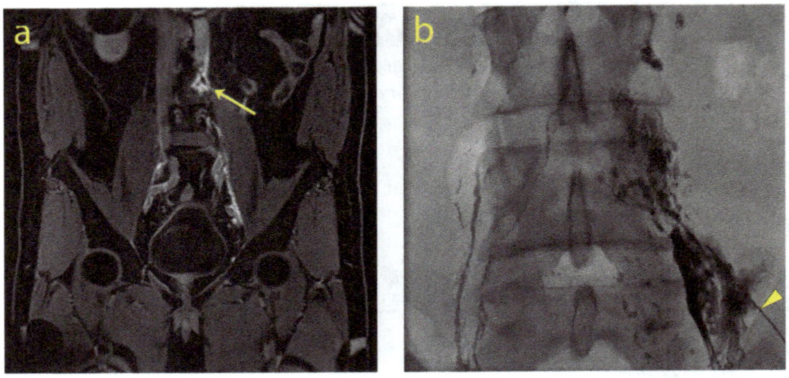

(a) (b)

Figure 3: Magnetic resonance lymphangiogram with Lipiodol. Dynamic contrast-enhanced magnetic resonance lymphangiogram (a) with maximum intensity projection and the subtraction of noncontrasted structures shows a leak site at the L4-L5 level (arrow). (b) Shows the percutaneous embolization with Histoacryl® (head arrow) after identifying the leakage point in the lymphography with Lipiodol.

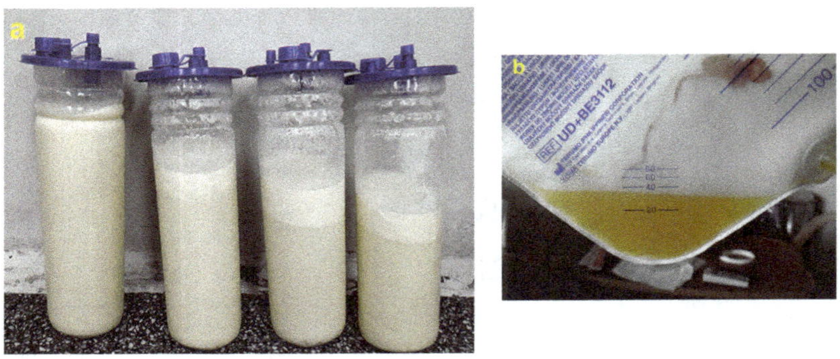

(a) (b)

Figure 4: Evolution of the appearance of the abdominal drainage fluid. Milky white ascites obtained during surgery can be seen in the suction receptacles (a). Since the first postoperative day, clear liquid can be seen in the intra-abdominal drainage collecting bag (b).

general physical examination, only a body mass index of 33.4 Kg/m^2 and scars of previous laparoscopic cholecystectomy are noted.

In January 2016, the patient underwent an elective left partial nephrectomy due to an incidental renal tumor (pT1a, clear cell renal cell carcinoma (ccRCC) with negative margins). Unfortunately, the patient presented local lymph node recurrence three years later, and an uneventful left laparoscopic radical nephrectomy (LRN) and lumbo-aortic lymphadenectomy (LALA) were carried out. Metastasis of ccRCC was found in two out of five lymph nodes without evidence of tumor in kidney tissue (pT0pN1). Figure 1 summarizes the timeline of interventions and outcomes.

In April 2019, the patient presented to the emergency service complaining of generalized abdominal pain, marked abdominal distension, nausea, and vomiting. Abdominopelvic computed tomography (AP-CT) scan revealed many intra-abdominal free fluids (Figure 2). The patient was diagnosed with CA based on the findings in both diagnostic paracentesis and dynamic contrast-enhanced magnetic resonance lymphangiogram (DCMRL) (Figure 3(a)). Percutaneous drainage was placed (12 L of chyle), and dietary modifications were applied (high-protein and low-fat diet with MCTs supplements). Due to the persistence of an active CL, the point of CL was identified using an intranodal lymphangiography with Lipiodol and embolized with Histoacryl® (Braun) in a 1 : 4 ratio (Figure 3(b)). During follow-up, despite dietary restrictions, the patient presented progressive abdominal distension. Therapeutic paracentesis was performed every 3-4 weeks, evacuating a maximum of four liters per session. A new Lipiodol lymphangiography and uneventful Histoacryl® embolization were performed at the beginning of June. The team underwent surgical treatment because CL remained active despite conservative measures and two embolizations.

In September 2019, the patient was hospitalized. Two days before the surgery, a high-fat diet was prescribed to increase CA production and identify the point of CL during surgical repair. Laparoscopy was performed in a right lateral decubitus position using two 12 mm and two 5 mm ports inserted in the scars of the previous ports' sites. Intraoperatively, nine liters of chyle was drained (Figure 4(a)). The left Toldt white line was opened, and the left colon was medialized. Despite colon dissection and meticulous observation of the retroperitoneum, the point of CL had not been identified. Subsequently, 20 mL of methylene blue was injected

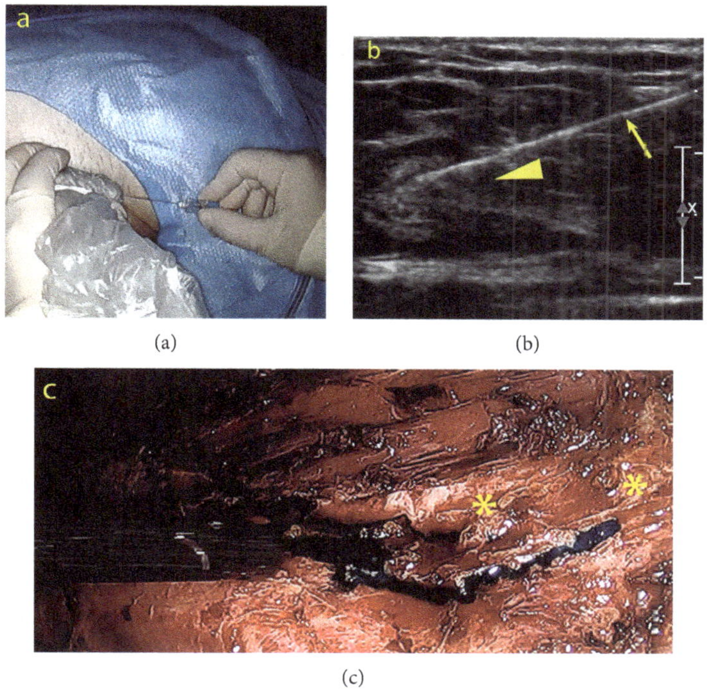

FIGURE 5: Identification of the point of chylous leakage. External (a) and ultrasound vision (b) of a transnodal injection of methylene blue under image guidance (lymph node, head arrow; needle, and arrow). Two leak points (stars) can be observed in the retroperitoneum (c) after seven minutes of percutaneous administration of methylene blue.

percutaneously in a left inguinal lymph node under ultrasound- (US-) guidance using a standard lymph node US access approach (Figures 5(a)–5(b)). Under sterile conditions, a linear 10-14 MHz probe was used to explore the inguinal region, identifying a lymph node with adequate size and depth for punction. Afterward, a 25G needle was used to access the lymph node under real-time US view. Seven minutes later, two methylene blue leak points into the retroperitoneum were identified in the para-aortic region, 4 cm below the old renal hilum (Figure 5(c)). Endosuturing of both leaking points was done from distal to proximal with a running barbed suture (3/0 Stratafix™, Ethicon) reinforced with titanium clips. A new injection of methylene blue ruled out the persistence of the CL. The procedure is summarized step-by-step in Video S1. First, an abdominal drain was placed (19 Ch Blake). The total operative time was 90 minutes, and the estimated blood loss was 20 mL.

To help the healing of the CL, the patient was under absolute fasting and parenteral nutrition during the first three postoperative days (POD). Additionally, from the third to the sixth PODs, he was fed a protein-rich, low-fat diet and MCT supplements. However, during the immediate postoperative period, the liquid coming from the drainage was clear (Figure 4(b)), and the biochemical analyses confirmed transudative fluid (low triglyceride and protein content). Therefore, the drain was withdrawn on the fourth POD, and the patient was discharged on the seventh POD.

After twelve months of follow-up, our patient had a complete resolution of CA, a good nutritional and performance status, and no immediate or delayed complications related to the procedure were recorded.

3. Discussion

We report a case of CA after LRN and LALA for kidney cancer successfully treated with laparoscopic repair after the failure of conservative treatment, where intranodal ultrasound-guided percutaneous methylene blue injection was crucial to identify the leakage point.

CA is an infrequent but significant complication to consider after abdominal surgery. CA may go unnoticed intraoperatively in laparoscopic surgery because the high intra-abdominal pressure created by the pneumoperitoneum can mask leakage from the low-pressure lymph vessels. Various algorithms have been reported [5–9], but no standardized treatment guidelines are available yet; thus, the optimal management of postoperative CA is unclear.

Surgical interventions are reserved for refractory patients. The most common procedure is to suture or clip the point of the CL in the retroperitoneum once it is localized. Direct glue application (e.g., Floseal), argon beam [2], intravenous heparin injection [10], and low-dose radiation therapy [11] have been described as alternatives to suturing. Laparoscopic suture of the point of CL has a success rate of up to 86% [1]. Still, the main pitfall in surgical repair is the failure to identify the point of CL, which is a significant determinant of its success. In this regard, Molina et al., who first reported the laparoscopic approach for CA secondary to lymphadenectomy, could not identify the CL point despite the administration of intravenous indigo carmine and prolonged laparoscopic observation [12]. Thus, the authors performed extensive blinded clipping (50 clips), argon beam coagulation, and fibrin glue (6 units) in the fibrous fatty tissue surrounding the renal hilum.

Some strategies have been described to help localize the point of CL by increasing the production or dyeing the CA [2, 12–16]:

(i) *Preoperative Strategies*. Ingestion of high-fat diet/milk one or two days before surgery

(ii) *Intraoperative Strategies*. Methylene blue or heavy cream administration through a gastric tube; injection of intravenous indigo carmine during surgery; mesenteric intranodal lymphangiography

In our case, we administered a high-fat diet on the days before surgery to increase chyle production. However, it was impossible to identify CL's point once the retroperitoneum was dissected. Therefore, we administered methylene blue through an inguinal node under ultrasound guidance, and two points of CL could be observed seven minutes later in the para-aortic region. Subsequently, we could perform a laparoscopic suture reinforced with titanium clips selectively on the points of CL. Finally, we administered methylene blue again to the same node, confirming the absence of CL.

Methylene blue is a very versatile drug. As a medication, it helps treat methemoglobinemia, vasoplegic syndrome, ifosfamide-induced encephalopathy, and cyanide poisoning. In addition, it is instrumental in many diagnostic (e.g., bacterial staining and fistula identification) and therapeutic procedures as a dye. However, it should be noted that methylene blue can cause serotonin syndrome in those patients who consume serotonergic psychiatric medications [17], probably because it is a potent reversible monoamine oxidase inhibitor. Therefore, its use should be avoided in these patients, even in small amounts.

It is important to highlight that chylous lymphatic fluid mostly forms after fat absorption in the small bowel and originate from the above part of the body and thus some refractory chylous ascites cannot be detected by lymphangiography from the below. In this scenario, mesenteric intranodal lymphangiography could be useful, as described by Lee et al. [16].

To conclude, identifying the point of the CL is of paramount importance to enable the success of the surgical treatment. In this regard, percutaneous image-guided intranodal methylene blue injection through an inguinal lymph node is an invaluable tool to identify the CL during surgical repair, allowing selective lymphatic ligation.

Abbreviations

AP-CT: Abdominopelvic computed tomography
CA: Chylous ascites
ccRCC: Clear cell renal cell carcinoma
CL: Chylous leakage
DCMRL: Dynamic contrast-enhanced magnetic resonance lymphangiogram
LALA: Lumbo-aortic lymphadenectomy
LCT: Long-chain triglycerides
LRN: Laparoscopic radical nephrectomy
MCT: Medium-chain triglycerides
POD: Postoperative day
US: Ultrasound.

Acknowledgments

The authors express their acknowledgments to Santiago Otaola.

References

[1] Z. Q. Ng and B. He, "A proposed classification system and therapeutic strategy for chyle leak after laparoscopic living-donor nephrectomy: a single-center experience and review of the literature," *Experimental and Clinical Transplantation*, vol. 16, no. 2, pp. 143–149, 2018.

[2] A. Seth, A. Sharma, D. B. Kenwar, and S. Singh, "Chylous ascites: complication of laparoscopic donor nephrectomy. Case report and review of literature," *Transplantation*, vol. 103, no. 4, pp. e74–e78, 2019.

[3] L.-A. Dale, P. R. Sandoval, and L. E. Ratner, "Chylous ascites following laparoscopic live donor nephrectomy: a new improved treatment paradigm," *Clinical Transplantation*, vol. 33, no. 3, article e13483, 2019.

[4] C. C. Pieper, S. Hur, C.-M. Sommer et al., "Back to the future: Lipiodol in lymphography-from diagnostics to theranostics," *Investigative Radiology*, vol. 54, no. 9, pp. 600–615, 2019.

[5] O. O. Aalami, D. B. Allen, and C. H. Organ, "Chylous ascites: A collective review," *Surgery*, vol. 128, no. 5, pp. 761–778, 2000.

[6] R. Bhardwaj, H. Vaziri, A. Gautam, E. Ballesteros, D. Karimeddini, and G. Y. Wu, "Chylous ascites: a review of pathogenesis, diagnosis and treatment," *Journal of Clinical and Translational Hepatology*, vol. 6, no. 1, pp. 105–113, 2018.

[7] B. Lizaola, A. Bonder, H. D. Trivedi, E. B. Tapper, and A. Cardenas, "Review article: the diagnostic approach and current management of chylous ascites," *Alimentary Pharmacology & Therapeutics*, vol. 46, no. 9, pp. 816–824, 2017.

[8] I. Leibovitch, Y. Mor, J. Golomb, and J. Ramon, "The diagnosis and management of postoperative chylous ascites," *The Journal of Urology*, vol. 167, 2 Part 1, pp. 449–457, 2002.

[9] A. Jairath, A. Singh, A. Ganpule, S. Mishra, R. Sabnis, and M. Desai, "Management protocol for chylous ascites after laparoscopic nephrectomy," *Urology*, vol. 86, no. 3, pp. 521–528, 2015.

[10] M. Soriano-Ramos, E. Orellana-Felis, M. T. Moral-Pumarega et al., "Heparin in congenital chylothorax and chylous ascites," *Indian Journal of Pediatrics*, vol. 86, no. 7, pp. 660-661, 2019.

[11] S. Brown, C. O. Abana, H. Hammad et al., "Low-dose radiation therapy is an effective treatment for refractory postoperative chylous ascites: a case report," *Practical Radiation Oncology*, vol. 9, no. 3, pp. 153–157, 2019.

[12] W. R. Molina, M. M. Desai, and I. S. Gill, "Laparoscopic management of chylous ascites after donor nephrectomy," *The Journal of Urology*, vol. 170, no. 5, p. 1938, 2003.

[13] B. D. Carr, C. N. Grant, R. E. Overman, S. K. Gadepalli, and J. D. Geiger, "Retroperitoneal exploration with Vicryl mesh and fibrin tissue sealant for refractory chylous ascites," *Journal of Pediatric Surgery*, vol. 54, no. 3, pp. 604–607, 2019.

[14] Q. Gao, W. Xie, Q. Wang et al., "Novel technique to manage refractory chylous ascites with carbon nanoparticle suspension in infants," *Journal of Pediatric Surgery*, vol. 55, no. 4, pp. 772–776, 2020.

[15] B. Geary, B. Wade, W. Wollmann, and R. El-Galley, "Laparoscopic repair of chylous ascites," *The Journal of Urology*, vol. 171, no. 3, pp. 1231-1232, 2004.

[16] H. Lee, S. J. Kim, S. Hur et al., "The feasibility of mesenteric intranodal lymphangiography: its clinical application for refractory postoperative chylous ascites," *Journal of Vascular and Interventional Radiology*, vol. 29, no. 9, pp. 1290–1292, 2018.

[17] FDA Drug Safety Communication, "Serious CNS reactions possible when methylene blue is given to patients taking certain psychiatric edications," 2019, https://www.fda.gov/drugs/drug-safety-and-availability/fda-drug-safety-communication-serious-cns-reactions-possible-when-methylene-blue-given-patients.

10

Metastasis to the Bladder: A Rare Site of Recurrence of Renal Cell Carcinoma

Amanda Smart,[1] **Michael Wynne**,[1] **Ezra Baraban**,[2] **Yasser Ged**,[3] **and Armine Smith**[4]

[1]*Department of Urology, George Washington University Hospital, Washington, DC, USA*
[2]*Department of Pathology, Johns Hopkins University School of Medicine, Baltimore, MD, USA*
[3]*Department of Oncology, Johns Hopkins University School of Medicine, Baltimore, MD, USA*
[4]*The James Buchanan Brady Urologic Institute and Department of Urology, Johns Hopkins University School of Medicine, Baltimore, MD, USA*

Correspondence should be addressed to Michael Wynne; mwynne@gwu.edu

Academic Editor: Tun-Chieh Chen

Renal cell carcinoma (RCC) is considered to be the deadliest urologic cancer with high rates of metastasis and recurrence after nephrectomy. RCC can metastasize to nearly any organ but most commonly metastasizes to the liver, lung, brain, and bone. To date, there are only about 40 reported cases of RCC with solitary bladder metastasis. The following report contributes to this limited data set of patients with RCC who develop solitary metastasis to the bladder. A 69-year-old male presented with occasional gross hematuria and was found to have a left renal mass infiltrating the collecting system. Ureteroscopic biopsy revealed clear cell RCC, and the patient subsequently underwent radical left nephrectomy. Eight months after nephrectomy, the patient presented to the clinic with gross hematuria. In-office cystoscopy demonstrated a nodular lesion in the bladder arising from the left ureteral orifice. The patient underwent transurethral resection of the bladder mass and pathology demonstrated clear cell RCC. Subsequent imaging showed no evidence of metastatic disease. Five months after transurethral resection, the patient was found to have a left distal ureteral mass and underwent left ureterectomy with partial cystectomy. Pathology again demonstrated clear cell RCC. RCC with solitary metastasis to the bladder is rare, and there are no targeted guideline recommendations for management. Per standard of care, patients with painless hematuria and risk factors for malignancy should undergo cystoscopy. In patients with a history of RCC, metastasis to the bladder should be considered in the differential diagnosis. Patients with metastatic RCC to the bladder should undergo a thorough work-up for additional sites of metastasis. In patients with RCC who develop solitary bladder metastasis amenable to resection following nephrectomy, there is a lack of evidence to guide therapy and a multidisciplinary discussion is warranted. However, if the tumor is amenable to resection, metastasectomy is a reasonable therapeutic approach and offers the patient an improved quality of life and an opportunity for remission.

1. Introduction

Renal cell carcinoma (RCC) accounts for 2% of global cancer diagnoses, and about 33% of patients have metastatic disease at the time of diagnosis [1, 2]. An estimated 20-40% of patients with RCC will progress after surgical resection and develop metastases [2]. Approximately 50% of recurrences occur within 2 years of resection [3]. The lung, bone, liver, and brain are the most frequent sites of metastasis for RCC; however, metastases can be found in nearly any organ. There are about 40 cases reported, including the largest series of 11 patients with solitary metastases to the bladder [4]. Our report adds to this limited data set of patients with RCC developing a solitary metastasis to the bladder.

2. Case Report

A 69-year-old male with hypertension, gastroesophageal reflux, and hepatitis presented with occasional gross hematuria for one month and was found to have a 9 cm left renal mass infiltrating the collecting system (Figure 1). He was a former smoker with a 12 pack-year history who quit over 30 years prior to presentation. He had no known family history of urologic malignancy; however, his father had metastatic cancer with unknown primary site. Ureteroscopic biopsy of the mass was performed and pathology demonstrated clear cell RCC, nucleolar grade 3. A laparoscopic left radical nephrectomy was performed. Intraoperatively, a portion of the adrenal gland was densely adherent to the kidney capsule, and thus, a partial adrenalectomy was also performed. Pathology demonstrated clear cell RCC nucleolar grade 3 with 10% necrosis. Histologically, the tumor showed classic areas of low-grade clear cell renal cell carcinoma, as well as higher grade areas that demonstrated invasion into renal sinus fibroadipose tissue and ureteral urothelium as well as lymphovascular invasion (Figures 2(a)–2(c)). Resection margins were uninvolved and the final pathologic stage was pT3aNx.

The patient was advised to follow up with labs and imaging every six months for the first three years and then annually. Imaging at six-month follow-up demonstrated no evidence of disease. Eight months after nephrectomy, the patient presented to the clinic with gross hematuria and was found to have a nodular bladder lesion on in-office cystoscopy. Cytology was negative for high-grade urothelial carcinoma. Transurethral resection of the bladder tumor was performed after identification of a 5 cm nodular lesion arising from the left ureteral orifice from a small stalk. Pathology demonstrated clear cell RCC (Figures 2(d) and 2(e)). Computed tomography imaging of the chest and magnetic resonance imaging of the abdomen and pelvis all demonstrated no evidence of metastatic disease. The case was discussed in genitourinary tumor board, and close follow-up was recommended with imaging every three months for one year, extending the interval from four to six months subsequently. Additionally, repeat cystoscopy was recommended if any recurrent gross hematuria developed.

Five months after transurethral resection of the bladder tumor, a left distal ureteral mass was identified on follow-up MRI (Figure 3). Left ureterectomy with partial cystectomy was performed and pathology again demonstrated metastatic clear cell RCC (Figures 2(f) and 2(g)).

Transcriptomic profiling and targeted gene sequencing data (BostonGene) of the primary renal tumor revealed *PBRM1* (Q167kfs*7) loss of function (LOF) mutation, *CDKN2A* (E120*) LOF mutation, high programmed death ligand 1(PD-L1) expression (94%), high immune active infiltrates (CD4+ T cells and B cells), and low angiogenesis signals.

3. Discussion

This case presents an early recurrence after nephrectomy of a metastatic RCC with a solitary metastasis to the bladder.

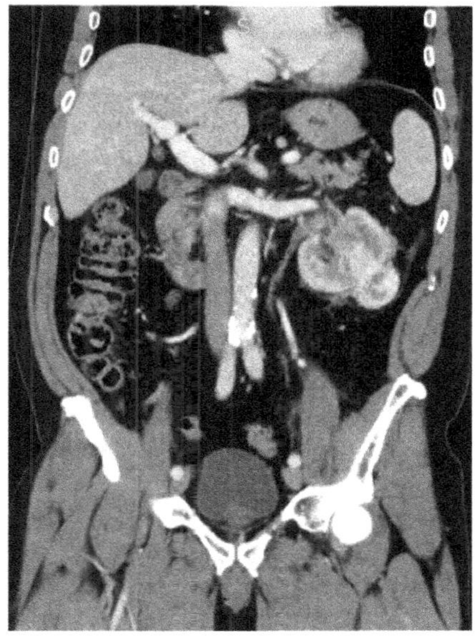

FIGURE 1: Computed tomography of renal mass demonstrating exophytic and infiltrative components of a 9 cm left interpole renal mass.

Higher tumor stage has been found to correlate with sooner recurrence after nephrectomy with T3 tumors generally recurring between 17 and 28 months [5]. In this case, recurrence occurred after less than one year and presented in the bladder, a rare site of recurrence for RCC. The mechanism for bladder metastasis has been debated and may vary between individual patients. Proposed mechanisms include direct spread and implantation, lymphatic spread, and vascular spread especially via retrograde venous emboli through connections between the left renal vein and the bladder [6]. Direct spread to the bladder via the collecting system and ureter seems likely in this case due to involvement of the left ureteral orifice, negative nephrectomy surgical margins, and lack of other metastases although lymphangitic spread along periureteral lymphatics is also a possibility. The additional RCC recurrence in the left ureter following transurethral resection of the bladder tumor further supports this route of metastasis. In contrast, other reported cases where metastasis to the bladder has occurred along with spread to additional sites such as the brain, liver, abdomen, and mediastinum seem to arise via vascular or lymphatic spread [4]. While the liver, lung, brain, and bone remain the most frequent sites of metastasis, RCC can metastasize to a number of other rare sites including the pancreas, spleen, thyroid, vagina, rectum, and breast which further complicates our understanding of the mechanism of RCC metastasis [7–11]. An analysis of isolated RCC metastases to the pancreas supports an underlying seed-and-soil mechanism in the metastasis of RCC to rare sites [7]. Further characterization of these mechanisms in metastatic renal cell carcinoma (mRCC) is required to better understand and predict sites of metastasis. Previous studies have implicated differential microRNA expression in metastasis of RCC to different sites, and investigation of gene expression profiles in mRCC remains an interesting active area of research [12–14].

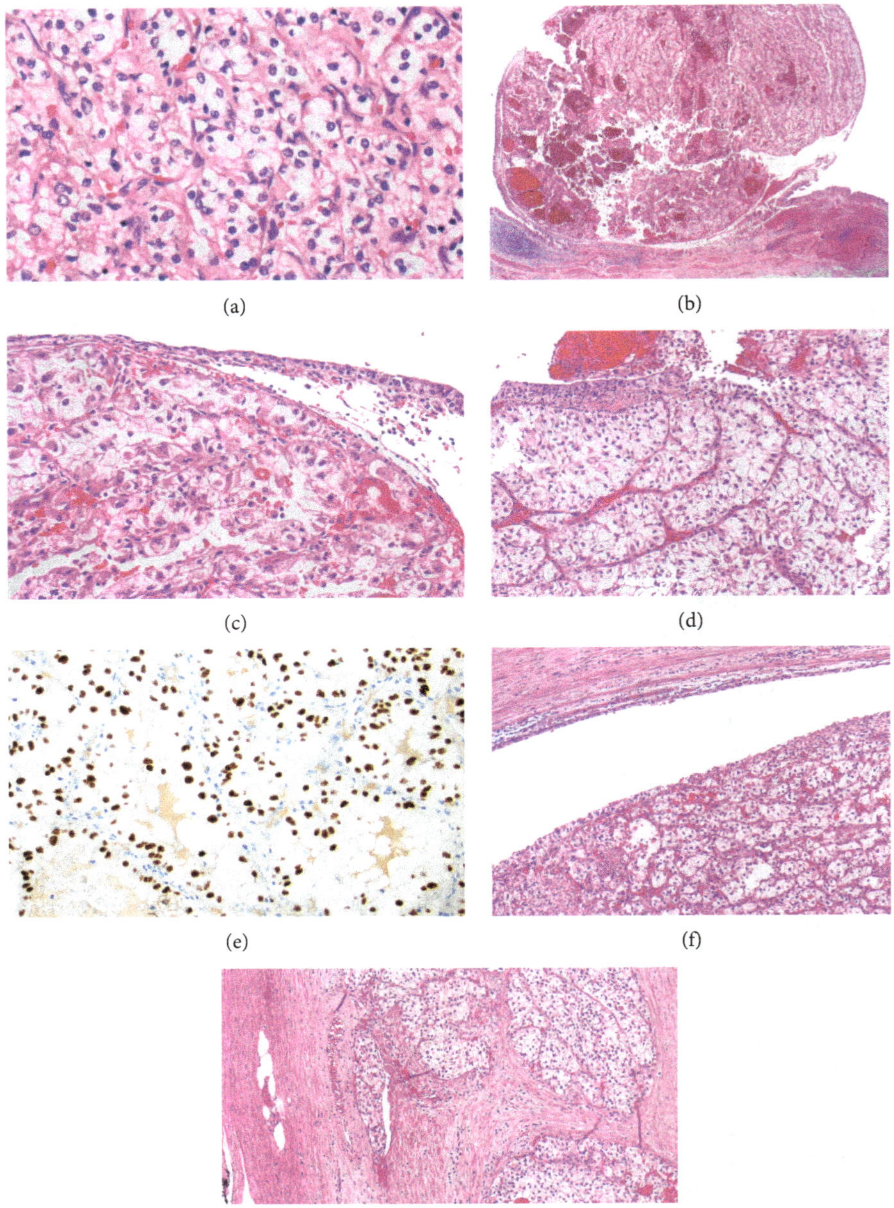

(a) (b) (c) (d) (e) (f) (g)

FIGURE 2: H&E-stained sections from the radical nephrectomy showed (a) areas of classic low-grade clear cell renal cell carcinoma (40x) and (b) an exophytic nodule of tumor undermining ureteral epithelium (2x). (c) Higher magnification of tumor invading the ureteral wall shows higher grade nuclei and tumor cells with voluminous and focally eosinophilic cytoplasm undermining urothelium (20x). (d) Transurethral resection of the subsequent bladder tumor showed tumor morphologically identical to that seen in the nephrectomy depicted in panel (c), undermining benign urothelium. (e) PAX8 shows diffuse nuclear labeling consistent with renal cell carcinoma metastatic to the bladder (20x). (f) Subsequent ureteral resection showed clear cell renal cell carcinoma forming an intraluminal mass with benign urothelium above (10x). (g) Focal lymphovascular invasion was noted within the ureteral wall (10x).

Molecular characterization of mRCC tumors, especially from rare metastatic sites such as the bladder, may aid in predicting specific sites of metastasis and contribute to improved diagnostic and therapeutic interventions. Our molecular analysis of the primary renal tumor showed low angiogenesis signal expression and higher immune signatures, which could have implications on treatment selection. Molecular characterization of the primary renal tumor and metastatic bladder lesions as part of a larger series would be helpful to understand bladder tropism in mRCC.

Treatment for oligometastatic RCC amenable to resection has long favored metastasectomy. In the more commonly observed setting of solitary pulmonary metastases, metastasectomy has demonstrated five year survival rates from 30-45% and a twofold decrease in risk of death [15]. The timing of solitary metastasis occurrence after definitive

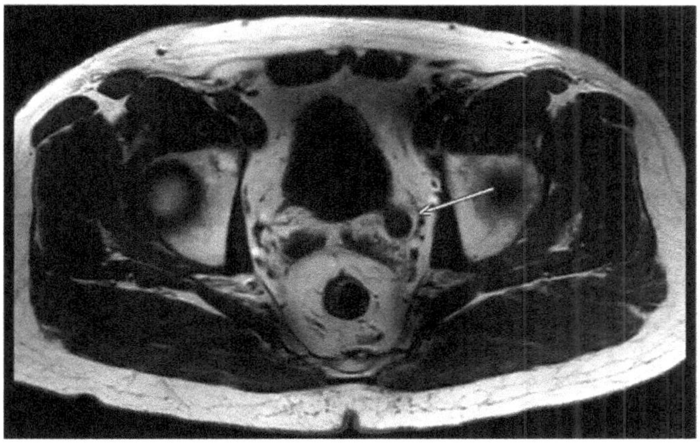

FIGURE 3: MRI with left distal ureteral recurrence (arrow).

RCC treatment has been shown to play a significant role in overall survival post metastasectomy. One study reported an overall survival of 31 months if metastasis occurred before 1 year compared to 63 months if metastasis occurred after 1 year [16]. Of note, the bladder was not a site of metastasis in any of the patients included in the aforementioned study. Site of metastasis likely plays an important role in survival as demonstrated by significant differences in survival between patients with lung and bone vs. liver and brain metastasis [16, 17]. Reports of RCC metastasizing to the bladder are sparse; however, a case report from 2002 examined 27 other such cases and identified an 80% three-year survival in 13 patients with solitary metastasis to the bladder and a 20% three-year survival rate in 15 patients with multiple metastases [6]. A 2015 systematic review of 65 reported cases of RCC metastasizing to the bladder identified a 71.1% 2-year cancer-specific survival rate in 36 patients with solitary bladder metastasis compared to 25.8% in 22 patients with additional metastases. The same review identified a 2-year cancer-specific survival of 34.6% in patients who developed bladder metastasis within 1 year of primary RCC diagnosis compared to 58.4% after 1 year of diagnosis. All bladder lesions in these cases were managed surgically [18]. In addition to reported data on timing and site of metastasis, use of risk stratification tools such as the International Metastatic Renal Cell Carcinoma Database Consortium criteria and Memorial Sloan Kettering Cancer Center criteria plays an important role in predicting prognosis in patients with mRCC.

Guidelines uniformly recommend metastasectomy for resectable single site RCC metastases [19]. Until recently, there was no role for postmetastasectomy adjuvant therapy as neither sorafenib nor pazopanib have demonstrated recurrence-free survival benefit in patients with mRCC [20, 21]. However, a recent phase III trial demonstrates improved disease-free survival with adjuvant pembrolizumab therapy following nephrectomy and metastasectomy in patients with oligometastatic RCC [22]. Due to the rare occurrence of metastatic RCC to the bladder, there are no targeted guideline recommendations for management. The limited data that is currently available suggests that postnephrectomy metastasectomy can afford a favorable prognosis, especially if the bladder is the sole site of metastasis as with the patient reported in this case. However, appearance of bladder metastasis sooner than one year postnephrectomy may be associated with worse survival, which complicates the prognosis of this patient. This patient's prognosis is further complicated by the additional ureteral recurrence following transurethral resection of the bladder tumor. While urothelial carcinomas comprise the vast majority of malignant bladder tumors, this case reinforces that in a patient with a history of RCC, discovery of a bladder tumor on cystoscopy should raise clinical suspicion for RCC recurrence. Additionally, in patients who develop metastatic RCC to the bladder, thorough work-up for additional sites of metastasis is essential for determining prognosis as well as the need for systemic therapy.

References

[1] S. A. Padala, A. Barsouk, K. C. Thandra et al., "Epidemiology of renal cell carcinoma," *World Journal of Oncology*, vol. 11, no. 3, pp. 79–87, 2020.

[2] A. M. Molina, "A multidisciplinary approach for the management of earlier stage renal cell carcinoma," *Urologic Oncology*, vol. 36, no. 1, pp. 15-16, 2018.

[3] M. D. Tyson and S. S. Chang, "Optimal surveillance strategies after surgery for renal cell carcinoma," *Journal of the National Comprehensive Cancer Network*, vol. 15, no. 6, pp. 835–840, 2017.

[4] M. Zhang, C. Wah, and J. I. Epstein, "Metastatic renal cell carcinoma to the urinary bladder: a report of 11 cases," *The American Journal of Surgical Pathology*, vol. 38, no. 11, pp. 1516–1531, 2014.

[5] A. I. Chin, J. S. Lam, R. A. Figlin, and A. S. Belldegrun, "Surveillance strategies for renal cell carcinoma patients following nephrectomy," *Revista de Urologia*, vol. 8, no. 1, pp. 1–7, 2006.

[6] M. Matsuo, S. Koga, M. Nishikido et al., "Renal cell carcinoma with solitary metachronous metastasis to the urinary bladder," *Urology*, vol. 60, no. 5, pp. 911-912, 2002.

[7] F. Sellner, "Isolated pancreatic metastases of renal cell carcinoma-a paradigm of a seed and soil mechanism: a literature analysis of 1,034 observations," *Frontiers in Oncology*, vol. 10, p. 709, 2020.

[8] M. Costantini, G. Tuderti, F. Minisola et al., "Metachronous isolated splenic metastasis in a young patient with renal cell carcinoma: case report and literature review," *Urology*, vol. 127, pp. 13–18, 2019.

[9] T. R. Geisbush, Z. Dymon, M. S. Gabriel, and V. Yedavalli, "A multimodal and pathological analysis of a renal cell carcinoma metastasis to the thyroid gland 11 years post nephrectomy," *Journal of Radiology Case Reports*, vol. 13, no. 4, pp. 1–9, 2019.

[10] H. O. E. Ali, T. Ghorab, I. R. Cameron, and A. M. S. M. Marzouk, "Renal cell carcinoma metastasis to the breast: a rare presentation," *Case Reports in Radiology*, vol. 2021, Article ID 6625689, 9 pages, 2021.

[11] S. Ouellet, A. Binette, A. Nguyen, P. Garde-Granger, and R. Sabbagh, "Metastatic renal cell carcinoma initially presenting with hematochezia and subsequently with vaginal bleeding: a case report," *BMC Urology*, vol. 18, no. 1, 2018.

[12] S. Gao, L. Yan, H. Zhang, X. Fan, X. Jiao, and F. Shao, "Identification of a metastasis-associated gene signature of clear cell renal cell carcinoma," *Frontiers in Genetics*, vol. 11, no. 11, article 603455, 2021.

[13] J. Heinzelmann, A. Unrein, U. Wickmann et al., "MicroRNAs with prognostic potential for metastasis in clear cell renal cell carcinoma: a comparison of primary tumors and distant metastases," *Annals of Surgical Oncology*, vol. 21, no. 3, pp. 1046–1054, 2014.

[14] L. Yu, L. Xiang, J. Feng et al., "miRNA-21 and miRNA-223 expression signature as a predictor for lymph node metastasis, distant metastasis and survival in kidney renal clear cell carcinoma," *Journal of Cancer*, vol. 9, no. 20, pp. 3651–3659, 2018.

[15] A. L. Alt, S. A. Boorjian, C. M. Lohse, B. A. Costello, B. C. Leibovich, and M. L. Blute, "Survival after complete surgical resection of multiple metastases from renal cell carcinoma," *Cancer*, vol. 117, no. 13, pp. 2873–2882, 2011.

[16] Y. B. Thyavihally, U. Mahantshetty, R. S. Chamarajanagar, S. G. Raibhattanavar, and H. B. Tongaonkar, "Management of renal cell carcinoma with solitary metastasis," *World Journal of Surgical Oncology*, vol. 3, no. 1, 2005.

[17] M. A. Kuczyk, A. G. Anastasiadis, R. Zimmermann, A. S. Merseburger, S. Corvin, and A. Stenzl, "Current aspects of the surgical management of organ-confined, metastatic, and recurrent renal cell cancer," *BJU International*, vol. 96, no. 5, pp. 721–727, 2005.

[18] K. Matsumoto, N. Hayakawa, S. Nakamura, and M. Oya, "Bladder metastasis from renal cell carcinoma: retrospective analysis of 65 reported cases," *Clinical & Experimental Metastasis*, vol. 32, no. 2, pp. 135–141, 2015.

[19] A. Bamias, B. Escudier, C. N. Sternberg et al., "Current clinical practice guidelines for the treatment of renal cell carcinoma: a systematic review and critical evaluation," *The Oncologist*, vol. 22, no. 6, pp. 667–679, 2017.

[20] G. Procopio, G. Apollonio, F. Cognetti et al., "Sorafenib versus observation following radical metastasectomy for clear-cell renal cell carcinoma: results from the phase 2 randomized open-label RESORT study," *European Urology Oncology*, vol. 2, no. 6, pp. 699–707, 2019.

[21] L. J. Appleman, M. Puligandla, S. K. Pal et al., "Randomized, double-blind phase III study of pazopanib versus placebo in patients with metastatic renal cell carcinoma who have no evidence of disease following metastasectomy: a trial of the ECOG-ACRIN cancer research group (E2810)," *Journal of Clinical Oncology*, vol. 37, 15_supplement, p. 4502, 2019.

[22] T. K. Choueiri, P. Tomczak, S. H. Park et al., "Adjuvant pembrolizumab after nephrectomy in renal-cell carcinoma," *The New England Journal of Medicine*, vol. 385, no. 8, pp. 683–694, 2021.

11

Laparoscopic Management of an Inflammatory Pseudotumor Mimicking a Locally Advanced Renal Carcinoma: A Diagnostic Pitfall

Imad Boualaoui,[1] Idriss Ziani,[1] Salma Marrakchi,[2] Mohammed Raiss,[3] Fouad Zouidia,[4] Ahmed Ibrahimi,[1] Hachem El Sayegh,[1] and Yassine Nouini[1]

[1]Department of Urology A, Mohammed V University in Rabat, Ibn Sina University Hospital, Rabat, Morocco
[2]Department of Radiology, Mohammed V University in Rabat, Ibn Sina University Hospital, Rabat, Morocco
[3]Surgical Department "C", Mohammed V University in Rabat, Ibn Sina University Hospital, Rabat, Morocco
[4]Department of Anatomopathology and Cytology, Mohammed V University in Rabat, Ibn Sina University Hospital, Rabat, Morocco

Correspondence should be addressed to Imad Boualaoui; imadboualaoui@gmail.com

Academic Editor: Tun-Chieh Chen

Inflammatory pseudotumors of the kidney are an infrequent entity. More frequently described in the lung, the genitourinary tract location is rare. Commonly described in the bladder, the kidney damage remains exceptional. Herein, we report the case of 60 years old man with a history of flank pain, initially diagnosed with a locally advanced left renal carcinoma invading the left colon. Then, after performing a laparoscopic radical nephrectomy, the histopathological diagnosis of inflammatory pseudotumor of the left kidney has been made.

1. Introduction

Inflammatory pseudotumors of the kidney are a rare entity. More frequently described in the lung, the genitourinary tract location is rare [1]. Commonly described in the bladder, the kidney damage remains exceptional. Few cases have been reported in the literature. Herein, we report the case of 60-year-old man with a history of flank pain, initially diagnosed with a locally advanced left renal carcinoma invading the left colon. Then, after performing a laparoscopic radical nephrectomy, the histopathological diagnosis of inflammatory pseudotumor of the left kidney has been made. This case discussion is aimed at bringing light to this rarely encountered entity. Inflammatory neoplasms of the kidney needed to be kept in mind in cases of atypical radiological presentation of a renal tumor. Appropriate management of renal pseudotumors allows avoiding an unnecessary radical nephrectomy.

2. Case Presentation

A 60-year-old man has been presented with a year history of apyretic left flank pain. The clinical exam was normal, and the urine was clear. The first computerized tomography has shown a pelvic and caliceal dilatation associated with an aerial content and a hydroaeric level in the left renal pelvis. Moreover, the excretory phase of the uro-CT shows a contrast medium not only in the renal pelvis but also in the left colic angle extending to the transverse colon. These findings confirmed the diagnosis of a left renocolic fistula (Figures 1(a)–1(c)).

To certify the confirmed etiology of the fistula and to understand its genesis, we performed a magnetic resonance urography. It has revealed a $41 \times 38 \times 41$ mm lower pole left renal mass, rounded with irregular contours, and low signal intensity in T2-weighted spin-echo images. Outwards, the renal mass invaded the left colic angle noting the gadolinium

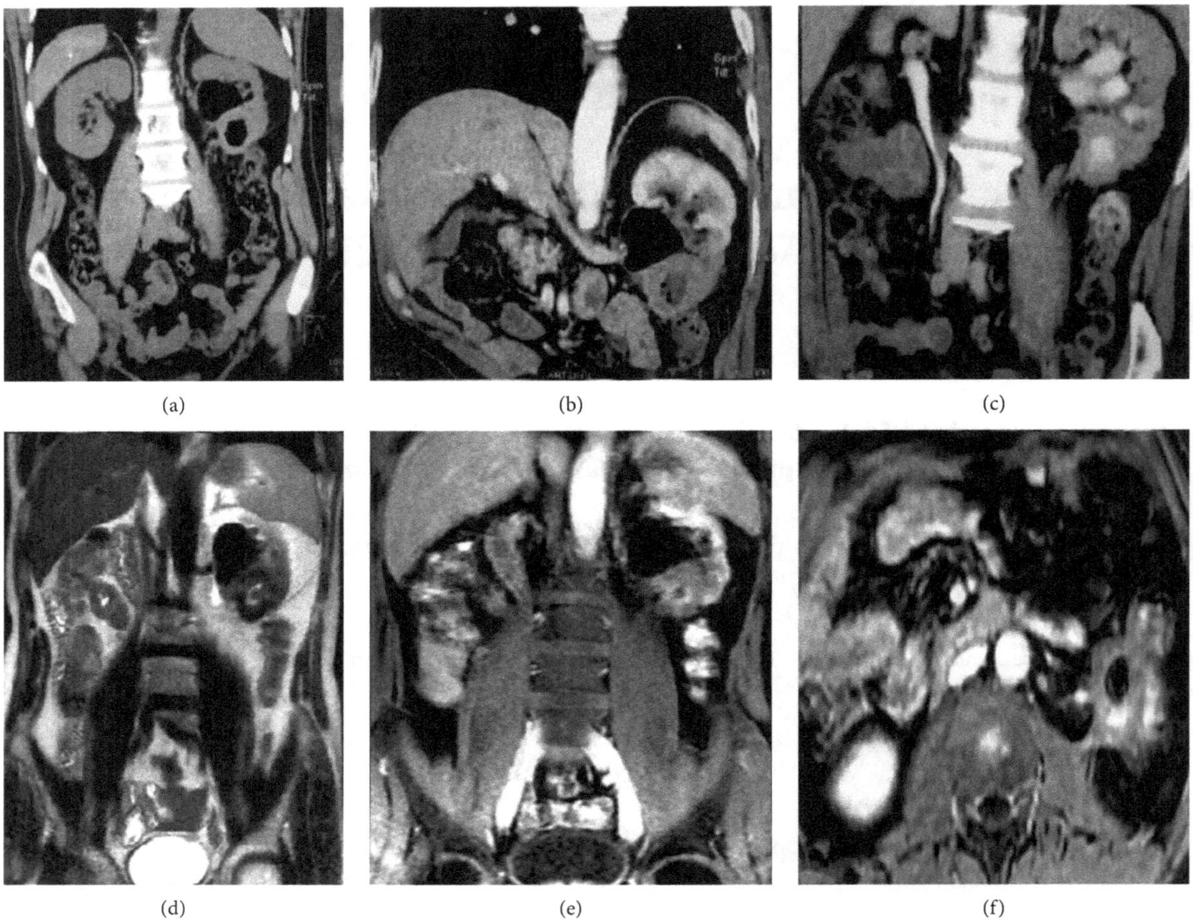

Figure 1: (a–c) Computed tomography; (a) pelvic hydroaeric level in the left kidney; (b) poorly enhanced lower pole in the left kidney; (c) contrast medium extending to the left colon. (d–f) Magnetic resonance imaging; (d) 41 × 38 × 41 mm T2 hypointense lower pole left renal mass associated with a pelvic hydroaeric level; (e) contrast medium extending to the left colon; (f) left renal mass invading the proximal ureter, the left colic angle, and the psoas muscle.

flow to the colic lumen certifying the renocolic fistula. Inner, it infiltrates the proximal ureter what is causing 37 mm hydronephrosis. Backward, the mass is closely adhering to the psoas muscle (Figures 1(d)–1(f)).

A 6 mm unique regional lymph node has also been demonstrated. The thoracic computed tomography did not reveal any metastasis. The tumor is then classified as a T4N1M0. We decided to perform a laparoscopic radical nephrectomy with a segmental colic resection.

After bowel preparation, we performed a left lateral and segmental colonic resection. We firstly proceed on lowering the left colon by performing an extensive dissection of the left colon and transverse to the tail of the pancreas medially and the spleen and stomach above. Then, we completed the resection by a total left nephrectomy extending to the perirenal fat and preserving the left adrenal (Figure 2).

The histopathologic study of the specimen using the Hemalin-Eosine coloration showed an inflammatory pseudotumor of the kidney. The inflammatory infiltrate is composed of lymphocytes, plasma cells, and fibrous backgrounds. The process invades the colic mucosa (Figure 3).

The intestinal transit resumption was effective on the second day after surgery, and the postoperative renal function was normal. The patient did not receive any specific treatment considering the histopathological diagnosis. An enhanced computed tomography has been performed after a month and shown an empty renal lodge without recurrence. We planned to perform an enhanced computed tomography once a year for five years.

3. Discussion

Renal inflammatory pseudotumor (RIPT) is an exceptional benign condition. It is also known as inflammatory myofibroblastic tumors, plasma cell granuloma, or myofibroblastoma. Inflammatory pseudotumors appear in the WHO classification as a distinct borderline lesion [2]. Different organs may be affected, especially the lung and orbit, which are the more common locations [1]. Few cases have been reported in the literature. The first urinary tract description was in the renal pelvis by Davides in 1972. However, the

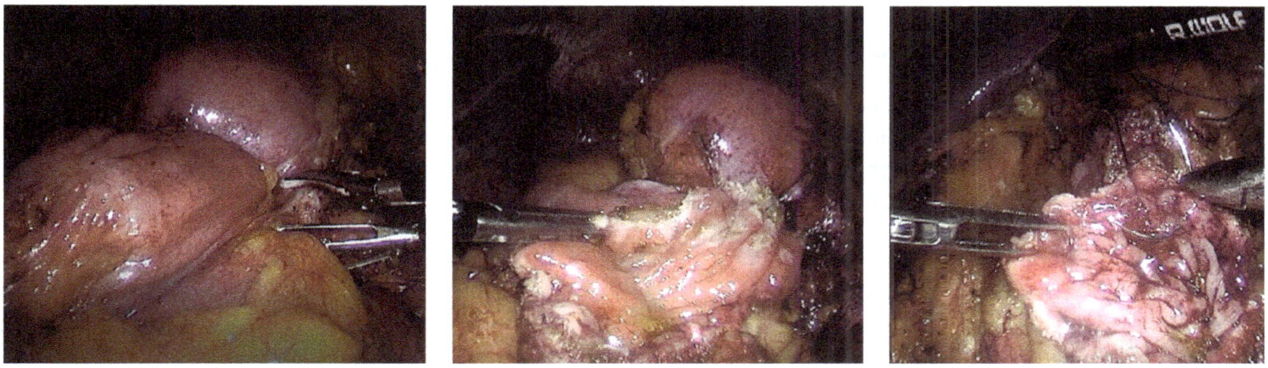

(a) (b) (c)

FIGURE 2: Laparoscopic images; (a) left renal tumor invading the left colon angle; (b) left lateral and segmental colonic resection began with opening the colonic mucosa in a healthy area; (c) closure of the colonic mucosa with a 4-0 vicryl thread.

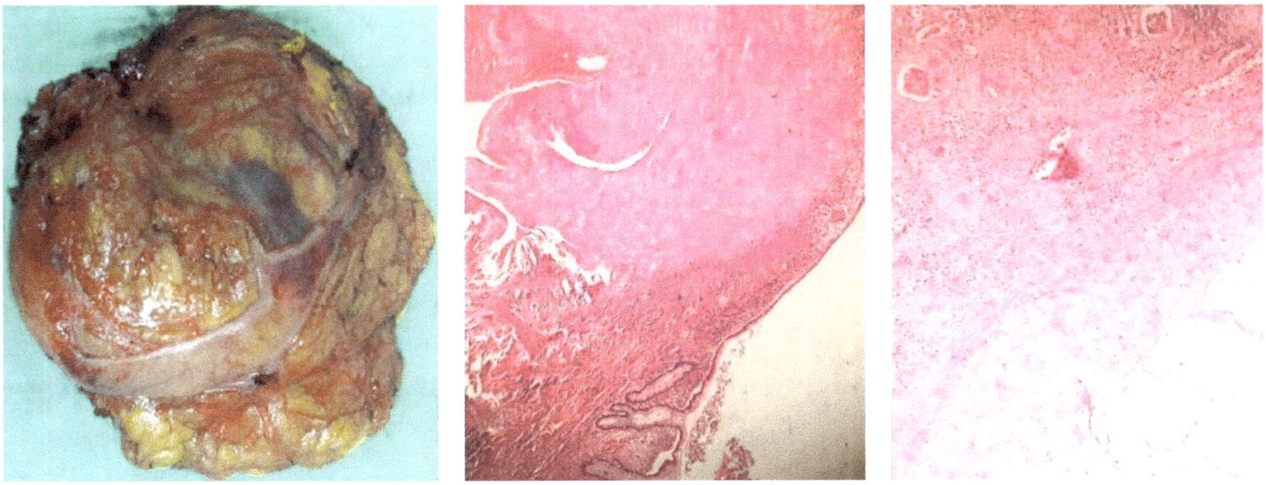

(a) (b) (c)

FIGURE 3: (a) Macroscopic image of the specimen; (b) inflammatory lesion infiltrating the intestinal mucosa (Hemalin-Eosine ×40); (c) renal tumor harboring an inflammatory lymphoplasmacytic infiltrate on a fibrous background (Hemalin-Eosine ×100).

bladder is the most commonly described location in the genitourinary tract [3, 4].

The disease occurs at all ages, predominately in children and young adults; both sexes are affected with a slight male predominance [5]. The pathophysiology of these tumors is not yet understood and remains controversial. It is still difficult to determine whether this is reactive hyperplasia or a natural tumor process. The discovery of chromosomal abnormalities suggests that there is also an oncogenetic theory [6].

The etiology of these tumors also remains to be discovered. Different theories have been suggested, including Epstein-Barr and hepatitis B virus infections, and traumatic, vascular, and autoimmune causes, among others. In addition, Schweckendiek et al. also raised the possibility of arrangements of the ALK gene (Anaplastic Lymphoma Kinase), which plays an essential role in the genesis of these tumors [7].

Our patient presented with left lumbar pain without irradiation. The clinical presentation is atypical. Symptoms could be localized pain in the lumbar region like our patient and also renal colic related to hydronephrosis due to ureteral or pelvic compression. However, hematuria is the most frequently described clinical sign in the literature. It can be micro or macroscopic, concomitant, or not with the painful symptoms. It should also be noted that inflammatory pseudotumors can be completely asymptomatic and therefore discovered fortuitously.

Imaging of inflammatory pseudotumors is also nonspecific. This fact explains why in almost all the writings on this subject, the diagnosis is only made on a piece of enlarged nephrectomy. In addition, the radiological signs are misleading, and the diagnosis of a malignant renal tumor is most often difficult to rule out due to the heterogeneous characteristics of the mass. Some characteristics have nevertheless been mentioned in the literature. On ultrasound, the lesion appears rather hypoechoic and heterogeneous, mimicking an atypical cyst. On CT, the lesion is rather hypodense and appears as T2 hypointense on MRI [3].

There is currently no consensus on the management and the follow-up of inflammatory pseudotumors. Due to the rarity of renal involvement, there are no prospective studies on this subject to date. The published articles relate only to case reports.

An atypical presentation for a renal tumor should attract the attention of clinicians, especially in cases of a unique kidney, to avoid unnecessary radical nephrectomies.

4. Conclusion

Inflammatory pseudotumors or inflammatory myofibroblastic kidney tumors remain rare, often confused with malignant kidney tumors. Larger-scale studies are needed to have more answers concerning the etiology and pathogenesis of this entity and establish diagnostic criteria in order to limit the number of unnecessary nephrectomies. The rarity of renal involvement, the heterogeneity of the clinical presentation, and the nonspecificity of the radiological signs make it a significant diagnostic and therapeutic challenge and a diagnostic pitfall to be avoided. The laparoscopic approach that we also lift allows a less invasive approach for these lesions whose neoplastic origin has not yet been demonstrated.

References

[1] C. M. Coffin, J. Watterson, J. R. Priest, and L. P. Dehner, "Extrapulmonary inflammatory myofibroblastic tumor (inflammatory pseudotumor) a clinicopathologic and immunohistochemical study of 84 cases," *The American Journal of Surgical Pathology*, vol. 19, no. 8, pp. 859–872, 1995.

[2] S. B. Park, K. S. Cho, J. K. Kim et al., "Inflammatory pseudotumor (myoblastic tumor) of the genitourinary tract," *AJR. American Journal of Roentgenology*, vol. 191, pp. 1255–1262, 2008.

[3] K. C. Davides, S. H. Johnson 3rd, M. Marshall Jr., S. E. Price Jr., and A. Stavrides, "Plasma cell granuloma of the renal pelvis," *The Journal of Urology*, vol. 107, no. 6, pp. 938-939, 1972.

[4] N. G. Lee, M. P. Alexander, H. Xu, and D. S. Wang, "Renal inflammatory myofibroblastic tumor: a case report and comprehensive review of literature," *World journal of oncology*, vol. 2, no. 2, pp. 85–88, 2011.

[5] M. Patnana, A. B. Sevrukov, K. M. Elsayes, C. Viswanathan, M. Lubner, and C. O. Menias, "Inflammatory pseudotumor: the great mimicker," *AJR. American Journal of Roentgenology*, vol. 198, no. 3, pp. W217–W227, 2012.

[6] C. M. Coffin, P. A. Humphrey, and L. P. Dehner, "Extrapulmonary inflammatory myofibroblastic tumor: a clinical and pathological survey," *Seminars in Diagnostic Pathology*, vol. 15, pp. 85–101, 1998.

[7] D. Schweckendiek, I. Inci, D. Schneiter, and W. Weder, "Inflammatory myofibroblastic tumor of the lung: two progressing pulmonary nodules in a 25-Year-Old adult with a Moraxella catharalis infection," *The Annals of Thoracic Surgery*, vol. 100, no. 6, pp. e123–e124, 2015.

[8] P. Babu, M. K. Kalpana Kumari, H. K. Nagaraj, and V. V. Mysorekar, "Inflammatory pseudotumor of kidney masquerading as renal carcinoma," *Journal of cancer research and therapeutics*, vol. 11, no. 3, article 143351, p. 668, 2015.

12

Bilateral Renal Colic as an Initial Presentation of Erdheim-Chester Disease

Julien Sarkis[1] **Fady Haddad,**[2] **Sarah Nasr,**[3] **Elie Hanna,**[1] **Ahmad Mroueh,**[4] **and Elie Nemr**[1]

[1]*Department of Urology, Hôtel-Dieu de France, Beirut, Lebanon*
[2]*Department of Internal Medicine, Hôtel-Dieu de France, Beirut, Lebanon*
[3]*Department of Pathology, Hôtel-Dieu de France, Beirut, Lebanon*
[4]*Department of Nephrology, Hôtel-Dieu de France, Beirut, Lebanon*

Correspondence should be addressed to Julien Sarkis; juliensarkis@live.com

Academic Editor: Sigurdur Gudjonsson

Erdheim-Chester disease (ECD) is a rare non-Langerhans cells histiocytosis characterized by multiorgan involvement, with renal-ECD documented in over one-third of patients. Renal disease is generally asymptomatic, rarely causing hydronephrosis and kidney impairment. In addition, the diverse clinical picture of Erdheim-Chester disease arises slowly with sequential manifestations. We present a rare case of a 75-year-old woman on long-term treatment for panhypopituitarism and steroid therapy for vasculitis, presenting to the emergency department with bilateral renal colic and acute kidney injury. Abdominopelvic CT scan revealed renal infiltration with signs of retroperitoneal fibrosis and hydronephrosis. Kidney CT-guided biopsy and 18-fluorodeoxyglucose (FDG) positron emission tomography whole body scan as well as the history of hypopituitarism and vasculitis confirmed the diagnosis of Erdheim-Chester disease. Proper therapy with interferon-α was started. This case describes the multifaced manifestation of this disease and the difficulty to establish the diagnosis, as well as the pivotal role that a urologist can play in its management.

1. Background

Erdheim-Chester disease (ECD) is a rare non-Langerhans histiocytic disorder with fewer than 600 cases reported in the literature [1]. It is characterized by a multiorgan involvement with a special affinity to the skeletal and the central nervous systems [2]. Asymptomatic retroperitoneal involvement is seen in more than one-third of patients with ECD [3]. However renal involvement with consequent hydronephrosis and impairment was described in only 6% of the population [4]. This diverse clinical picture of ECD arises as a slowly forming mosaic with sequential manifestations, leading to frequent delay in diagnosis.

Here, we present a rare case of a 75-year-old woman on long-term treatment for panhypopituitarism and steroid therapy for vasculitis, diagnosed of ECD following bilateral renal colic.

2. Case Presentation

It is the case of a 75-year-old Caucasian woman with a medical history of central diabetes insipidus and central hypothyroidism, both diagnosed in 2005. Six years ago, she was diagnosed with large vessel vasculitis following symptoms of headache associated to elevated C-reactive protein (CRP) and aortic involvement on PET/CT scan. Steroid-based immunosuppressive therapy was started. Methotrexate was first given in adjunction to prednisone but later discontinued due to severe myelosuppression. Both temporal artery biopsies were negative for Horton's disease. Patient is hypertensive and obese with recurrent osteoporotic vertebral compression fractures requiring cementoplasty and a sedentary lifestyle due to lower limb pain limiting her daily activity.

She presented to our emergency department due to increasing bilateral flank pain that started several weeks

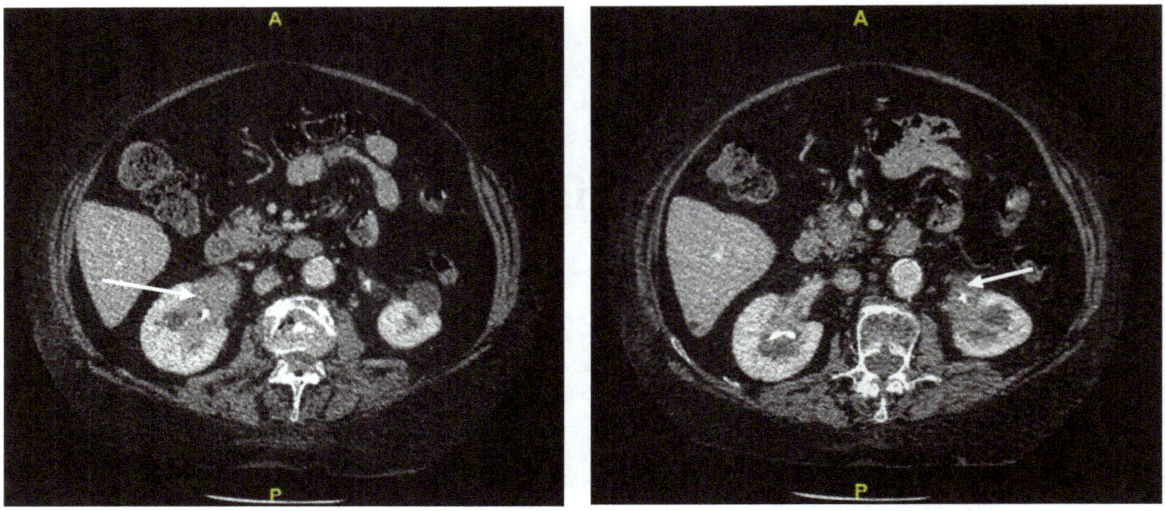

(a) (b)

Figure 1: Injected computed tomography of the abdomen after bilateral ureteral stent insertion: *arrows* showing the infiltration of the right (a) and left (b) kidneys by a homogeneous tissue enclosing the pelvis, signs of retroperitoneal fibrosis. No characteristic "hairy kidney" appearance and no signs of aortic involvement.

ago, associated to recent episodes of vomiting and general weakness. On physical exam, patient was alert and conscious, afebrile with stable vital signs. Abdomen was soft without any point tenderness. Lumbar punch was positive bilaterally. Investigations revealed acute kidney injury with a creatinine of 308 μmol/L (3.8 mg/dL), and bilateral hydronephrosis with renal pelvic thickening on imaging. The patient underwent urgent bilateral ureteral stent insertion, resulting in an improved renal function (creatinine of 65 μmol/L or 0.73 mg/dL on day 5 after surgery).

Due to the unusual renal involvement on imaging, as well as the patient's medical history of panhypopituitarism and vasculitis, a diagnosis of histiocytosis was suggested. An injected thoraco-abdominopelvic CT scan showed infiltration of both the kidney sinus by a homogeneous tissue enclosing the pelvis and the proximal ureters as well as the vascular structures of the renal hilum suggestive of retroperitoneal fibrosis (Figure 1). On bone windows, iliac wings were seen containing poorly defined sclerotic plaques, associated to bone lysis and fracture on the right side.

In coordination with our interventional radiology team, multiple CT-guided Tru-Cut biopsies of the left thickened renal pelvis were obtained. The diagnosis of ECD was confirmed by pathology, with signs of retroperitoneal fibrosis, as well as histiocytosis associated to lymphocytic and monocellular invasion (Figure 2(a)). On immunohistochemical staining, histiocytes were CD68 positive (Figure 2(b)) but negative for CD1a antigen (Figure 2(c)). Multinucleated giant Touton cells were also visible (Figures 2(b) and 2(d)). IgG4 testing results on pathology and serology were both negative, ruling out IgG4-related retroperitoneal fibrosis.

An 18-fluorodeoxyglucose (FDG) positron emission tomography whole body scan was realized to assess the extension of the disease revealed an intensely FDG-avid suprasellar soft tissue lesion, as well multiple FDG-avid sclerotic bone lesions in the distal femoral metadiaphysis bilaterally. An uptake of 18-FDG was also notable in the fractured right iliac bone (Figure 3). The diagnosis of ECD was confirmed, followed by negative BRAF mutation testing. The patient was discharged on interferon-α at day 17 after her admission, with a creatinine of 72 μmol/L (0.81 mg/dL). An echocardiogram ruled out heart involvement. Her hospital course was complicated by a nonmassive pulmonary embolism with normal right ventricular function, treated by therapeutic anticoagulation.

3. Discussion and Conclusion

Histiocytosis is a group of rare diseases characterized by abnormal accumulation of macrophages, dendritic cells, or monocyte-derived cells in different tissues causing highly heterogenous clinical findings [5]. Erdheim-Chester disease (ECD) is an uncommon non-Langerhans cell histiocytosis distinguished on pathology by the presence of lipid-laden histiocytes that are immunochemically CD68 (histiocyte marker) positive but negative for CD1a and S100 (Langerhans cell markers). Multinucleated Touton giant cell's presence also favors the disease [6]. Like all histiocytosis, ECD has a multiorgan implication, but it is typically characterized by skeletal and central nervous system involvement. Skeletal lesions occur in 74% of patients with characteristic multifocal osteosclerotic lesions of the long bones [7]. The central nervous system is involved in half of the cases, with central diabetes insipidus being the most common manifestation of neuro-ECD [3]. Renally, a recent systematic review of the literature described asymptomatic retroperitoneal involvement in more than one third of patients [3]. However, renal involvement with consequent hydronephrosis and impairment was present in only 6% of the population, generally with the characteristic appearance of "hairy kidneys" on the CT scan [4].

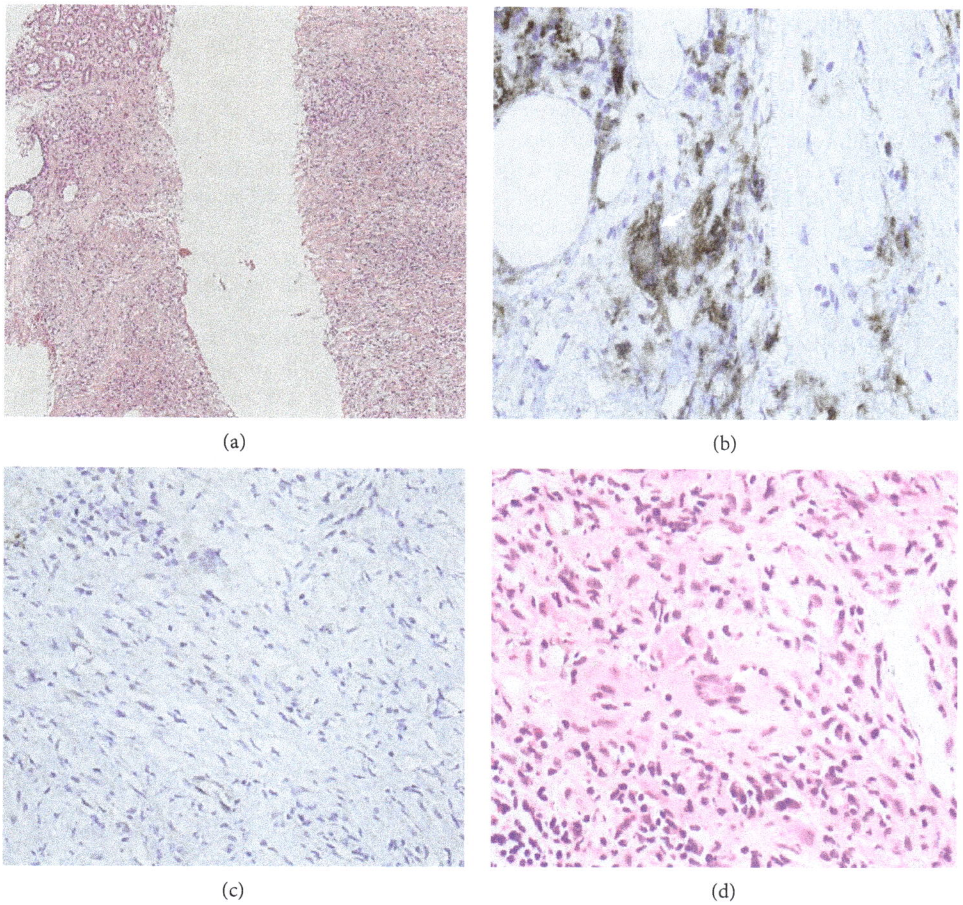

FIGURE 2: Histopathological finding of the renal specimen resected by CT-guided Tru-Cut biopsies: hematoxylin-eosin staining revealed a diffuse proliferation of histiocytes associated to lymphocytic and monocellular invasion, as well as important fibrotic involvement ((a) original magnification ×100). Immunochemistry demonstrated that histiocytes were strongly positive for CD68 (b) and negative for CD1a antigen (c) ((b, c) original magnification ×400). Touton-like multinucleated giant cells (arrowheads) are visible on both CD68 (b) and hematoxylin-eosin staining ((d) original magnification ×400).

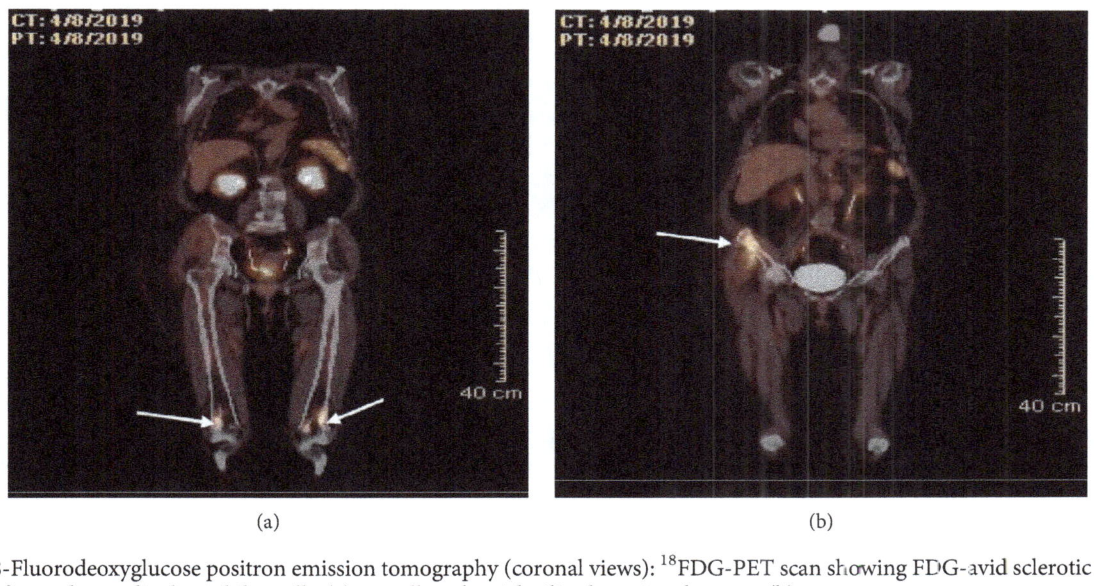

FIGURE 3: 18-Fluorodeoxyglucose positron emission tomography (coronal views): ^{18}FDG-PET scan showing FDG-avid sclerotic bone lesions in the distal femoral metadiaphysis bilaterally (a) as well as the right iliac bone involvement (b).

The protean manifestations of ECD as well as its slow progression render its diagnosis challenging. Patients frequently face a delay in initiation of therapy often due to a difficulty in diagnosis. Our patient has suffered a delay of over 10 years since her initial diagnosis of central diabetes insipidus and hypothyroidism. Steroid and methotrexate started as treatment of her vascular involvement were the consequence of morbid drug side effects: corticosteroid-induced obesity and osteoporosis, as well as methotrexate-induced myelosuppression. Skeletal involvement was also present in our patient, leading to two episodes of vertebral fractures requiring cementoplasty as well as chronic lower limbs pain. However, bone disease was underlooked, and linked to chronic prednisone therapy. The presence of osteosclerosis of the iliac crests on CT as well as the history of vascular and central nervous disease, with the new image of signs of retroperitoneal fibrosis causing acute kidney injury finally pointed to ECD. Renal involvement in this case is atypical, consisting of symptomatic retroperitoneal fibrosis without the characteristic "hairy kidneys" on CT scan. Pathology is mandatory in confirming the diagnosis. In our case, CT-guided biopsies were of little morbidity and sufficient, showing the characteristic lipid-laden histiocytosis and monocellular invasion as well as signs of retroperitoneal fibrosis. The search of BRAF mutation was negative, rendering the use of BRAF-inhibitors impossible. Considered as first-line therapy in BRAF-negative patients, Interferon-α was started and response evaluation programmed.

This case typically describes the multifaced manifestation of ECD, as well as the difficulty to establish the diagnosis. Even though its clinical manifestations are well described in the literature, the diverse and multi-system involvement render the diagnosis challenging. Therefore, physicians should be familiar with this disease, sparing patients years of unnecessary treatments.

Consent

Written informed consent was obtained from the patient for publication of this case report and any accompanying images.

Disclosure

The work has been reported in line with the CARE criteria for case reports.

References

[1] M. Adawi, B. Bisharat, and A. Bowirrat, "Erdheim-Chester disease (ECD): case report, clinical and basic investigations, and review of literature," *Medicine (Baltimore)*, vol. 95, no. 42, article e5167, 2016.

[2] M. V. Shah, T. G. Call, C. C. Hook et al., "Clinical presentation, diagnosis, treatment, and outcome of patients with Erdheim-Chester disease: the Mayo Clinic experience," *Blood*, vol. 124, no. 21, pp. 1405–1405, 2014.

[3] M. Cives, V. Simone, F. M. Rizzo et al., "Erdheim-Chester disease: a systematic review," *Critical Reviews in Oncology/-Hematology*, vol. 95, no. 1, pp. 1–11, 2015.

[4] J. C. Scolaro and A. N. Peiris, "The hairy kidney of Erdheim-Chester disease," *Mayo Clinic Proceedings*, vol. 93, no. 5, p. 671, 2018.

[5] P. Zhu, N. Li, L. Yu, M. N. Miranda, G. Wang, and Y. Duan, "Erdheim-Chester disease with emperipolesis: a unique case involving the heart," *Cancer research and treatment: official journal of Korean Cancer Association*, vol. 49, no. 2, pp. 553–558, 2017.

[6] J. Liersch, J. A. Carlson, and J. Schaller, "Histopathological and clinical findings in cutaneous manifestation of Erdheim-Chester disease and Langerhans cell histiocytosis overlap syndrome associated with the BRAFV600E mutation," *The American Journal of Dermatopathology*, vol. 39, no. 7, pp. 493–503, 2017.

[7] H. Hashmi, D. Murray, J. Greenwell, M. Shaikh, S. Basu, and M. Krem, "A rare case of Erdheim-Chester disease (non-Langerhans cell histiocytosis) with concurrent Langerhans cell histiocytosis: a diagnostic and therapeutic challenge," *Case Reports in Hematology*, vol. 2018, Article ID 7865325, 6 pages, 2018.

13

Indocyanine Green Near-Infrared Fluorescence Imaging-Guided Laparoscopic Heminephrectomy for Left Ureteral Cancer in Patient with Horseshoe Kidney

Takao Natsuyama,[1] Yozo Mitsui,[1,2] Masato Uetani,[1] Shigeyuki Ohta,[1] and Shin-ichi Hisasue[1]

[1]*Department of Urology, Chiba-Nishi General Hospital, 270-2251 Chiba, Japan*
[2]*Department of Urology, Toho University Faculty of Medicine, 143-8540 Tokyo, Japan*

Correspondence should be addressed to Yozo Mitsui; yozo_321@yahoo.co.jp

Academic Editor: Apul Goel

Laparoscopic surgery for patients with a horseshoe kidney is challenging because of the location, aberrant vasculature, and difficulty with division of the isthmus with adequate hemostasis. We herein report performance of a laparoscopic heminephrectomy for left ureteral cancer in a patient with a horseshoe kidney under guidance from near-infrared fluorescence (NIRF) imaging using indocyanine green (ICG). A 62-year-old male was referred to our hospital for treatment of left ureteral cancer associated with a horseshoe kidney. We performed a laparoscopic left nephroureterectomy and bladder resection in June 2017. During the operation, the NIRF imaging system was used to evaluate the border of the kidney parenchyma isthmus after ligation of the left kidney vasculature supply. Interestingly, the dominant region of the right kidney showed strong ICG fluorescence as compared to the left kidney region. With the assistance of ICG-based NIRF imaging, isthmus division was performed with monopolar scissors and adequate hemostasis was obtained by electrocautery coagulation. This is the first report of use of an ICG-based NIRF imaging system and this novel approach can help to demarcate the left moiety isthmus from right one with more certainty.

1. Introduction

A horseshoe kidney, one of the most common renal fusion anomalies, is associated with various urological diseases, such as urolithiasis, ureteropelvic junction obstruction, and urinary infection, though rarely malignant, which may require a surgical procedure for treatment. A laparoscopic approach in a case with a horseshoe kidney is challenging because of location, as well as vascular anomalies and the kidney parenchyma isthmus that connects the two sides. Good preoperative understanding of the anatomical structure of a horseshoe kidney based on radiological imaging as well as functional intraoperative visualization may contribute to more safe and reliable laparoscopic surgery.

Near-infrared fluorescence (NIRF) imaging with indocyanine green (ICG) is a novel intraoperative technique that can be applied in a variety of clinical settings, such as for confirmation of blood flow and detection of sentinel lymph nodes, as well as cancer detection. We previously reported that normal kidney tissues showed high fluorescence with ICG administration [1, 2], which led us to speculate that this novel technology could be applied for intraoperative discrimination of the isthmus of a horseshoe kidney. We herein report a case of left ureteral cancer in a patient with a horseshoe kidney who was successfully treated for the first time by a laparoscopic heminephrectomy under the aid of intraoperative ICG-based NIRF imaging.

2. Case Presentation

A 62-year-old Japanese male with a horseshoe kidney was referred to our hospital for further examination of left hydronephrosis. The patient was obese with a body mass index of 32.0 kg/m^2 (height 170 cm, body weight 92 kg) and

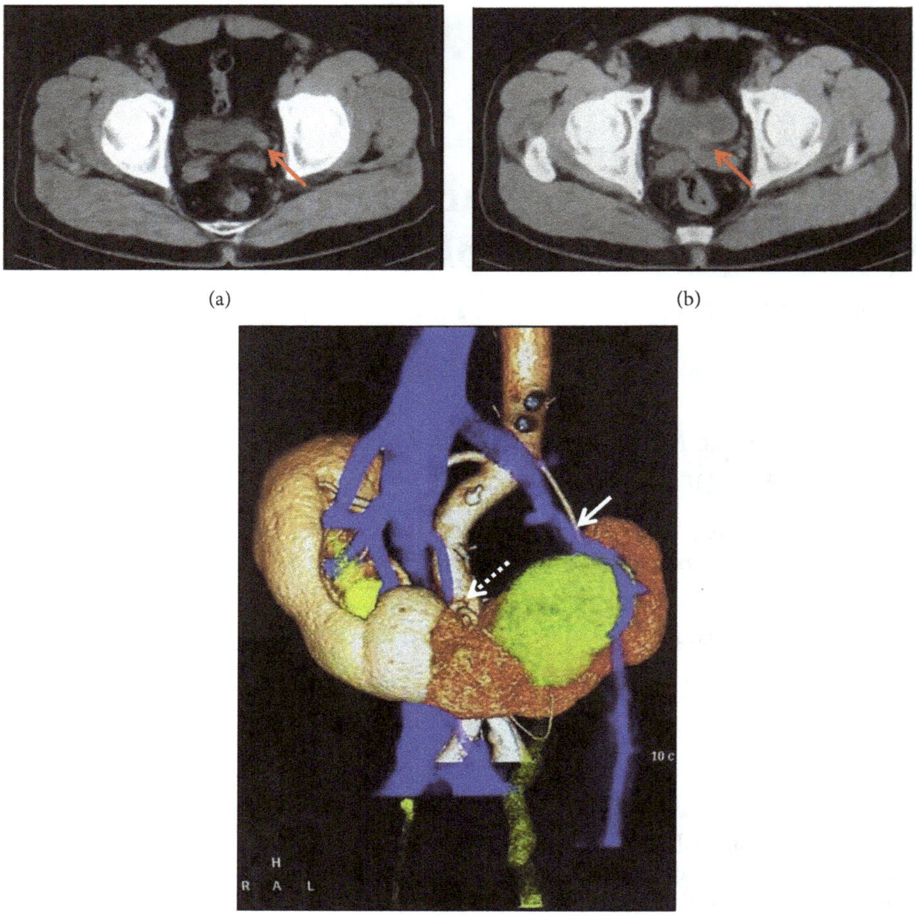

(a) (b) (c)

FIGURE 1: (a), (b) Pelvic CT images showing a left lower ureteral tumor near the ureteral orifice (red arrows). (c) Three-D CT imaging. The left renal artery (white arrow) and an aberrant renal artery (white dotted arrow) supplied the left part of the horseshoe kidney.

had undergone medical treatment for hypertension. Laboratory examination results showed mild renal dysfunction with a serum creatinine level of 1.21 mg/dL and estimate glomerular filtration rate of 48.2 mL/minute. Computed tomography (CT) revealed a left lower ureteral mass near the ureteral orifice, resulting in renal hydronephrosis (Figures 1(a) and 1(b)). Furthermore, three-dimensional (3-D) CT imaging showed a normal renal vascular system, while an aberrant renal artery located just below the root of the inferior mesenteric artery (IMA) was found to supply the bilateral sides of the lower part of the horseshoe kidney (Figure 1(c)). In addition, urine cytology findings were positive for malignancy. Based on these findings, we diagnosed a left lower ureteral tumor associated with a horseshoe kidney.

In June 2017, laparoscopic left nephroureterectomy and bladder resection procedures were performed with 5 laparoscopic ports, with the port schema shown in Figure 2(a). Using an intraperitoneal approach, we cut the peritoneum and dislocated the intestine to approach the renal helium. After visualizing the left renal vascular system, the main renal artery supplying the left side of the upper part of the horseshoe kidney and left branch of the aberrant renal artery passing under the IMA were ligated by use of a Hem-o-lok® polymer clip and divided, after which the left renal vein was ligated and divided in the same manner (Figure 2(b)). Next, we were able to observe the renal isthmus using an NIRF system (da Vinci Xi FireFlyTM®) at 1 minute after intravenous administration of 1 mL of ICG (Diagnogreen 0.25%; Daiichi Pharmaceutical, Tokyo, Japan). Strong ICG fluorescence was observed in the dominant region of the right part of the kidney, while no fluorescence was noted in the left kidney region (Figure 3(d)). These findings indicated that blood supply to the left side of the kidney was completely blocked, which was more apparent as compared to white light images (Figure 3(a)). Subsequently, the heminephrectomy was started under the assistance of NIRF imaging using cold scissors. During excision, visualization with white light and the NIRF was switched at the discretion of the operator in order to confirm the plane of excision between the right and left parts of the kidney (Figures 3(b) and 3(e)). Adequate hemostasis from the resected area could be obtained by electrocautery bipolar coagulation and use of a TacoSil®

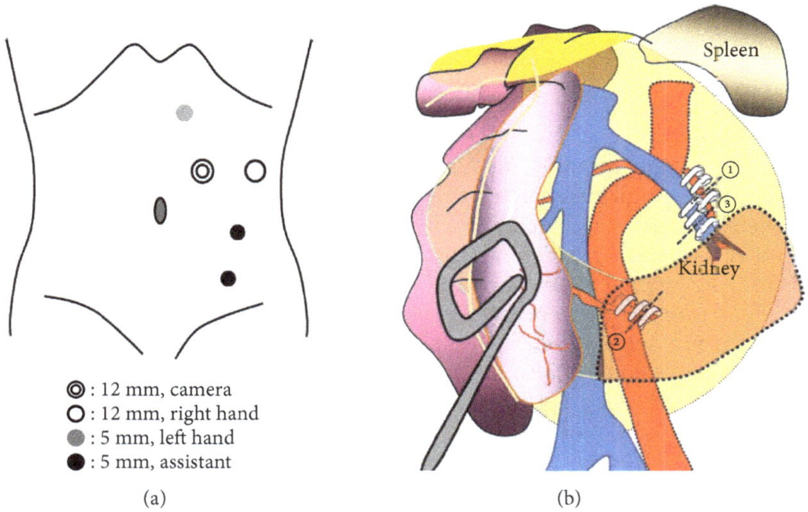

FIGURE 2: (a) Laparoscopic ports used in this case. (b) Schema of procedure for ligation of the left renal vascular system. The main renal artery and an aberrant renal artery were ligated and divided in that order; then the renal vein was cut.

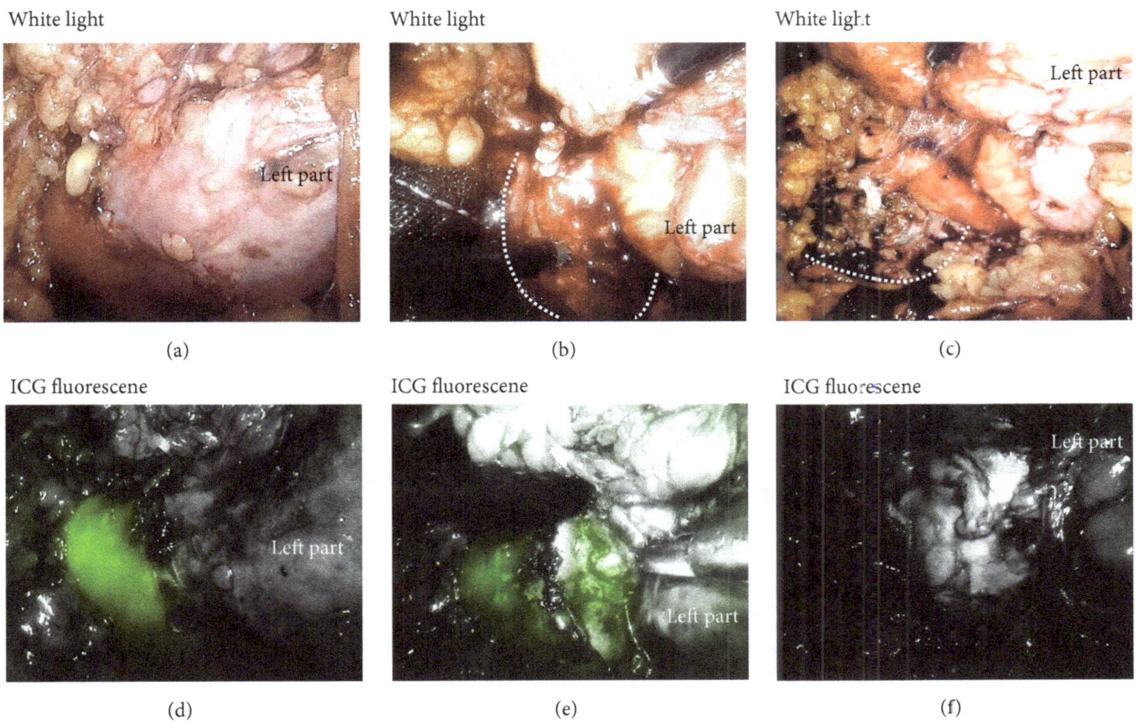

FIGURE 3: (a) Gross appearance of horseshoe kidney under white light after blockage of blood supply to the left kidney. (b) Resection of the renal isthmus under white light. Dotted circle indicates renal isthmus border. (c) Resected surface of right part of kidney under white light. Adequate hemostasis was obtained by bipolar coagulation and a fibrin patch. Dotted circle indicates renal isthmus border. (d) ICG-based NIRF images showing strong ICG fluorescence in the dominant region of the right part of the kidney after blockage of blood supply to the left kidney. (e) Proper resection of the renal isthmus could be performed with assistance from NIRF imaging. (f) Adequate hemostasis of the resected surface of the right part of the kidney was confirmed using ICG-based NIRF imaging.

tissue sealing sheet, with no suturing required (Figures 3(c) and 3(f)). Following completion of the laparoscopic heminephrectomy, the patient was placed in a supine position and partial resection of the bladder was performed. The total operation time was 5 hours 21 minutes and blood loss was 410 mL (obtained in urine from the bladder). A histopathological examination revealed an invasive urothelial carcinoma (grade 2>1, INFβ, pT2a, ly0, v0, u-lt0, RM0).

There were no perioperative complications and the patient was discharged 9 days after surgery.

3. Discussion

A horseshoe kidney is one of the most commonly encountered kidney fusion anomalies, with an incidence rate estimated to be 1 in 400 in the general population. This condition is often accompanied by other urologic disorders and a surgical procedure such as a heminephrectomy may be necessary in some cases. Recently, minimally invasive surgical techniques including a laparoscopic approach have been widely applied for urological surgery, a trend that also applies to diseases associated with a horseshoe kidney. For example, Tuncel et al. reported the efficacy and safety of a laparoscopic heminephrectomy in a case of horseshoe kidney [3]. To enhance the utility and safety of such an approach, we used an ICG-based NIRF imaging system during performance of a laparoscopic heminephrectomy for left ureteral cancer associated with a horseshoe kidney. Our results are the first to show that this system may be a promising intraoperative imaging technique to facilitate laparoscopic attempts for performance of a heminephrectomy.

NIRF imaging technology, which can be utilized in real time during surgery, has been applied for a variety of surgical specialties over the past decade. Several fluorescent tracers can be used, of which ICG is most widely selected because it has few side effects and its pharmacokinetics are well understood. Following an intravenous injection, most of the ICG binds to serum protein, which allows fluorescence to be visualized throughout the vascular system, while in well-perfused normal renal parenchyma, fluorescence can be observed from approximately 1 minute after ICG administration [1, 2]. In the present case, the dominant region of the right kidney showed strong green fluorescence with NIRF imaging, while no fluorescence was seen in the ischemic region of the left kidney, suggesting that all renal arteries in the left side were completely blocked. Preoperative 3D CT images are very useful to identify horseshoe kidney vessels [4–6], though the complicated vessel anatomy associated with this condition can sometimes lead to overlooked small aberrant vessels. We consider that use of an ICG-based NIRF imaging system complements preoperative radiological imaging by providing real-time intraoperative renal angiogram images.

A successful heminephrectomy requires not entering the renal collecting system of the contralateral kidney and achievement of adequate bleeding control [3]. When dividing the isthmus, we repeatedly referred to images from the ICG-based NIRF system, as they assisted in determining the proper direction of the incision. As shown in Figure 3(e), this system enabled intraoperative discrimination between the ischemic and well-perfused renal parenchyma and helped to avoid entering the right kidney renal collecting system. Also, sufficient hemostasis was obtained by use of bipolar coagulation and a fibrin patch, indicating that proper resection of the isthmus with assistance from ICG-based NIRF imaging contributed to reducing the amount of bleeding in our case. In addition, the technique was not difficult and did not affect the time needed for division of the isthmus. Based on our findings, we concluded that the ICG-based NIRF imaging system enhances the safety and reliability of a laparoscopic heminephrectomy procedure.

The urological surgery procedure that most often utilizes the ICG-based NIRF imaging system is robotic-assisted partial nephrectomy for renal tumors [7]. Under guidance provided by the system, a renal tumor appears hypofluorescent as compared to the normal kidney parenchyma because of an absence in the tumor of bilitranslocase, a carrier protein of ICG present in normal proximal tubule cells [8], allowing for clear discrimination between cancer and normal kidney tissues. In general, renal tumors associated with a horseshoe kidney are more rare than upper urinary tract urothelial tumors, though approximately 200 cases have been described thus far and robotic approaches have recently been attempted [6, 9, 10]. We speculate that the ICG-based NIRF imaging system can also help with minimally invasive surgery for renal tumors associated with a horseshoe kidney.

In conclusion, a laparoscopic heminephrectomy for left ureteral cancer in a patient with a horseshoe kidney was performed safely and reliably with guidance from ICG-based NIRF imaging. This novel system may play an important role in minimally invasive surgery for various horseshoe kidney-associated diseases.

References

[1] Y. Mitsui, H. Shiina, N. Arichi et al., "Indocyanine green (ICG)-based fluorescence navigation system for discrimination of kidney cancer from normal parenchyma: Application during partial nephrectomy," *International Urology and Nephrology*, vol. 44, no. 3, pp. 753–759, 2012.

[2] N. Arichi, Y. Mitsui, K. Ogawa et al., "Intraoperative fluorescence vascular imaging using indocyanine green for assessment of transplanted kidney perfusion," *Transplantation Proceedings*, vol. 46, no. 2, pp. 342–345, 2014.

[3] A. Tuncel, A. Erkan, M. Sofikerim et al., "Laparoscopic heminephrectomy for benign and malignant diseases if the horseshoe kidney," *Archivio Italiano di Urologia e Andrologia*, vol. 88, no. 4, pp. 255–257, 2016.

[4] Y. Maeda, T. Shinohara, A. Nagatsu, N. Futakawa, and T. Hamada, "Laparoscopic resection aided by preoperative 3-D CT angiography for rectosigmoid colon cancer associated with a horseshoe kidney: A case report," *Asian Journal of Endoscopic Surgery*, vol. 7, no. 4, pp. 317–319, 2014.

[5] S. I. Ohtake, T. I. Kawahara, G. Noguchi et al., "Renal cell carcinoma in a horseshoe kidney treated with laparoscopic partial nephrectomy," *Case Reports in Oncological Medicine*, vol. 2018, Article ID 7135180, 3 pages, 2018.

[6] A. Raman, T. Kuusk, E. R. Hyde, L. U. Berger, A. Bex, and F. Mumtaz, "Robotic-assisted Laparoscopic Partial Nephrectomy in a Horseshoe Kidney. a case report and review of the literature," *Urology*, vol. 114, pp. e3–e5, 2018.

[7] M. A. Bjurlin, T. R. McClintock, and M. D. Stifelman, "Near-infrared fluorescence imaging with intraoperative administration of indocyanine green for robotic partial nephrectomy," *Current Urology Reports*, vol. 16, no. 4, 2015.

[8] D. J. Golijanin, J. Marshall, A. Cardin et al., "Passamonti S, Messing EM. Bilitranslocase (BTL) is immunolocalised in proximal and distal renal tubules and absent in renal cortical tumors accurately corresponding to intraoperative near infrared fluorescence (NIRF) expression of renal cortical tumors using intravenous indocyanin green (ICG)," *The Journal of Urology*, vol. 179, no. 4S, p. 137, 2008.

[9] C. G. Rogers, W. M. Linehan, and P. A. Pinto, "Robotic nephrectomy for kidney cancer in a horseshoe kidney with renal vein tumor thrombus: Novel technique for thrombectomy," *Journal of Endourology*, vol. 22, no. 8, pp. 1561–1563, 2008.

[10] S. Kumar, S. Singh, S. Jain, G. S. Bora, and S. K. Singh, "Robot-assisted heminephrectomy for chromophobe renal cell carcinoma in L-shaped crossed ectopia: Surgical challenge," *Korean Journal of Urology*, vol. 56, no. 10, pp. 729–732, 2015.

14

Laparoscopic Nephroureterectomy with Heminephrectomy for Urothelial Carcinoma of the Upper Renal Pelvis on the Left Side of the Horseshoe Kidney

Taro Ikeda,[1] Kazunori Matsumoto,[2] Go Hasegawa,[3] Yohei Ikeda,[4] Noboru Hara,[1] and Tsutomu Nishiyama[1]

[1]*Department of Urology, Uonuma Institute of Community Medicine, Niigata University Medical and Dental Hospital, Minamiuonuma, Niigata, Japan*
[2]*Department of Radiation Engineering, Uonuma Institute of Community Medicine, Niigata University Medical and Dental Hospital, Minamiuonuma, Niigata, Japan*
[3]*Department of Pathology, Uonuma Institute of Community Medicine, Niigata University Medical and Dental Hospital, Minamiuonuma, Niigata, Japan*
[4]*Department of Diagnostic Radiology, Uonuma Institute of Community Medicine, Niigata University Medical and Dental Hospital, Minamiuonuma, Niigata, Japan*

Correspondence should be addressed to Tsutomu Nishiyama; nisiyama@med.niigata-u.ac.jp

Academic Editor: Fumitaka Koga

A 70-year-old male was diagnosed with urothelial carcinoma of the upper renal pelvis on the left side of the horseshoe kidney. Preoperative thin-slice contrast-enhanced CT with three-dimensional reconstruction of the images revealed that two arteries arising from the aorta supplied the left moiety of the horseshoe kidney. He underwent laparoscopic transperitoneal nephroureterectomy with heminephrectomy on the left side of the horseshoe kidney visualized by indocyanine green fluorescence system. The histopathological findings of the renal pelvic tumor revealed invasive urothelial carcinoma with squamous differentiation, high grade, and pT3.

1. Introduction

Upper tract urothelial carcinoma represents a small proportion (5%-10%) of all urothelial cancers [1]. Horseshoe kidney is a congenital abnormality in which the two kidneys are fused at their lower poles by a region of parenchymal and fibrous tissue called the isthmus [2]. There is no known association of horseshoe kidney with urothelial cancer; however, there are several case reports describing surgical management of tumors in patients with horseshoe kidney [3–7]. Herein, we present a case of urothelial carcinoma in the left renal pelvis of the horseshoe kidney. The patient underwent laparoscopic left nephroureterectomy with heminephrectomy for urothelial carcinoma of the upper renal pelvis on the left side of the horseshoe kidney.

2. Case Report

The patient, a 70-year-old male, was treated with laparoscopic radical prostatectomy and salvage radiotherapy for localized prostate cancer in 2016 and 2017.

Atypical urothelial cells were found in urine cytology in 2019 on a prostate cancer follow-up. There was no evidence of urothelial cancer on repeated computed tomography (CT) and cystoscopy; however, atypical urothelial cells in urine cytology continued to be detected. In May 2021, CT and magnetic resonance image (MRI) revealed a mass lesion of the upper pelvis of the left side of the horseshoe kidney (Figures 1(a) and 1(b)). A urine sample collected from the left side of the renal pelvis was suspicious for high-grade urothelial carcinoma in cytology. Thus, he was diagnosed

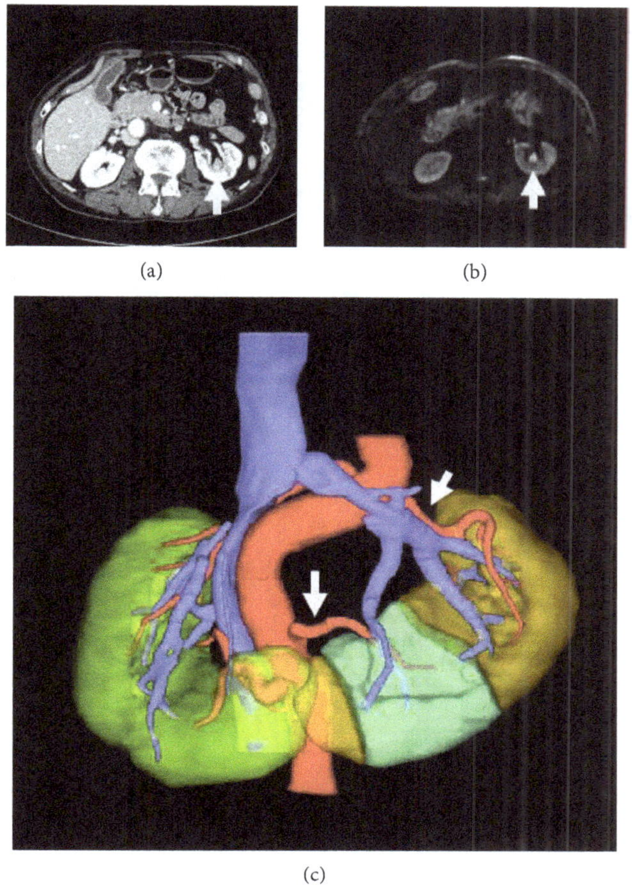

FIGURE 1: (a) CT findings. CT reveals a mass lesion of upper pelvis of the left side of the horseshoe kidney (arrow). (b) MRI findings. MRI reveals a high signal intensity on diffusion-weighted imaging (arrow). (c) Reconstruction of three-dimensional analysis of the images of thin-slice contrast-enhanced CT. Three-dimensional reconstruction reveals two renal arteries arising from the aorta that supplied to the left side of the horseshoe kidney (arrow).

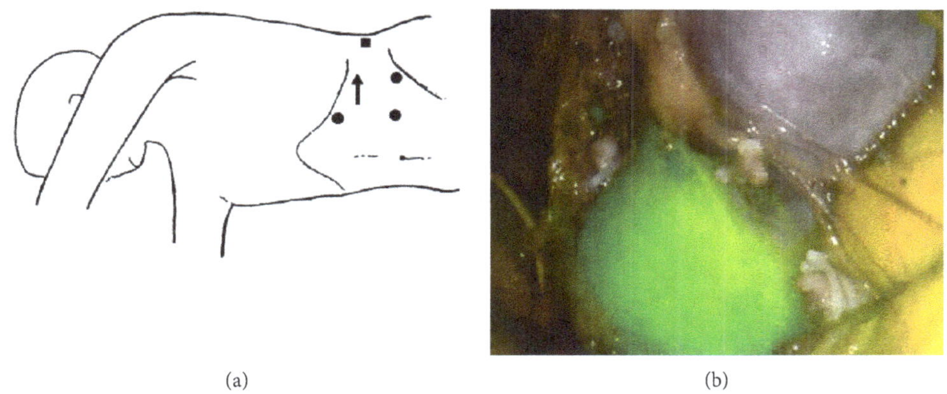

FIGURE 2: (a) The placement of the trocar port and an incision for removal of the extirpating organs. Black circle: operator's port. Black triangle: camera port. Black square: assistant's port. Black rectangle: six cm incision for removal of extirpating organs. (b) Interruption of blood flow is confirmed between the left moiety and the right moiety visualized by indocyanine green (ICG) fluorescence system. The green region shows blood flow to the right moiety.

with urothelial carcinoma of the upper renal pelvis on the left side of the horseshoe kidney. Preoperative thin-slice contrast-enhanced CT was performed with reconstruction of three-dimensional analysis of the images (SYNAPSE

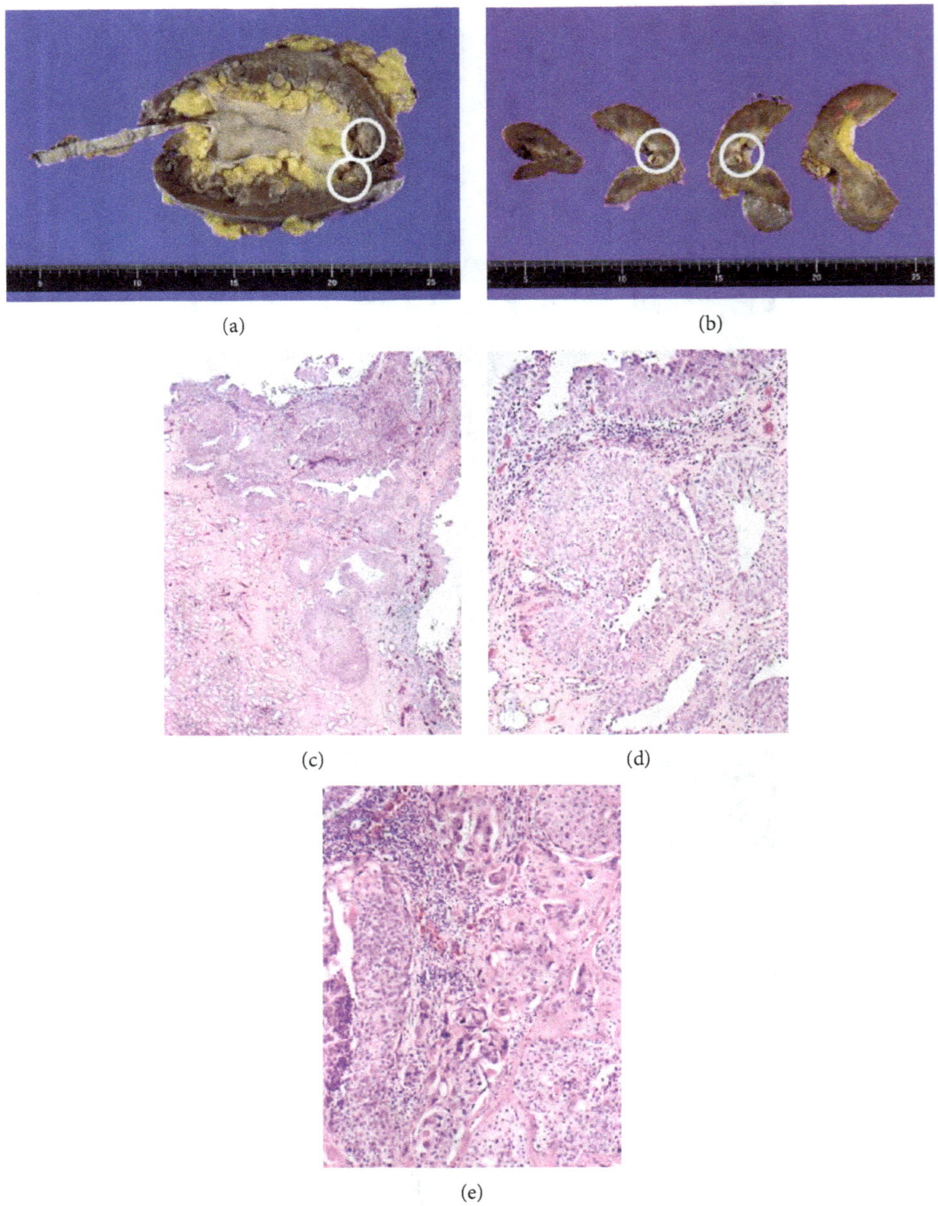

Figure 3: Pathological findings. The macroscopic specimen reveals the tumor was a 30 × 15 mm mass in the upper renal pelvis ((a, b), circle). The histopathological findings of the renal pelvic tumor reveal invasive high grade urothelial carcinoma (c, d) with squamous differentiation (e). The tumor invades renal papilla and there is no lymphovascular invasion.

VINCENT, FUJIFILM, Tokyo, Japan), which revealed that two arteries arising from the aorta supplied the left moiety of the horseshoe kidney (Figure 1(c)).

2.1. Operational Findings. The patient underwent laparoscopic transperitoneal nephroureterectomy with heminephrectomy on the left side of the horseshoe kidney in the right decubitus position in July 2021 (Figure 2(a)). We ligated two arteries with arising from the aorta that supplied the left moiety using Hem-o-loc (Teleflex Incorporated, Morrisville, North Carolina, USA). We confirmed interruption of blood flow to the left moiety and blood flow to the right moiety visualized by indocyanine green (ICG) fluorescence system (PINPOINT Endoscopic fluorescence imaging system, Stryker, Michigan, USA) (Figure 2(b)). Then, we ligated the vein of the left moiety flowing into the vena cava with Hem-o-loc. A splitting operation was performed on the renal tissue without blood flow between the interruption of blood flow to the left moiety and blood flow to the right moiety. Little bleeding was encountered during and after the separation. The ureter was ligated with Hem-o-loc not to implant cancer cells in lower urinary tract following confirming left ureter. After performing left heminephrectomy, we performed an en-bloc left nephroureterectomy including the left ureter close to the bladder cuff. We cut the ureter at the tenting site of ureter at the vesicoureteral junction laparoscopically without opening the bladder. The excised organ was removed from the abdominal space. The operating time was six hours 21 minutes and estimated total blood loss was 250 ml. No post-operative complication occurred.

2.2. Pathological Findings (Figure 3). The excised organ revealed the tumor was a 30×15 mm mass in the upper renal pelvis. The histopathological findings of the renal pelvic tumor revealed invasive urothelial carcinoma with squamous differentiation, high grade, and pT3.

He was discharged from the hospital on postoperative four days. In February 2022, there was no evidence of recurrence.

3. Discussion

Horseshoe kidney represents one of the most frequent renal malformations, with an incidence of 0.25% among the general population, being twice as frequent in males [2]. The fusion prevents normal rotation of the kidney so that the ureter arises anteriorly and crosses over the isthmus.

It has been reported that the incidence of carcinoma of the renal pelvis is at least three times greater in horseshoe kidney patients [3]. The higher incidence has been attributed to chronic noxious stimulation associated with infection, stasis, and stones; however, the pathological features are unclear. Mizusawa et al. reviewed 24 cases of renal pelvic tumor in horseshoe kidneys previously reported in Japan [8]. Seven cases (30%) included components of squamous cell carcinoma. The renal pelvic tumor of the present patient also showed invasive high-grade urothelial carcinoma with squamous differentiation. Voided urine cytology performances are worse for upper urinary tract urothelial carcinoma than for urothelial carcinoma of bladder [1]. Because of its low sensitivity, urine samples are collected from the upper urinary tracts before injection of contrast medium for retrograde pyelography.

Variable blood supply is one of the anatomical features of horseshoe kidney. Majos et al. reported that horseshoe kidneys had nearly twice as many renal arteries as normal kidneys (4.57 vs. 2.4 per patient) [9]. Preoperative thin-slice contrast-enhanced CT with reconstruction of three-dimensional analysis of the images is extremely useful for detailed analysis of blood supply. We used a three-dimensional analyzer of the images. Intraoperative ICG fluorescence navigation system is used for laparoscopic partial nephrectomy to conserve more normal renal tissue without increasing the rate of positive surgical margins [10]. Moreover, we revealed that blood flow evaluation by ICG system is also useful for performing laparoscopic heminephrectomy for a horseshoe kidney. We have not been detected previously published case reports of upper urinary tract cancer arising from horseshoe kidney treated with laparoscopic nephroureterectomy with 3D-reconstructed images or intraoperative ICG fluorescence navigation system.

4. Conclusion

We performed laparoscopic transperitoneal nephroureterectomy with heminephrectomy for urothelial carcinoma of the renal pelvis on the left side of the horseshoe kidney. Preoperative thin-slice contrast-enhanced CT with reconstruction of three-dimensional analysis of the images and intraoperative ICG fluorescence navigation system were useful for performing heminephrectomy.

References

[1] F. Soria, S. F. Shariat, S. P. Lerner et al., "Epidemiology, diagnosis, preoperative evaluation and prognostic assessment of upper-tract urothelial carcinoma (UTUC)," *World Journal of Urology*, vol. 35, no. 3, pp. 379–387, 2017.

[2] G. Schiappacasse, J. Aguirre, P. Soffia, C. S. Silva, and N. Zilleruelo, "CT findings of the main pathological conditions associated with horseshoe kidneys," *The British Journal of Radiology*, vol. 88, no. 1045, article 20140456, 2015.

[3] H. M. Reed and N. D. Robinson, "Horseshoe kidney with simultaneous occurrence of calculi, transitional cell and squamous cell carcinoma," *Urology*, vol. 23, no. 1, pp. 62–64, 1984.

[4] A. Brant, N. Almassi, S. J. Sirintrapun, and P. Russo, "Upper tract urothelial carcinoma in a patient with horseshoe kidney," *Urology*, vol. 142, pp. e20–e24, 2020.

[5] E. R. Latif, I. Ahmed, M. Thomas, and B. Eddy, "Robotic nephroureterectomy in a horseshoe kidney for upper tract urothelial carcinoma," *BML Case Reports*, vol. 14, no. 6, article e234901, 2021.

[6] J. Fikri, A. M. Almalki, S. A. Almalki, M. Murad, S. Makhdoum, and F. Hassan, "Upper urinary tract urothelial carcinoma with squamous, glandular, and sarcomatoid variants in a horseshoe kidney: a novel case report and literature review," *Cureus*, vol. 13, no. 11, article e19627, 2021.

[7] H. Suzuki, K. Takemura, K. Sakamoto et al., "A case of renal pelvic cancer complicated by horseshoe kidney treated with RoboSurgeon gasless single-port retroperitoneoscopic nephroureterectomy," *Case Reports in Urology*, vol. 2018, Article ID 3231480, 4 pages, 2018.

[8] H. Mizusawa, I. Komiyama, Y. Ueno, T. Maejima, and H. Kato, "Squamous cell carcinoma in the renal pelvis of a horseshoe kidney," *International Journal of Urology*, vol. 11, no. 9, pp. 782–784, 2004.

[9] M. Majos, M. Polguj, Z. Szemraj-Rogucka, A. Arazińska, and L. Stefańczyk, "The level of origin of renal arteries in horseshoe kidney vs. in separated kidneys: CT-based study," *Surgical and Radiologic Anatomy*, vol. 40, no. 10, pp. 1185–1191, 2018.

[10] R. Wang, J. Tang, Y. Chen, Z. Fang, and J. Shen, "The clinical value of indocyanine green fluorescence navigation system for laparoscopic partial nephrectomy in the case of complex renal clear cell carcinoma (R.E.N.A.L score ≥7)," *Journal of Cancer*, vol. 12, no. 6, pp. 1764–1769, 2021.

15

A Case of Heterotopic Ossification in Papillary Renal Cell Carcinoma Type 2

Facundo Davaro,[1] **Elizabeth Davaro,**[2] **Amna Qureshi,**[2] **and Lindsay Lombardo**[1]

[1]*Division of Urology, Department of Surgery, Saint Louis University, 3635 Vista Ave, 3rd Floor Desloge Towers, St. Louis, MO 63110, USA*
[2]*Department of Pathology, Saint Louis University, 3635 Vista Ave, 4th Floor Desloge Towers, St. Louis, MO 63110, USA*

Correspondence should be addressed to Facundo Davaro; facundo.davarocomas@health.slu.edu

Academic Editor: Fumitaka Koga

Renal cell carcinoma (RCC) is associated with a variety of different histopathologic subtypes in which each subtype may be further subclassified. These entities carry with them unique prognoses and necessitate treatment with specific immunotherapy agents should advanced disease be uncovered. Meanwhile, aberrant physiologic processes may lead to unique histologic findings within these subtypes, further complicating management and prognostication. Heterotopic ossification within RCC is one of these rare occurrences and was once thought to have favorable prognostic implications. We report a case of a young female with papillary type 2 RCC with heterotopic ossification.

1. Introduction

The process of osseous metaplasia is a rare histopathologic manifestation within renal cell carcinoma (RCC) believed to be a product of ischemia, necrosis, and/or inflammation [1]. Consequently, heterotopic ossification within RCC is thought to arise in hypovascular regions within the tumor [2]. Its presence is presumably associated with a more favorable prognosis, owing to the decreased vasculature associated with this finding [1]. Meanwhile, papillary RCC (PRCC) is the second most common subtype of RCC accounting for 10-15% of all RCCs, with type 2 carrying with it a poorer prognosis [3]. The occurrence of both histopathologic findings in a single case has been an infrequently reported phenomenon in the literature [1, 4]. We report a rare case of papillary type 2 RCC with heterotopic ossification.

2. Case Presentation

An otherwise healthy 39-year-old African-American female with a history of migraines, sickle cell trait, and morbid obesity (body mass index 37.08 kg/m^2) presented to the emergency department with nausea, emesis, and nonbloody diarrhea. Her physical exam revealed mild abdominal tenderness to palpation on the right side. No costovertebral angle tenderness was elicited. The laboratory work indicated a normal white blood cell count and baseline renal function as evidenced by a creatinine of 0.8 mg/dL. Food poisoning was suspected due to her reporting recent consumption of an "uncooked burger"; however, a computed tomography (CT) scan without contrast was performed to rule out more serious pathology. In doing so, an incidental right renal lesion was found. She was discharged with oral ondansetron 5 mg as needed for nausea and a scheduled follow-up with urology. To further characterize the mass, a renal protocol computed tomography scan with contrast was performed prior to her outpatient follow-up. This revealed a 2.5 cm renal mass located in the posterior, upper pole of the right kidney with post contrast enhancement, suspicious for malignancy. The R.E.N.A.L. nephrometry score was calculated at 7p (Figure 1). Given her young age, the patient opted for definitive treatment after risks, benefits, and alternatives of the procedure were discussed. She subsequently underwent a right

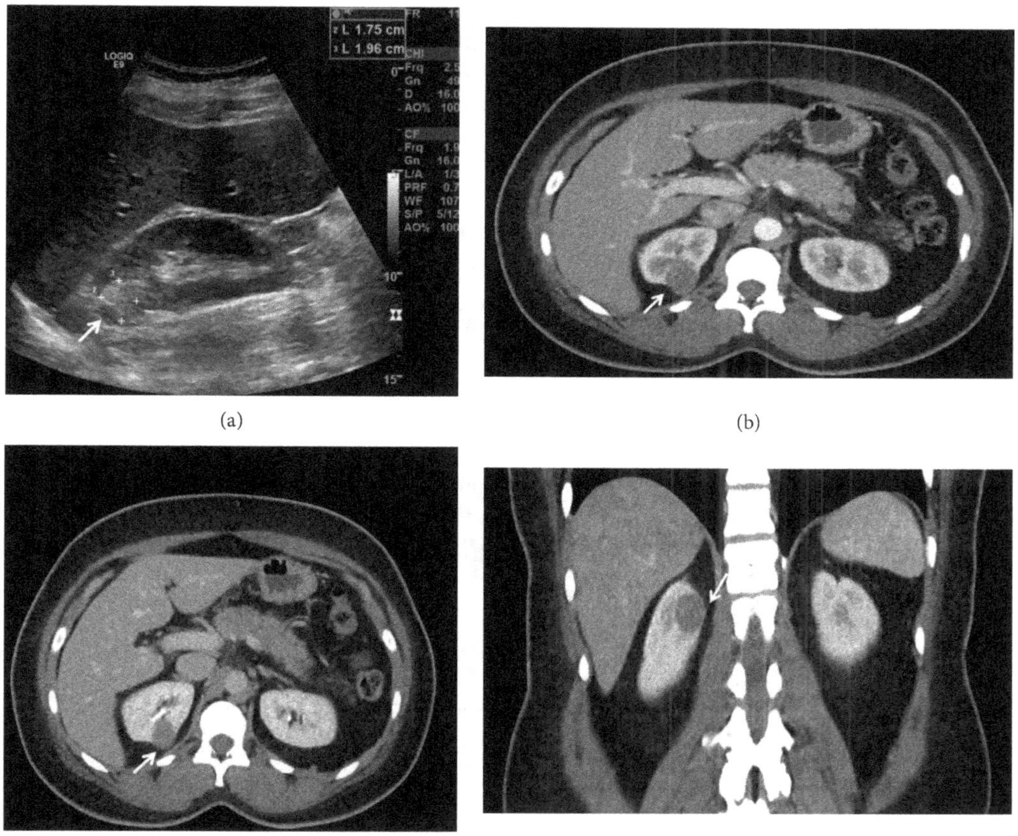

FIGURE 1: Patient preoperative imaging revealing the renal mass (white arrows). (a) Sagittal ultrasound image of the echogenic, solid renal mass measuring 1.75 cm by 1.96 cm. (b, c) Axial CT images with contrast highlighting the posterior location of the mass, its enhancing posterior wall, and nearness to the collecting system. (d) Coronal CT image of the same mass and its upper pole location. No calcifications were noted throughout the mass.

robotic partial nephrectomy. The patient's hospital course was uncomplicated, and she was discharged on postoperative day one.

Gross pathologic examination demonstrated a well-circumscribed tumor, the cut surface of which showed a variegated yellow-tan 2.1 × 1.9 cm mass with punctate hemorrhages. The patient staged with pT1a disease. Microscopic examination confirmed a papillary renal cell carcinoma, type 2, with an associated International Society of Urologic Pathologist (ISUP) grade 2 as evidenced by Figure 2(a). Irregular deposits of bone could be seen intermixed with the tumor cells (Figures 2(b)–2(d)).

Postoperatively, the patient was instructed to return to the clinic in 2 weeks for a wound check and counseling over her diagnosis. The patient appeared well at this time with resolution of pain and increasing appetite and energy. Her 18-month follow-up imaging did not demonstrate any evidence of locoregional or distant recurrence, and her creatinine remained near her baseline at 1.0 mg/dL.

3. Discussion

Renal cell carcinoma has been categorized into 16 histologic subtypes by the 2016 World Health Organization (WHO) [3]. Within these subtypes, further classification occurs helping clinicians determine evidence-based management decisions and prognostication information used in patient counseling. A classic example of this substratification is seen in PRCC, as patients are labeled as having type 1 or type 2 disease. Clinically, type 1 disease is associated with superior survival outcomes relative to type 2 [5]. Microscopically, type 1 is characterized by having simple cuboidal epithelium distinguishing it from type 2 which demonstrates true cellular pseudostratification with eosinophilic cytoplasm [3]. In a histopathologic review of PRCC at their institution, Warrick et al. retrospectively examined 56 cases of PRCC attempting to elucidate histomorphologic features that distinguish the two papillary subtypes from one another. The presence of psammoma bodies, foamy macrophages, and eosinophilic cytoplasm along with several other histologic features was catalogued within the tumors. They found that although classic features of type 1 and type 2 tended to cluster together, no singular characteristics were able to reliably differentiate one from the other [6].

Beyond the classic differences in histologic architecture, other rare, nuanced microscopic findings have unclear implications and may complicate this substratification even further. Histopathologic findings such as bone marrow within a RCC or solitary fibrous tumor of the kidney have been reported

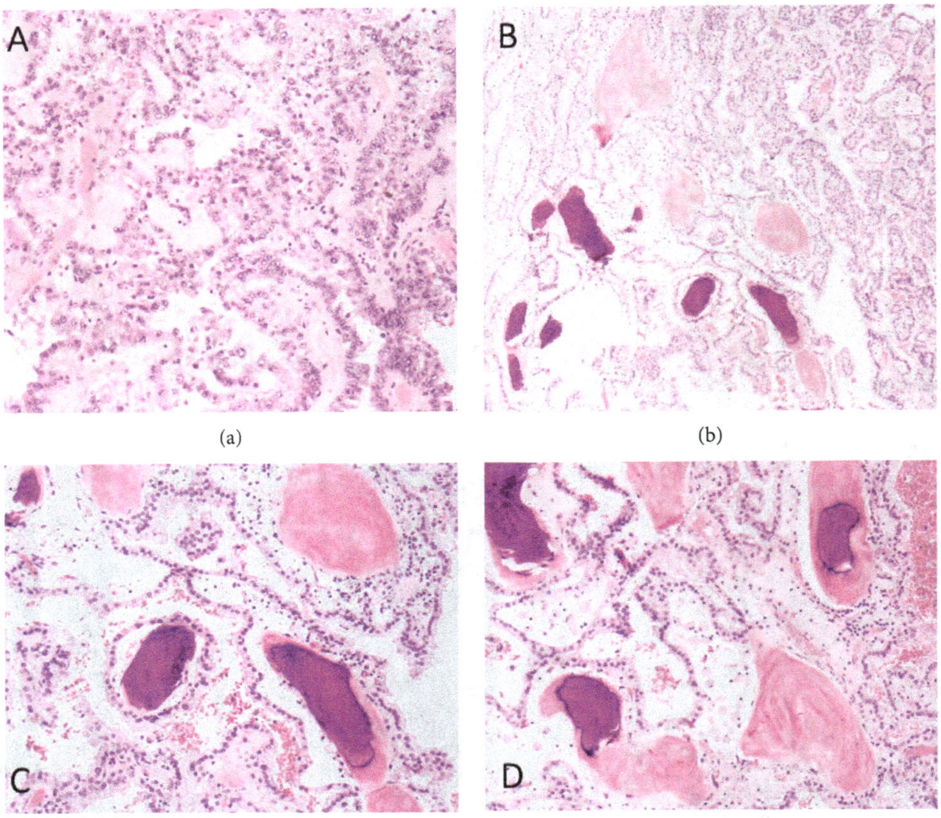

(a) (b) (c) (d)

Figure 2: (a) Hematoxylin and eosin-stained sections representative of tumor with nuclear pseudostratification and nuclear enlargement consistent with papillary renal cell carcinoma type 2. Granular to eosinophilic cytoplasm is also seen. (b) A low power view with heterotopic ossification with intervening tumor. (c, d) On higher power, focal osteoblastic rimming is seen surrounding trabecular woven bone.

[7, 8]. Heterotopic ossification is another, even rarer microscopic finding within RCC. It is the formation of extraskeletal bone in muscle or soft tissue as defined by Meyers et al. [9]. Several case reports discussing the finding have been published in varying types of RCC; however, to date, there have been few case reports describing this histopathologic finding in type 2 PRCC [1, 4].

Investigations into molecular pathways contributing to heterotopic ossification have been undertaken in order to elucidate the prognostic implications of its presence. For example, hypoxia-inducible factor and mammalian target of rapamycin signaling pathways are involved in heterotopic ossification [9]. These are known aberrant pathways in RCC that have been targeted with immunotherapy for treatment. In vitro experiments inhibiting hypoxia-inducible factor have been conducted revealing an increase in the expression of bone morphogenetic proteins, a family of proteins involved in osseous metaplasia [10]. In their research, Wang et al. corroborate the dogma that heterotopic ossification is a process that predominantly occurs in hypoxic environments. Furthermore, when they performed in vivo stimulation of bone morphogenetic protein-2 in certain mouse cell lines with RCC, they noted an arrest in tumor growth. Unfortunately, this response was not uniform throughout all mouse cell lines indicating the need for further research in the underlying signaling pathways [11].

Given the significant rarity of this histopathologic occurrence, any conclusions about the etiology of heterotopic ossification in type 2 PRCC, or RCC as a whole, are purely conjecture.

4. Conclusion

Heterotopic ossification is an atypical phenomenon infrequently encountered in RCC. Although presumed to have favorable prognostic implications, its rarity makes it difficult to establish any true associations.

Abbreviations

RCC: Renal cell carcinoma
PRCC: Papillary renal cell carcinoma
R.E.N.A.L.: Radius, endophytic/exophytic, nearness, anterior/posterior, location
ISUP: International Society of Urologic Pathologists
WHO: World Health Organization.

References

[1] T. Jindal, N. Jain, and A. Agarwal, "Type II papillary renal cell carcinoma with heterotrophic ossification: a case report," *Annals of the Royal College of Surgeons of England*, vol. 100, no. 3, pp. e49–e50, 2018.

[2] C. Kwak, Y. H. Park, I. Y. Kim, K. C. Moon, and J. H. Ku, "Expression of bone morphogenetic proteins, the subfamily of the transforming growth factor-β superfamily, in renal cell carcinoma," *The Journal of Urology*, vol. 178, no. 3, pp. 1062–1067, 2007.

[3] K. Inamura, "Renal cell tumors: understanding their molecular pathological epidemiology and the 2016 WHO classification," *International Journal of Molecular Sciences*, vol. 18, no. 10, article e2195, 2017.

[4] A. Ahmed, "Chondroid and osseous metaplasia in an incidental type II papillary renal cell carcinoma with extensive solid areas: an unraveled molecular character," *The Pan African Medical Journal*, vol. 31, p. 26, 2018.

[5] G. Pignot, C. Elie, S. Conquy et al., "Survival analysis of 130 patients with papillary renal cell carcinoma: prognostic utility of type 1 and type 2 subclassification," *Urology*, vol. 69, no. 2, pp. 230–235, 2007.

[6] J. I. Warrick, A. Tsodikov, L. P. Kunju et al., "Papillary renal cell carcinoma revisited: a comprehensive histomorphologic study with outcome correlations," *Human Pathology*, vol. 45, no. 6, pp. 1139–1146, 2014.

[7] S. Ozkanli, A. Yildirim, E. Zemheri, S. K. Keskin, and E. K. Basok, "Osseous metaplasia and bone marrow elements in a case of renal cell carcinoma," *Case Reports in Urology*, vol. 2012, Article ID 649257, 3 pages, 2012.

[8] S. P. Raman, R. H. Hruban, and E. K. Fishman, "Beyond renal cell carcinoma: rare and unusual renal masses," *Abdominal Radiology*, vol. 37, no. 5, pp. 873–884, 2012.

[9] C. Meyers, J. Lisiecki, S. Miller et al., "Heterotopic ossification: a comprehensive review," *JBMR Plus*, vol. 3, no. 4, article e10172, 2019.

[10] H. Wang, C. Lindborg, V. Lounev et al., "Cellular hypoxia promotes heterotopic ossification by amplifying BMP signaling," *Journal of Bone and Mineral Research*, vol. 31, no. 9, pp. 1652–1665, 2016.

[11] L. Wang, P. Park, F. la Marca, K. D. Than, and C. Y. Lin, "BMP-2 inhibits tumor-initiating ability in human renal cancer stem cells and induces bone formation," *Journal of Cancer Research and Clinical Oncology*, vol. 141, no. 6, pp. 1013–1024, 2015.

16

Percutaneous Nephrolithotripsy in Morbidly Obese Patient: A Case Report

Fadhel Yusuf, Amr Elmekresh, Senthil Kumar, and Fariborz Bagheri

Department of Urology, Dubai Hospital, Dubai, UAE

Correspondence should be addressed to Fariborz Bagheri; fbagheri@dha.gov.ae

Academic Editor: Tun-Chieh Chen

A 50-year old male patient with morbid obesity was admitted for removal of large staghorn calculi and multiple small stones in the left kidney. The patient was managed by Percutaneous Nephrolithotomy (PCNL). Surgery was carried out in prone position and Alken's metal dilators were used for tract dilation. Alken dilators were inserted without any challenges, and the procedure was completed in a shorter span of time than anticipated with total operative time of 2 hours, including the change of positioning from lithotomy to prone. No intra-operative or post-operative complications were encountered. The patient has been followed up for 6 months post-operatively, without any complications or any evidence of stone recurrence.

1. Introduction

The incidence of obesity has been dramatically increasing globally, in both developed and developing countries [1]. Consequently, there has been a significant rise in the number of obesity-related conditions, where obesity is the primary cause or is a vital contributing factor.

Obesity has been linked to the occurrence of several comorbidities such as diabetes mellitus, hypertension, and atherosclerosis. Insulin resistance, which is a significant consequence of obesity, constitutes one of the most important risk factors for renal stone formation [2].

Extracorporeal Shock Wave Lithotripsy (ESWL), Percutaneous Nephrolithotomy (PCNL), and Ureteroscopy (URS) are the most frequent current treatments for renal stones [3]. However, in obese patients, the use of ESWL is restricted due to the skin to stone distance. Alternatively, RIRS is a safe and effective method for treating renal stones in obese people, although it takes a long time to perform and multiple sessions is needed depending on the size, quantity, and location of the stones.

For renal stones greater than 2 cm, PCNL is the gold standard first-line treatment, particularly for obese people [3]. It is a minimally invasive technique which is successfully being used for the management of multiple calculi, staghorn calculi, or large calculi in lower calyx [4, 5].

Management of renal stones in morbidly obese patients can be challenging for the surgeon and anesthesia team. PCNL is a particularly important therapeutic modality for obese individuals and has revealed similar outcomes for obese and nonobese patients, although some technical modifications are suggested for treating morbidly obese patients [6]. This article is a case report of a morbidly obese patient presenting with a large kidney stone which was managed by PCNL using Alken technique for tract dilatation.

2. Case Presentation

A 50 years old Russian gentleman was referred to our facility from another hospital due to large left renal stone seen on ultrasound study, following active complaint of left flank pain for more than 1 year. He was a known case of recurrent kidney stones, and type II diabetes mellitus (DM). Additionally, he acquires a morbidly obese body habitus, with weight of 185 kg, height of 172 cm, and a BMI of 62 kg/m^2. To assess further risk factors, when asked about his social habits and lifestyle, he stated has lives a normal active lifestyle, with a career in company management. Additionally, he stated that he tries to drink about 3 liters of water on a daily basis. His creatinine level and glomerular filtration rate (GFR) were within normal range during his multiple office visits.

CT abdomen and pelvis with contrast was carried which showed small left kidney with staghorn stone of about 7 cm in diameter and multiple smaller stone in the calyces (Figure 1). Right kidney and ureter were free of stones. He was then offered to undergo PCNL, as the ultimate therapy for his renal stone (Figure 2).

A major challenge faced intraoperatively, was safe positioning of the patient due to his body habitus, which required additional care and time. Intraoperatively, in lithotomy position, left retrograde pyelography was done which showed large staghorn stone in the left renal pelvis and the calyces. Ureteral catheter was inserted and fixed externally. This was connected to normal saline and 1% methylene blue.

He was shifted to prone position. Under fluoroscopy guidance, the lower calyx was punctured, and a guide wire (Sensor from Boston Scientific) was inserted down to the left lower ureter.

A 10/8 French Teflon dilator was inserted down to the renal pelvis. Accordingly, a stiff guide wire could be placed next to the sensor guide wire which was used for dilatation of the tract by the Alken technique. The sensor guide wire was kept as a safety wire. Finally, the nephroscope was inserted through the stiff guide wire. All the stones were easily fragmented and aspirated by ultrasound probe of lithoclast machine (from EMS). Nephroscopy and fluoroscopy did not reveal any residual stones. There was no any difficulty in stone fragmentation and clearance comparing to other PCNL cases in prone position. Additionally, there was no need for extra long nephroscope or flexible nephoscope. An 18 Fr. Malecot nephrostomy tube was inserted. The total operative time was about 2 hours (Total operative time counts from the moment when cystoscope was inserted into the bladder in lithotomy position, continues with shifting the patient to prone position, and finishing with closure of skin incision) (Figure 2). Similar padding was used for this procedure as any other prone PCNL procedures and there was no need for any extra padding. The whole procedure was performed by an endourologist expert with 25 years of experience in urology and more than 500 cases of prone PCNL procedures.

Intra- and postoperative periods were uneventful.

He remained hospitalized for a total of four days, nephrostomy tube was clamped on day three, and as he was afebrile and pain-free, it was removed prior to discharge. Throughout the admission, creatinine followed a normal trend. Furthermore, his kidney stone analysis revealed uric acid stone composition.

He was further followed up after 2 weeks postoperatively. Bedside ultrasonography was done and showed unremarkable left kidney with no hydronephrosis or stones.

3. Discussion

In the recent decades, a significant rise in obesity has been observed worldwide. An increase in BMI has been positively associated with nephrolithiasis as well, with varying preva-

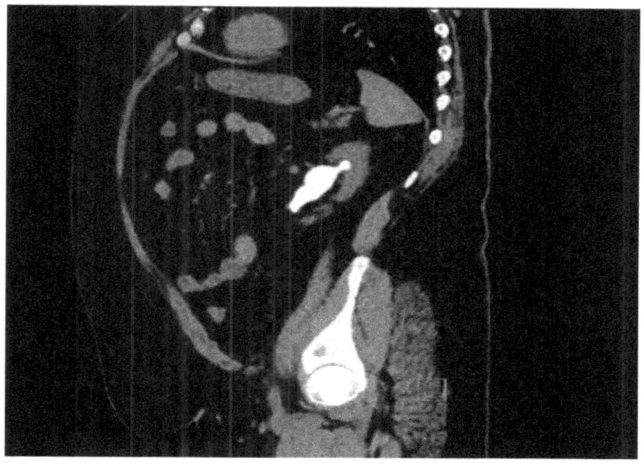

FIGURE 1: CT KUB demonstrating left staghorn kidney stone.

lence ranging from 3-20% reported across the literature, with majority of the stones identified as oxalate and uric acid stones [7–9]. In a study conducted by Taylor and Curhan which investigated the corelation of BMI on stone composition, observing for urinary excretion of various stone compositions, participants with higher BMI had a positive association with excretion of both oxalate and uric acid [10]. This complements uric acid stone analysis finding on our patient. The exact reason behind this association is multifactorial, however, the most hypothesized causes are failure of following a balanced dietary habit which leads to excess consumption of lithogenic food, and insulin resistance, as was the case in our patient who had a background of type II diabetes as well [11].

The most common surgical procedures currently in practice are ESWL, PCNL, and URS [3]. Amongst the aforementioned procedures, ESWL is the least-invasive procedure, which is more popular amongst eligible patients. However, this procedure carries a low feasibility amongst obese and morbidly obese patients. Several studies have reported on high rates of failure of stone removal with ESWL technique, particularly with increased skin-to-stone distance (SSD), leaving residual stone fragments behind [12–14].

RIRS is a preferable alternative option for obese and morbidly obese patient as there are no contraindications for, with no safety concerns [15]. However, in our case, the patient had a renal stone size of about 7 cm which is not an indication for RIRS, and is a candidate for PCNL [3].

The application of PCNL in obese patients may be challenging for surgeons. Obese patients present several technical challenges including anesthesia, patient positioning, imaging for access, longer skin-to-collecting-system distances, and nephrostomy tube dislodgement [16]. Traditionally, prone position is preferred for PCNL as it allows a direct access to the posterior calyx, and provides a safer procedure regarding the location of the bowel [17, 18]. Although a supine approach is suggested for obese patients due to a risk of ventilatory compromise in them, this position increases the working distance making it particularly difficult to rupture the upper pole. It also decreases the filling of the collecting system, making it constantly collapsed, and thus

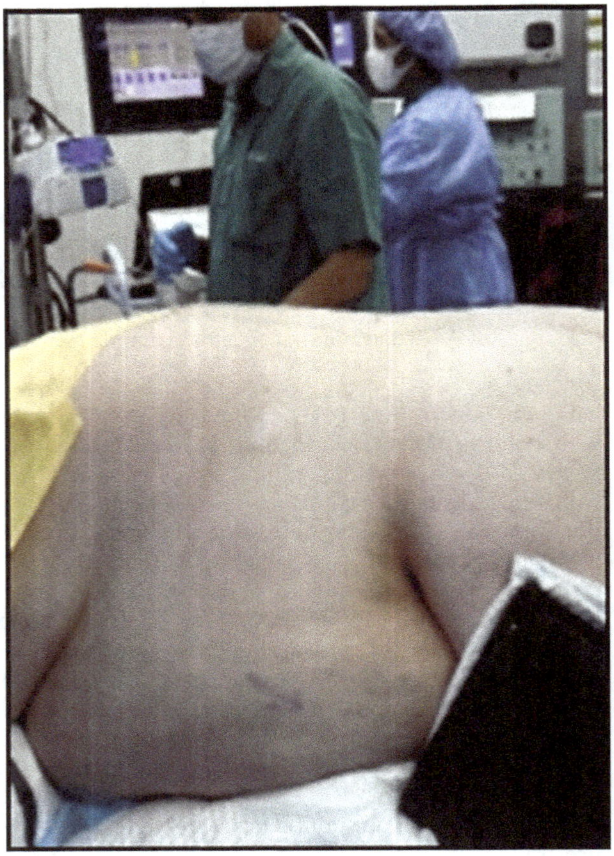

(a)

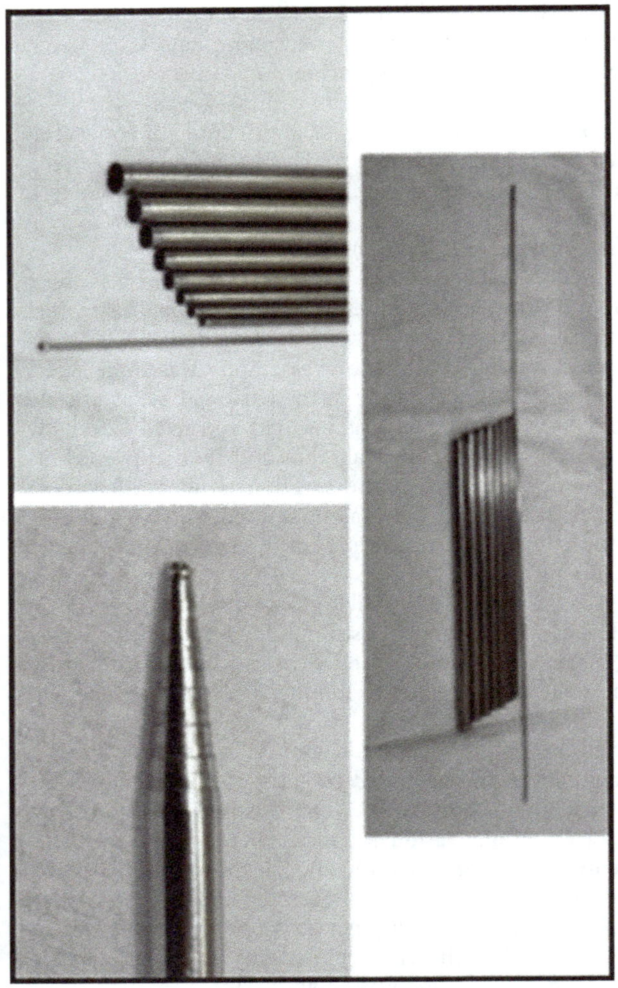

(b)

Figure 2: Continued.

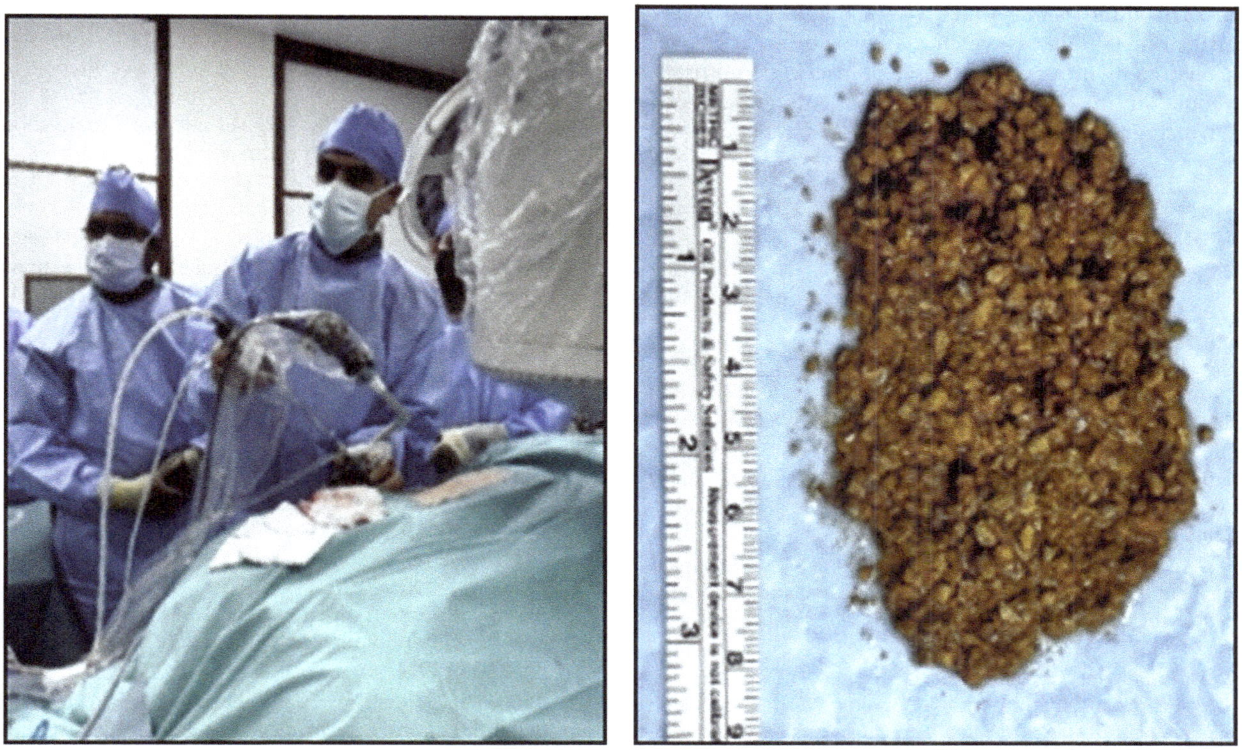

(c) (d)

FIGURE 2: (a) Patient in prone positioning. (b) Alken dilators. (c) PCNL procedure. (d) Patient's stone fragments.

nephroscopy tends to be more difficult [19–21]. Hence, the use of supine position is still debatable. In the present case, PCNL was carried out in prone position and did not lead to any untoward respiratory events. Although most studies have noted similar outcomes in terms of stone-free rate, complications, and length of stay in obese versus nonobese patients, the only exception found was longer operative time in obese patients [6, 16]. Thus, minimizing surgical time in these patients may help prevent any cardiopulmonary complications that are anticipated to arise.

Dilatation of the percutaneous access tract is a critical step in PCNL procedure as it can lead to postoperative complications including bleeding and sepsis [20]. Dilation can be achieved by three standard techniques: semirigid (plastic or elastic) Amplatz dilatation, metal telescopic dilatation of the Alken type, and balloon dilatation. Balloon dilatation although has advantages of reduced complication rates and shorter durations of X-ray exposure, its application is limited due to high cost [19].

Plastic and metal dilators are inexpensive and have a higher chance of successful tract creation thus; these are widely used for tract dilation in PCNL. Studies comparing the use of plastic versus metal dilators revealed similar efficacy for both Alken dilator and Amplatz dilators [19, 22], commonly noted complications with metal dilators were the presence of more postoperative fevers >38.5°C and a higher rate of urosepsis. Amongst those with plastic dilators were more pleural injuries and subsequent blood loss, most likely occurring on withdrawal for insertion of the next larger dilator, leading to loss of compression, leading to subsequent bloos loss. On the other hand, telescopic Alken dilators exert pressure continuously, hence blood loss may be lower [19].

Another reported difference is the shorter tract formation time using Alken dilation was noted as compared to the plastic ones [22]. In our case too, the procedure was completed in a total of about two hours even though the patient was morbidly obese. Surgeon expertise certainly is a determining factor for the length of procedure however, the shorter duration of procedure can also be attributed to the use of Alken's telescopic metal dilators which are easier to insert and sequentially fit over the central metal rod to allow step wise dilation. The most challenging part of the procedure was changing the patient's position from lithotomy to prone position, which was managed safely and properly with help of 4 muscular messengers.

Although, there is no definite distinction as to which could be the best dilation technique to use in obese patients and surgeons may select different methods depending on their familiarity or experience with certain techniques, the use of metal dilators in the present case revealed positive results with no evidence of postop complications and a long stone free rate as determined endoscopically.

4. Conclusion

Obesity is a major risk factor for nephrolithiasis. In this case report we present a case of 50-year-old male with large staghorn left kidney stone which was managed with PCNL using Alken metal dilators which may provide an edge over plastic dilators by means of their ease of insertion and probable reduction in surgical time for patients undergoing PCNL which are critical, especially in obese patients.

References

[1] Who, *Obesity and overweight*, 2009, https://www.who.int/news-room/fact-sheets/detail/obesity-and-overweight.

[2] C. P. Kovesdy, S. L. Furth, C. Zoccali, and on behalf of the World Kidney Day Steering Committee, "Obesity and kidney disease: hidden consequences of the epidemic," *Journal of Renal Care*, vol. 43, no. 1, pp. 3–10, 2017.

[3] D. Assimos, A. Krambeck, N. L. Miller et al., "Surgical management of stones: American urological association/endourological society guideline, part I," *Journal of Urology*, vol. 196, no. 4, pp. 1153–1160, 2016.

[4] G. M. Preminger, D. G. Assimos, J. E. Lingeman, S. Y. Nakada, M. S. Pearle, and J. S. Wolf Jr., "Chapter 1: AUA guideline on management of staghorn calculi: diagnosis and treatment recommendations," *The Journal of Urology*, vol. 173, no. 6, pp. 1991–2000, 2005.

[5] I. M. Sabler, I. Katafigiotis, O. N. Gofrit, and M. Duvdevani, "Present indications and techniques of percutaneous nephrolithotomy: what the future holds?," *Asian Journal of Urology*, vol. 5, no. 4, pp. 287–294, 2018.

[6] X. Zhou, X. Sun, X. Chen et al., "Effect of obesity on outcomes of percutaneous nephrolithotomy in renal stone management: a systematic review and meta-analysis," *Urologia Internationalis*, vol. 98, no. 4, pp. 382–390, 2017.

[7] A. L. Negri, F. R. Spivacow, E. E. Del Valle, M. Forrester, G. Rosende, and I. Pinduli, "Role of overweight and obesity on the urinary excretion of promoters and inhibitors of stone formation in stone formers," *Urological Research*, vol. 36, no. 6, pp. 303–307, 2008.

[8] M. Daudon, B. Lacour, and P. Jungers, "Influence of body size on urinary stone composition in men and women," *Urological Research*, vol. 34, no. 3, pp. 193–199, 2006.

[9] G. C. Curhan, W. C. Willett, E. B. Rimm, F. E. Speizer, and M. J. Stampfer, "Body size and risk of kidney stones," *Journal of American Society of Nephrology*, vol. 9, no. 9, pp. 1645–1652, 1998.

[10] E. N. Taylor and G. C. Curhan, "Body size and 24-hour urine composition," *American Journal of Kidney Diseases*, vol. 48, no. 6, pp. 905–915, 2006.

[11] A. Carbone, Y. Al Salhi, A. Tasca, G. Palleschi, A. Fuschi, and C. De Nunzio, "Obesity and kidney stone disease: a systematic review," *Minerva Urologica e Nefrologica*, vol. 70, no. 4, pp. 393–400, 2018.

[12] D. Delakas, I. Karyotis, G. Daskalopoulos, E. Lianos, and E. Mavromanolakis, "Independent predictors of failure of shockwave lithotripsy for ureteral stones employing a second-generation lithotripter," *Journal of Endourology*, vol. 17, no. 4, pp. 201–205, 2003.

[13] G. Pareek, S. P. Hedican, F. T. Lee Jr., and S. Y. Nakada, "Shock wave lithotripsy success determined by skin-to-stone distance on computed tomography," *Urology*, vol. 66, no. 5, pp. 941–944, 2005.

[14] A. E. Perks, T. D. Schuler, J. Lee et al., "Stone attenuation and skin-to-stone distance on computed tomography predicts for stone fragmentation by shock wave lithotripsy," *Urology*, vol. 72, no. 4, pp. 765–769, 2008.

[15] F. Laclergerie, B. Jacquemet, G. Guichard et al., "Flexible ureterorenoscopy in obese patients: results from a large monocenter cohort," *Progrès en Urologie*, vol. 24, no. 10, pp. 634–639, 2014.

[16] M. Keheila, D. Leavitt, R. Galli et al., "Percutaneous nephrolithotomy in super obese patients (body mass index ≥ 50 kg/m2): overcoming the challenges," *BJU International*, vol. 117, no. 2, pp. 300–306, 2016.

[17] D. Yuan, Y. Liu, H. Rao et al., "Supine versus prone position in percutaneous Nephrolithotomy for kidney calculi: a meta-analysis," *Journal of Endourology*, vol. 30, no. 7, pp. 754–763, 2016.

[18] X. Zhang, L. Xia, T. Xu, X. Wang, S. Zhong, and Z. Shen, "Is the supine position superior to the prone position for percutaneous nephrolithotomy (PCNL)?," *Urolithiasis.*, vol. 42, no. 1, pp. 87–93, 2014.

[19] P. Bryniarski, P. Stelmach, P. Taborowski et al., "Percutaneous nephrolithotomy with Amplatz and Alken dilators: an eight-year single tertiary care centre experience," *Medical Science Monitor*, vol. 22, pp. 4918–4923, 2016.

[20] R. K. Handa, B. R. Matlaga, B. A. Connors et al., "Acute effects of percutaneous tract dilation on renal function and structure," *Journal of Endourology*, vol. 20, no. 12, pp. 1030–1040, 2006.

[21] H. H. Nour, A. M. Kamal, S. E. Ghobashi, A. S. Zayed, M. M. Rushdy, and A. G. El-Baz, "Percutaneous nephrolithotomy in the supine position: safety and outcomes in a single-centre experience," *Arab Journal of Urology*, vol. 11, no. 1, pp. 62–67, 2013.

[22] H. U. Ozok, L. Sagnak, A. B. Senturk, N. Karakoyunlu, H. Topaloglu, and H. Ersoy, "A comparison of metal telescopic dilators and Amplatz dilators for nephrostomy tract dilation in percutaneous nephrolithotomy," *Journal of Endourology*, vol. 26, no. 6, pp. 630–634, 2012.

17

Palpable Abdominal Mass is a Renal Oncocytoma: Not All Large Renal Masses are Malignant

Sumi Dey,[1] Sabrina L. Noyes,[1] Ghayas Uddin,[2] and Brian R. Lane[1,3]

[1]*Spectrum Health, Department of Urology, Grand Rapids, MI, USA*
[2]*Spectrum Health, Department of Pathology, MI, USA*
[3]*Michigan State University College of Human Medicine, Grand Rapids, MI, USA*

Correspondence should be addressed to Brian R. Lane; brian.lane@spectrumhealth.org

Academic Editor: Fumitaka Koga

A 59-year-old woman presented with abdominal pain and a palpable abdominal mass. Initial imaging revealed a 14cm solid, enhancing renal mass and suspicion for liver and bone metastases. Family history included a brother with clear cell renal cell carcinoma and mother with glioblastoma multiforme. After liver biopsy was inconclusive, she underwent radical nephrectomy with final pathologic diagnosis of oncocytoma. Renal oncocytoma is the most common benign renal tumor but remains difficult to distinguish clinically and radiographically from renal cell carcinoma. Should urologists use renal mass biopsy even more frequently prior to surgical intervention?

1. Introduction

Renal oncocytoma is the most common benign renal neoplasm [1, 2], accounting for 3% to 7% of kidney tumors and more common in men than women [3]. The radiographic features of oncocytoma on all forms of conventional imaging are similar to renal cell carcinoma (RCC), making the differential diagnosis particularly challenging [1]. In this case report, we present a patient with family history of RCC and a 14 cm solid, enhancing renal mass with clinical suspicion for metastatic disease that was treated as a malignancy, but found to be an oncocytoma at final pathology.

2. Case Presentation

A 59-year-old woman had a palpable mass in the right midabdomen during routine physical examination by her primary care physician. Other than abdominal pain, she had no signs or symptoms of urogenital disorders, such as hematuria or irritative voiding symptoms. She had no prior history of renal disease or trauma. Family history included a brother who underwent nephrectomy for RCC at age 62.

An abdominopelvic computed tomography (CT) scan revealed a large, solid, right renal mass (14x13x12 cm) and several hypoenhancing liver lesions suspicious for metastases. CT also identified a focal, slightly lucent lesion with sclerotic rim in the T10 vertebral body which was felt to represent a small hemangioma of bone or metastatic lesion, but a subsequent bone scan was negative. CT thorax revealed no metastases. There was significant enhancement of the solid components of the tumor and finger-like extensions of absent enhancement throughout the renal mass consistent with areas of necrosis or acute inflammation (Figure 1(a)). The mass arose from the mid and upper pole of the right kidney and extended superiorly displacing the right lobe of the liver and inferior vena cava (IVC) anteriorly, making the liver palpable (Figure 1(b)). The liver, in fact, extended down to her right iliac crest and below her umbilicus on both sides of her abdomen (Figure 1(c)). There was no evidence of tumor thrombus in the right renal vein or IVC. A diagnosis of likely malignancy with potential liver metastases was made and she was scheduled with interventional radiology for biopsy for pathologic confirmation.

CT scan revealed multiple indeterminate lesions on her liver, the largest of which was 12x10 mm. She was referred for percutaneous biopsy of the kidney and liver lesions for tissue pathology and staging. As well-defined liver lesions were identified, the interventional radiologist

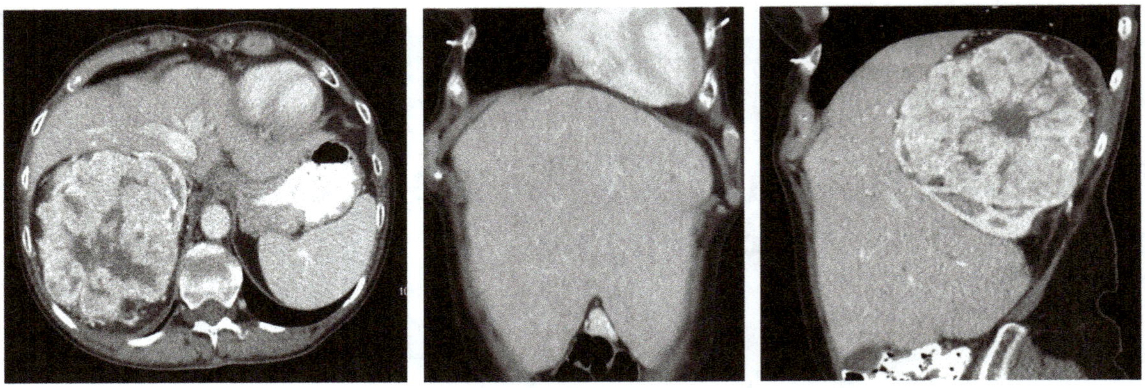

FIGURE 1: Abdominopelvic CT with IV contrast demonstrates a 14 cm enhancing mass in the right kidney. (a) Axial image shows there was significant enhancement of the solid components of the tumor with finger-like extensions of absent enhancement consistent with necrosis or inflammation. (b) Coronal image demonstrates the enlarged liver that filled all four abdominal quadrants. (c) In sagittal view, the liver is seen to be anteriorly displaced by the large renal mass and to extend down to the right iliac crest.

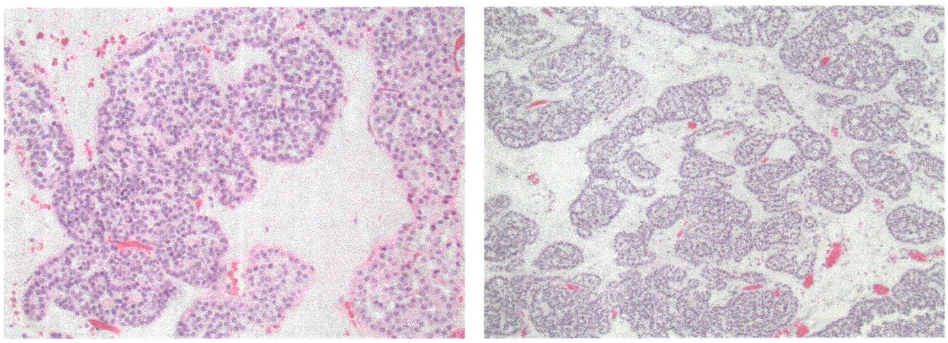

FIGURE 2: Histological findings of oncocytoma with large eosinophilic cells arranged in distinct nests.

performed liver mass biopsy only based on the perceived additional risk of biopsy of the hypervascular renal tumor. Pathology revealed liver parenchyma with fatty deposits, negative for malignancy. Given the negative liver biopsies and normal bone scan, an open radical nephrectomy with right retroperitoneal lymph node dissection was performed for suspected localized RCC using a subcostal incision. With a fixed retractor for the bowel and manual retraction of the liver, exposure of the renal hilum was quite good. No blood transfusion was necessary (estimated blood loss = 100 ml) and the patient was discharged home on postoperative day four without complication. According to final pathologic analysis, including a panel of immunochemical stains which excluded RCC and metanephric adenoma, the diagnosis was renal oncocytoma (Figure 2). Preoperative glomerular filtration rate (GFR) was 101 ml/min/1.73m^2 and new baseline GFR was 58 ml/min/1.73m^2. The liver and bone lesions identified prior to surgery have been stable and no local or distant metastases have been seen now nearly four years postoperatively.

3. Discussion

Renal oncocytomas were first described in 1942 and the first large series of 13 cases appeared in 1976 from Klein and Valensi [9]. Oncocytoma may coexist with primary RCC, most commonly clear cell and chromophobe RCC. The distinction between oncocytoma and RCC is difficult based on imaging features and generally requires histopathological analysis with a panel of immunochemical stains [10–12]. Oncocytoma has been associated with multiple chromosomal abnormalities including monosomy, trisomy, and loss of heterozygosity [13]. Though benign, renal oncocytomas can grow to very large size with associated symptoms (Table 1). Despite being benign in nature, recent studies have mentioned oncocytic cells integrating with perinephric fat [14, 15] and in rare cases, oncocytoma can invade the renal vein or vein branches [16]. They are generally well-encapsulated and are rarely invasive or associated with metastases [17]. In our case, nephrectomy was indicated for palliation of her abdominal pain and prevention of bleeding from this hypervascular tumor. The presence of only benign histology after surgery indicates that surgery may have been potentially avoided by a renal mass biopsy, but our opinion is that no change in management would have occurred given its large size and the potential of misclassification of an oncocytic RCC because of sampling error [18]. This patient's family history of RCC contributed to our suspicion of RCC, but the specific history in this patient's family was not typical for

Table 1: Largest reported renal oncocytomas.

References	Age (years)	Sex	Tumor size (cm)	Presenting Complaint	Treatment	Metastasis/Recurrences
Demos et al. [4]	64	Male	27x20x15	Palpable abdominal mass	Right open radical nephrectomy	None found
Ahmad et al. [5]	61	Male	25x16x16	Lower back/ flank pain	Right open radical nephrectomy	None found
Banks et al. [6]	57	Male	21x18x15	Abdominal discomfort and distension	Right open radical nephrectomy	1.7 cm left lung nodule and several indeterminate liver lesions at diagnosis. Metastasis could not be excluded.
Kilic et al. [7]	65	Male	20x15x10	Abdominal pain	Left open radical nephrectomy	None found
Sundararajan et al. [8]	37	Male	20	Abdominal mass and moderate hypertension	Right open radical nephrectomy	On follow up at 3 months hypertension had resolved.
Current case	59	Female	14x13x12	Palpable mass	Right open radical nephrectomy	Multiple indeterminate liver, bone and lung lesions at diagnosis with benign liver biopsy

any known syndrome given the diagnosis of clear cell RCC in a first-degree relative in his 50s and another first-degree relative with a cancer type not known to be associated with any RCC syndromes (glioblastoma multiforme) [19–21]. In this case, genetic evaluation was pursued but did not identify a deleterious mutation in any potentially causative genes. Our plan is to continue follow-up annually with this patient as there have been rare reports of malignant transformation of oncocytoma and she is at moderate risk for progression of CKD [22]. For this reason, surveillance for patients with a histologic diagnosis of oncocytoma from biopsy has been recommended as well [23, 24].

4. Conclusion

Renal oncocytoma has a benign clinical course with excellent long term outcomes. Unfortunately, most renal oncocytomas cannot be differentiated from malignant RCC by clinical or radiographic criteria. For this reason, renal mass biopsy is often recommended for small renal masses, as the result may lead such patients to choose surveillance over definitive treatment. For larger masses, such as this report of the sixth largest oncocytoma, radical nephrectomy will remain the preferred management strategy. When metastatic cancer is suspected, biopsy of a metastatic lesion is commonly performed. The primary tumor is occasionally biopsied, but often omitted as malignancy is assumed and the histology of the metastatic lesion establishes the diagnosis and stage. Even in the setting of presumed metastases, renal mass biopsy may be of value because the histologies may not match and the best management strategy may occasionally be altered.

Ethical Approval

The study was reviewed by the Spectrum Health Institution Review Board and determined that the activity did not meet the definition of research as defined by DHHS or FDA.

Consent

As the Spectrum Health Institution Review Board determined this activity is not research, waiver of informed consent for human study subjects is not necessary.

Authors' Contributions

Dey S researched the literature, compiled the data, and wrote the paper; Uddin G performed the pathology review of this case; Noyes SL reviewed and revised the paper; Lane BR supervised and critically reviewed and approved the manuscript.

Acknowledgments

The corresponding author would like to thank the Betz Family Endowment for Cancer Research for their support. Funding was provided in part by the Spectrum Health Foundation.

References

[1] B. Perez-Ordonez, G. Hamed, S. Campbell et al., "Renal oncocytoma: a clinicopathologic study of 70 cases," *The American Journal of Surgical Pathology*, vol. 21, no. 8, pp. 871–883, 1997.

[2] M. B. Amin, T. B. Crotty, S. K. Tickoo, and G. M. Farrow, "Renal oncocytoma: a reappraisal of morphologic features with clinicopathologic findings in 80 cases," *The American Journal of Surgical Pathology*, vol. 12, no. 1, pp. 1–12, 1997.

[3] J. Mauermann, M. de Martino, M. Waldert et al., "Gender differences in benign renal masses," *World Journal of Urology*, vol. 31, no. 5, pp. 1051–1057, 2013.

[4] T. C. Demos and A. J. Malone, "Computed tomography of a giant renal oncocytoma," *Journal of Computer Assisted Tomography*, vol. 12, no. 5, pp. 899-900, 1988.

[5] S. Ahmad, R. Manecksha, B. D. Hayes, and R. Grainger, "Case report of a symptomatic giant renal oncocytoma," *International Journal of Surgery Case Reports*, vol. 2, no. 6, pp. 83–85, 2011.

[6] K. L. Banks, E. E. Cherullo, and A. C. Novick, "Giant renal oncocytoma," *Urology*, vol. 57, no. 2, p. 365, 2001.

[7] S. Kılıç, M. T. Altinoki, D. İpek, and H. Ergin, "Case report of a giant renal oncocytoma," *International Urology and Nephrology*, vol. 35, no. 1, pp. 83-84, 2003.

[8] S. Sundararajan, J. Dyer, R. Pemberton, and R. J. Cohen, "Asymptomatic giant renal oncocytoma presenting with hypertension," *Pathology*, vol. 40, no. 7, pp. 723-724, 2008.

[9] M. J. Klein and Q. J. Valensi, "Proximal tubular adenomas of kidney with so-called oncocytic features. A clinicopathologic study of 13 cases of a rarely reported neoplasm," *Cancer*, vol. 38, no. 2, pp. 906–914, 1976.

[10] M. A. Gorin, S. P. Rowe, and M. E. Allaf, "Oncocytic neoplasm on renal mass biopsy: a diagnostic conundrum," *Oncology (Williston Park)*, vol. 30, no. 5, pp. 426–435, 2016.

[11] S. R. Williamson, R. Gadde, K. Trpkov et al., "Diagnostic criteria for oncocytic renal neoplasms: a survey of urologic pathologists," *Human Pathology*, vol. 63, pp. 149–156, 2017.

[12] C. Alamara, E. M. Karapanagiotou, I. Tourkantonis et al., "Renal oncocytoma: A case report and short review of the literature," *European Journal of Internal Medicine*, vol. 19, no. 7, pp. e67–e69, 2008.

[13] K. Junker, G. Weirich, P. Moravek et al., "Familial and sporadic renal oncocytomas–a comparative molecular–genetic analysis," *European Urology*, vol. 40, no. 3, pp. 330–336, 2001.

[14] S. R. Williamson, "Renal oncocytoma with perinephric fat invasion," *International Journal of Surgical Pathology*, vol. 24, no. 7, pp. 625-626, 2016.

[15] K. Trpkov, A. Yilmaz, D. Uzer et al., "Renal oncocytoma revisited: a clinicopathological study of 109 cases with emphasis on problematic diagnostic features," *Histopathology*, vol. 57, no. 6, pp. 893–906, 2010.

[16] O. Hes, M. Michal, R. Šíma et al., "Renal oncocytoma with and without intravascular extension into the branches of renal vein have the same morphological, immunohistochemical and genetic features," *Virchows Archiv*, vol. 452, no. 3, pp. 285–293, 2008.

[17] C. B. Dechet, D. G. Bostwick, M. L. Blute, S. C. Bryant, and H. Zincke, "Renal oncocytoma: multifocality, bilateralism, meatachronous tumor development and coexistent renal cell carcinoma," *The Journal of Urology*, vol. 162, no. 1, pp. 40–42, 1999.

[18] S. Campbell, R. G. Uzzo, M. E. Allaf et al., "Renal mass and localized renal cancer: AUA guideline," *The Journal of Urology*, vol. 198, no. 3, pp. 520–529, 2017.

[19] PDQ Cancer Genetics Editorial Board, *Health Professional Version*, PDQ Cancer Information Summaries, 2002.

[20] N. C. C. Network, *NCCN Guideline with NCCN Evidence Blocks - Kidney Cancer (Version 3.2019)*, 2019.

[21] V. M. Raymond, C. M. Herron, T. J. Giordano, and S. B. Gruber, "Familial renal cancer as an indicator of hereditary leiomyomatosis and renal cell cancer syndrome," *Familial Cancer*, vol. 11, no. 1, pp. 115–121, 2012.

[22] S. J. Sirintrapun, K. R. Geisinger, A. Cimic et al., "Oncocytoma-like renal tumor with transformation toward high-grade oncocytic carcinoma," *Medicine (Baltimore)*, vol. 93, no. 15, article e81, 2014.

[23] S. Liu, S. Lee, P. Rashid et al., "Active surveillance is suitable for intermediate term follow-up of renal oncocytoma diagnosed by percutaneous core biopsy," *BJU International*, vol. 118, pp. 30–34, 2016.

[24] M. Haifler, L. Copel, J. Sandbank et al., "Renal oncocytoma—are there sufficient grounds to consider surveillance following prenephrectomy histologic diagnosis," *Urologic Oncology: Seminars and Original Investigations*, vol. 30, no. 4, pp. 362–368, 2012.

18

Kidney Salvage with Renal Artery Reconstruction after Blunt Traumatic Injury

David G. Jackson,[1] Phillipe Abreu,[2] Manuel Anthony Moutinho,[3] Antonio Marttos,[3] George W. Burke III,[4] Nicholas Namias,[3] and Gaetano Ciancio[4]

[1]*Department of Surgery, University of Miami Miller School of Medicine, USA*
[2]*Multi-Organ Transplant Program, University of Toronto, Canada*
[3]*Ryder Trauma Center, Jackson Memorial Hospital, University of Miami Miller School of Medicine, USA*
[4]*Miami Transplant Institute, Jackson Memorial Hospital, University of Miami Miller School of Medicine, USA*

Correspondence should be addressed to Gaetano Ciancio; gciancio@med.miami.edu

Academic Editor: Tun-Chieh Chen

Renal artery injury from blunt abdominal trauma is a rare condition that is typically managed nonoperatively in hemodynamically stable patients. Revascularization can be achieved by stenting or surgical reconstruction of the renal artery. All attempts at revascularization should minimize warm ischemic time. Here, we discuss a patient postmotor vehicle accident who presented to Ryder Trauma Center with intra-abdominal bleeding. He underwent emergency exploratory laparotomy with splenectomy and abdominal packing. Postoperative CT scan revealed a contrast nonenhancing left kidney. The patient then returned to the operating room and underwent in situ renal artery reconstruction after >4 hours of warm ischemia. The patient survived a 2-month hospital course and was discharged home after prolonged in-hospital stay and intensive care treatment. Nuclear medicine scan showed scarring and atrophy of the reattached kidney with 16.3% of overall function attributed to the affected kidney. This case shows that patients with renal artery injury can be managed operatively with arterial reconstruction. Reducing warm ischemic time is critical in preserving kidney function.

1. Introduction

One rare consequence of blunt abdominal trauma is renal artery injury (incidence 0.05-0.1%) [1, 2]. Awareness of blunt renal artery trauma has increased due to improved detection by CT scan [3]. Blunt renal artery trauma can cause renal artery aneurysm, dissection, or rupture with subsequent renal infarction [4]. Renal trauma is graded on a spectrum (Grades I-V) [5]. Management of blunt renal artery injury can be nonoperative or operative, with the latter usually accomplished through endovascular stenting [6]. Nonoperative vs. operative management of blunt renal trauma depends on the severity of the trauma and laterality of the injury [1].

Conservative approaches are typically attempted in patients with unilateral renal injury who do not undergo exploratory laparotomy, while bilateral renal injury necessitates surgical revascularization. In cases with complications such as renal artery thrombosis, surgical revascularization is essential [7]. If the patient is unstable, more lethal injuries should be ameliorated prior to renal revascularization [1]. Even after revascularization, the patient may experience posttraumatic acute kidney injury (AKI) from renal crush injury and hemorrhagic shock [8].

Many revascularization attempts have been unsuccessful, with 26% of success rate as published by Haas and Spirnak [9]. The incidence of chronic complications such as decreased renal function and hypertension depends on factors including age, comorbidities, length of ischemic time, and prehospital trauma life support. Here, we present a patient who sustained blunt renal artery injury and underwent surgical revascularization at our institution.

Table 1: List of Injuries sustained by the patient during MVA. CT scan aided in the diagnosis of many of these injuries.

(1) Pulmonary contusions and pneumomediastinum
(2) Bilateral pneumothoraces
(3) Multiple bilateral rib fractures
(4) Manubrium fracture
(5) Bilateral clavicle fractures
(6) Left scapula fracture
(7) Multiple cervical spine fractures: left occipital condyle fracture, left C1 facet fracture, left C2 lateral mass fracture, and left C6-C7 laminar fracture
(8) Cortical irregularity at the superior endplates of T1, T3, T4, and T5 likely representing compression fractures
(9) Left T1 transverse process fracture
(10) Minimally displaced T3 and T7 spinous process fractures
(11) Comminuted displaced basicervical fracture of the right proximal femur, underwent open reduction internal fixation with proximal tibia traction pin
(12) Comminuted displaced subtrochanteric fracture of the left proximal femur, underwent open reduction internal fixation
(13) Extensive subcutaneous emphysema
(14) Scalp injury and suspected traumatic brain injury upon admission
(15) Noncontrast enhancing left kidney

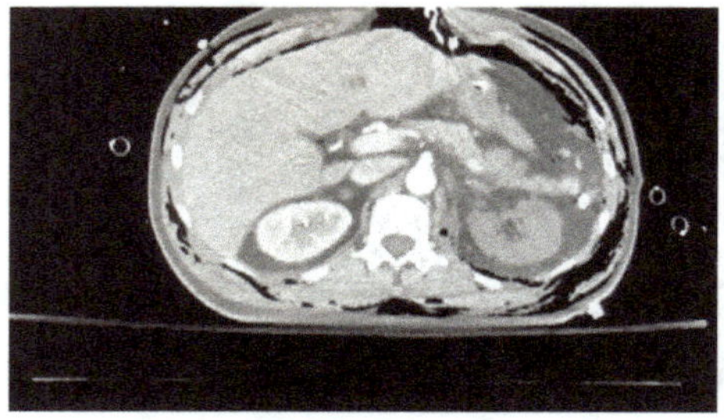

Figure 1: CT scan with contrast showing nonenhancing left kidney consistent with left renal artery injury.

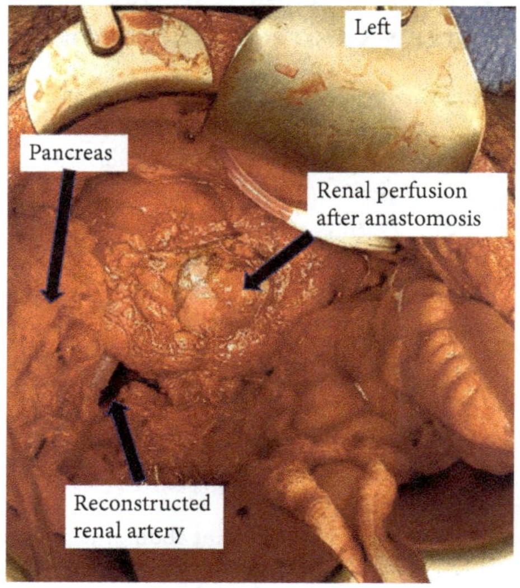

Figure 2: Surgical photography demonstrating renal parenchymal perfusion after reconstruction and anastomosis.

2. Case Report

A 48-year-old male with no significant past medical history who was a restrained driver in a motor vehicle accident sustained multiple injuries in the crash (Table 1) and had a prolonged and difficult extrication from the crash site before being brought to Ryder Trauma Center with a Glasgow Coma Scale of 15 approximately 1-2 hours after his accident. While in the resuscitation bay, bilateral chest tubes were placed for bilateral pneumothoraces and he had a positive FAST exam with tachycardia and severe hypotension (HR 128, BP 69/50). He was immediately brought to the operating room (OR) for emergency exploratory laparotomy, and splenectomy was performed for Grade V splenic injury, followed by abdominal packing without complete abdominal closure. His condition stabilized intraoperatively; no active abdominal bleeding or hematoma could be identified at that moment.

A full-body CT scan was then requested to investigate other injuries. A list of numerous bone fractures that demonstrate the serious extent of the traumatic injury is shown in Table 1. The patient had also a scalp injury and needed additional workup to rule out traumatic brain injury. Head CT was negative. Chest CT demonstrated no further injuries other than minor pulmonary contusions and pneumothoraxes already being treated by the previously placed chest tubes. Abdominal contrasted CT identified a left renal artery injury and a nonenhancing ischemic left kidney but no other abdominal organ injuries (Figure 1). In an attempt to salvage left kidney function despite over 4 hours of warm ischemia at that point, the patient was taken back to the OR for emergent repair of his left renal artery/in situ autotransplantation.

An occlusive 2 cm intra-arterial thrombus was removed, and a corresponding 2 cm damaged segment of the renal artery was excised. The kidney was flushed through the renal vein with histidine-tryptophan-ketoglutarate perfusion solution during the anastomosis of the renal artery. The left kidney was adequately perfused postreconstruction of the left renal artery (Figure 2).

During the two operations, the patient received a total of 7 units of packed red blood cells, 6 units of fresh frozen plasma, 2 units of cryoprecipitate, and 2 platelet transfusions. The patient was subsequently admitted to the Trauma Intensive Care Unit (TICU) for postoperative care. His hospital course was significant for worsening azotemia in the setting of decreased kidney function and falling urine output with a peak creatinine above 8 mg/dL. Dialysis and pressors were started on postoperative day 4. Eventually, his renal function improved, and his creatinine fell, and urinary output increased. He exhibited hypertension 2-3 weeks postrenal artery repair, but his systolic blood pressures eventually stabilized between 110 and 130 mmHg. He recovered in our TICU after multiple episodes of fungemia and bacteremia, was transferred to the trauma floor, and was discharged

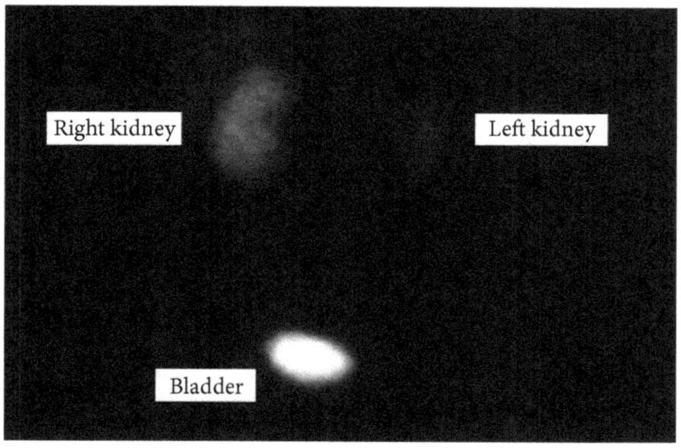

FIGURE 3: Follow-up nuclear scan (11 mCi technetium-99 m MAG3) demonstrating right kidney perfusion dominance at 6 months postsurgery.

two months after admission. He is currently being followed in an outpatient clinic. After 18 months of follow-up, his serum creatinine level is 1.3 mg/dL and vital signs were within normal limits, without hypertension.

Outpatient nuclear medicine renal scan indicated partial preservation of left renal function with a shrunken left kidney, and 16.3% (Figure 3) of split renal function attributed to the left kidney. Renal biopsy of the revascularized kidney was not performed. Left renal artery stenosis was not noted after its reattachment.

3. Discussion

Blunt renal artery trauma can be managed conservatively or surgically [1]. This patient presented with intra-abdominal bleeding and needed an emergent exploratory laparotomy prior to further abdominal investigation. Our patient's renal artery injury was severe. This is in contrast to what renal artery injury patients have who generally had minor renal artery injuries and underwent conservative management [1, 2, 10]. In a cohort published by Sangthong et al., only 8.7% of patients underwent operative renal artery reconstruction [2]. The open operative technique we used (in situ renal artery reconstruction) was also unlike most operative management of renal artery trauma treated elsewhere with endovascular approach [6]. In this case, endovascular repair would very likely not have been possible due to the degree of damage to the renal artery. However, where endovascular treatment is not available for trauma patients, open repair must be considered an option for the treatment of arterial injuries.

Thrombosis of end arterial supply is an uncommon indication for exploratory laparotomy in trauma, followed by renal artery surgical repair [7]. Our patient had two episodes of postoperative AKI. This may have resulted from prolonged ischemia to both kidneys due to hemorrhagic shock after difficult extrication and delayed prehospital trauma life support [8]. Salvage of an affected kidney may be of lower priority than more critical injuries including severe splenic hemorrhage and other abdominal organ injuries leading to major bleeding [1]. Renal artery injury bleeding may be contained and controlled within Gerota's fascia. We attempted renal revascularization only after his hemodynamic condition was stabilized. Surgical revascularization should be attempted soon after hemodynamic stabilization to minimize warm ischemic time. In addition, the patient would have to return to the OR after CT was performed at the least to remove abdominal packing.

This patient was initially managed in the TICU, which is the common management for up to 70% of blunt renal artery injury patients [2]. The intraoperative revascularization of the renal artery was however associated with longer ICU stay. Renal artery injury patients may develop hypertension as a long-term consequence of their injury/repair [9]. This patient sustained other injuries that caused him significant associated morbidity and pain. His blood pressure will need to be followed closely in order to diagnose and treat possible hypertension that may follow this injury to the left kidney.

An important question would be whether 16.3% of renal function at follow-up could be justified as acceptable renal salvage and justify the approach used in our case. The salvage of this kidney via arterial reconstruction was performed in order to optimize the patient's total physiologic capacity; while the degree of total functional return could not be estimated at the time, we felt that this justified the approach used in our case. Indeed, the question whether there is an upper limit of ischemic/traumatic injury beyond which a kidney should be considered unsalvageable remains incompletely answered [11]. The potential harm of a renal artery reconstruction should be weighed against the loss of function after arterial thrombosis or even nephrectomy. Better results in terms of long-term kidney function may be achieved in patients with lower prehospital trauma life support time and faster transportation to definitive care. Although clinically less harmful for young patients, radical nephrectomy was associated with double the loss of eGFR and 2.2-fold increased mortality when compared with partial nephrectomy in CKD patients, so radical nephrectomy may carry its own factors that increase mortality [12]. On the other hand, data from renal transplant donors demonstrates that risk of end-stage renal disease after surgically removing the kidneys was comparable to the general population [13].

The present case demonstrates that open operative renal artery reconstruction with autotransplantation is a viable method for managing severe blunt renal artery trauma with associated thrombosis and that special attention must be paid to warm ischemic time leading to posttraumatic AKI [1, 8].

4. Conclusion

Patients with high-grade renal injury and thrombosis of the affected renal artery can be managed with resection of the damaged portions of the renal artery and in situ arterial reconstruction of the affected kidney. Caution must be taken to minimize excessive warm ischemic time that would exacerbate postoperative AKI. Patients may have long-term loss of function of the revascularized kidney and/or hypertension.

Consent

Verbal informed consent was obtained from the patient.

Authors' Contributions

David G. Jackson and Phillipe Abreu contributed equally to this work.

References

[1] A. Jawas and F. M. Abu-Zidan, "Management algorithm for complete blunt renal artery occlusion in multiple trauma patients: case series," *International Journal of Surgery*, vol. 6, no. 4, pp. 317–322, 2008.

[2] B. Sangthong, D. Demetriades, M. Martin et al., "Management and hospital outcomes of blunt renal artery injuries: analysis of 517 patients from the National Trauma Data Bank," *Journal of the American College of Surgeons*, vol. 203, no. 5, pp. 612–617, 2006.

[3] S. J. D. Chow, K. J. Thompson, J. F. Hartman, and M. L. Wright, "A 10-year review of blunt renal artery injuries at an urban level I trauma centre," *Injury*, vol. 40, no. 8, pp. 844–850, 2009.

[4] K. P. Kang, S. Lee, W. Kim et al., "Renal infarction resulting from traumatic renal artery dissection," *The Korean Journal of Internal Medicine*, vol. 23, no. 2, pp. 103–105, 2008.

[5] E. E. Moore, S. R. Shackford, H. L. Pachter et al., "Organ injury Scaling," *The Journal of Trauma: Injury, Infection, and Critical Care*, vol. 29, no. 12, pp. 1664–1666, 1989.

[6] J. E. Lopera, R. Suri, G. Kroma, S. Gadani, and B. Dolmatch, "Traumatic occlusion and dissection of the main renal artery: endovascular treatment," *Journal of Vascular and Interventional Radiology*, vol. 22, no. 11, pp. 1570–1574, 2011.

[7] S. B. Dharap, J. Noronha, and V. Kumar, "Laparotomy for blunt abdominal trauma-some uncommon indications," *Journal of Emergencies, Trauma, and Shock*, vol. 9, no. 1, pp. 32–36, 2016.

[8] K. L. de Abreu, G. Jínior, A. Barreto et al., "Acute kidney injury after trauma: prevalence, clinical characteristics and RIFLE classification," *Indian Journal of Critical Care Medicine*, vol. 14, no. 3, pp. 121–128, 2010.

[9] C. A. Haas and J. P. Spirnak, "Traumatic renal artery occlusion: a review of the literature," *Techniques in Urology*, vol. 4, no. 1, pp. 1–11, 1998.

[10] Z. Ahmed, S. Nabir, M. N. Ahmed, S. Al Hilli, V. Ravikumar, and U. Z. Momin, "Renal artery injury secondary to blunt abdominal trauma – two case reports," *Polish Journal of Radiology*, vol. 81, pp. 572–577, 2016.

[11] M. Angelis, J. S. Augenstein, G. Ciancio et al., "Ex vivo repair and renal autotransplantation after penetrating trauma: is there an upper limit of ischemic/traumatic injury beyond which a kidney is unsalvageable?," *The Journal of Trauma: Injury, Infection, and Critical Care*, vol. 54, no. 3, pp. 606–609, 2003.

[12] E. Streja, K. Kalantar-Zadeh, M. Z. Molnar, J. Landman, O. A. Arah, and C. P. Kovesdy, "Radical versus partial nephrectomy, chronic kidney disease progression and mortality in US veterans," *Nephrology Dialysis Transplantation*, vol. 33, pp. 95–101, 2016.

[13] H. N. Ibrahim, R. Foley, L. Tan et al., "Long-term consequences of kidney donation," *The New England Journal of Medicine*, vol. 360, no. 5, pp. 459–469, 2009.

19

A Rare Presentation of Renal Papillary Necrosis in a COVID-19-Positive Patient

Bela Tallai,[1] Tawiz Gul Gulistan,[1] Maged Nasser Aa B. Alrayashi,[1] Salah Abdulhabeb Abdulwali Al Mughalles,[2] Hatem Mostari Kamkoum,[1] Mohamed Ali A. Ebrahim,[1] Mohamed Abdelkarim Ali Abdelkarim,[1] and Morshed Ali Salah[1]

[1]*Urology Division of Surgery Department, Hazm Mebaireek General Hospital, Hamad Medical Corporation, Industrial Area Street No. 33, PO Box 3050, Doha, Qatar*
[2]*Clinical Imaging Department, Hazm Mebaireek General Hospital, Hamad Medical Corporation, Industrial Area Street No. 33, PO Box 3050, Doha, Qatar*

Correspondence should be addressed to Bela Tallai; belatallai@gmail.com

Academic Editor: Apul Goel

In this case report we describe an unusual presentation of severe acute papillary necrosis in a COVID-19-positive patient. An emergency flexible ureteroscopy greatly helped in the establishment of the diagnosis. In the international literature, there is a paucity of intraoperative endoscopic images representing severe renal papillary necrosis. We present a case of severe acute renal papillary necrosis in a 49-year-old south-Asian, COVID-19-positive male patient who needed emergency urological intervention for macroscopic hematuria and urinary retention due to clot formation in the urinary bladder. The patient underwent emergency cystoscopy, clot evacuation, and by rigid and flexible ureteroscopy. The diagnosis was only confirmed in the postoperative period, retrospectively. Finally, the patient fully recovered due to the multidisciplinary management. Diagnosis of rare clinical entities can be sometimes challenging in the everyday routine practice. Having atypical clinical course, the surgeon should be prepared and sometimes must take responsible decisions promptly, even if needed intraoperatively, to manage unexpected findings in order to get the right diagnosis without compromising the patient's safety.

1. Introduction

Renal papillary necrosis is defined as an ischemic coagulative necrosis of the papillae in the kidneys. In most patients, diagnosis can be confirmed based on clinical symptoms and renal imaging [1]. A variety of etiological factors are known which can contribute to the process [2]. Clinical presentation can vary from an incidental finding in an asymptomatic patient to a severe, life-threatening condition. In the international literature, we did not find such intraoperative endoscopic images representing severe renal papillary necrosis we had obtained during the surgery.

In this case report, we describe a challenging clinical presentation of an acute papillary necrosis in a COVID-19-positive patient.

2. Case Presentation

A 49-year-old male patient with recent history of faint hematuria was admitted to a private outpatient clinic due to acute urinary retention. Apart from diabetes mellitus, his past medical and surgical histories were unremarkable. Foley catheter was smoothly inserted then frank bloody urine output could be observed. Therefore, he was referred to the governmental tertiary hospital as a urology emergency for further investigations and management. Besides faint hematuria and urinary retention, he did not have any other symptom. The patient was vitally stable and afebrile.

Physical examination of the genitourinary system was unremarkable. Among the initial laboratory investigations, mild anemia (hemoglobin 9.5 g/dL, hematocrit 29.5%) and azotemia (creatinine 153 μmL/L) were noted. C-reactive protein (CRP) was also elevated (185 mg/L). Regarding imaging, kidney-ureter-bladder (KUB) ultrasound did not report any pathology at the level of the kidneys; only a large blood clot was described on the trigone of the bladder. Due to the elevated kidney function test, only a noncontrast computer tomography (CT) scan was carried out, which reported the same clot, suggesting some sort of bladder wall origin. The patient was admitted for emergency surgical procedure. The plan was to do cystoscopy, clot evacuation, and probably transurethral resection of the urinary bladder (TURB) or bladder biopsy with appropriate hemostasis. A COVID-19 polymerase chain reaction (PCR) swab test was ordered as well preoperatively showing positive result. Nevertheless, the patient did not have any symptoms suggestive of ongoing COVID-19 infection. Due to the positive swab test result, the patient was transferred to our designated COVID-19 hospital where only coronavirus-positive patients were hospitalized, and all emergency procedures were carried according to established local pathways and protocols. Upon the patient's arrival, Hgb dropped to 7.5 g/dL. In the operation theater, under spinal anesthesia, the clot was evacuated cystoscopically. Surprisingly, no source of bleeding could be observed during meticulous cystoscopy. At the final moments of cystoscopy, a thick bloody jet was expulsed from the left ureteric orifice which appeared repeatedly.

Having realized the unexpected intraoperative situation, left rigid and flexible ureteroscopy (FURS) were carried out. Rigid ureteroscopy was negative up to the pelvi-ureteric junction. Multiple filling defects in several caliceal endings were seen during retrograde pyelography (Figure 1).

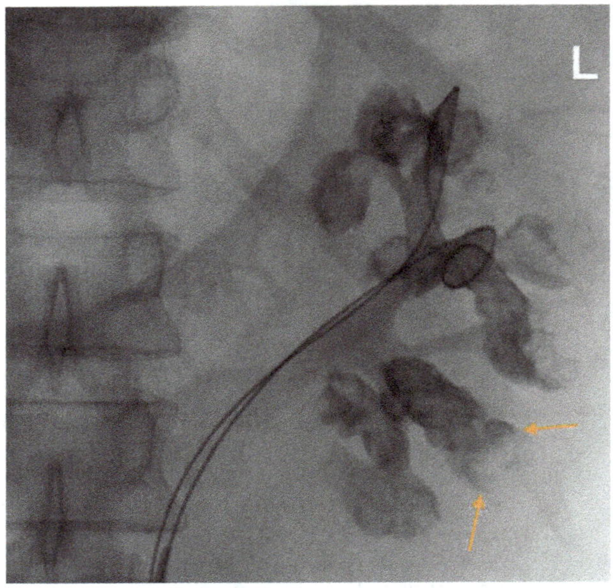

Figure 1: Left retrograde pyelography showing multiple filling defects in almost all caliceal ends. Arrows demonstrate the lobster claw sign as the characteristic radiology feature of renal papillary necrosis.

During FURS, along with diffuse inflammatory and hemorrhagic mucosal changes in the calyces, whitish, fluffy substance was sitting in almost all renal calyceal ends (Figures 2(a) and 2(b)).

The renal pelvis was intact. Due to the bizarre intraoperative finding, multiple biopsies and urine cytology samples followed. By the end of the procedure, only a simple ureteral catheter was left behind for 24 hours to avoid further mucosal irritation and bleeding.

The surgery went without any complication, and the postoperative period was uneventful as well. Finally, postoperative CT scan with contrast confirmed the diagnosis; however, it was already obvious for the radiologist when he received the images of intraoperative retrograde pyelography (Figure 3).

Later, the patient's condition continually improved, hematuria disappeared and the renal function became normal. The patient received 4 units of packed red blood cells during his hospital course. Both histology and cytology samples were negative for malignancy, showing necrotic debris with extensive neutrophilic infiltration, fibrin deposition, and acute inflammatory exudate. Investigations towards sickle cell anemia or tuberculosis were also negative. Nephrology was involved in the management in the postoperative period. However, though the patient's COVID-19 swab test was positive, he did not require any specific medication according to our infectious disease team. Finally, the patient was discharged into quarantine facility in fair general condition and with clear urine output.

During the multidisciplinary regular follow-up, the patient's urine has been clear, renal function has been maintained within the normal range, and blood sugar homeostasis has been controlled as well.

3. Discussion

Renal papillary necrosis is basically a rare medical disease. Several systemic factors can contribute in the development of the process, some of them might present simultaneously, synergizing each other [2]. The well-known underlying conditions are diabetes mellitus, analgesic abuse, sickle cell anemia, urinary tract obstruction, liver cirrhosis, and tuberculosis. The most common symptoms include flank and/or abdominal pain, various degrees of hematuria, dysuria, and chills and fever as signs of consecutive upper urinary tract infection [3]. In the presence of any clinical suspicion, usually, CT scan with contrast confirms the diagnosis and no further diagnostic or therapeutic interventions are required to be performed. In particular, during the COVID-19 pandemic, in selected patients, according to the individual institutional protocol, chest CT, in addition to abdominal scans, might have an important role in patients with the symptomatology of acute abdomen, even without respiratory symptoms [4].

The process of renal papillary necrosis can also show a chronic, slowly progressing course. Many of the patients can be treated conservatively without surgical intervention, and hematuria usually does not require blood transfusion. The single indication for urological intervention is acute ureteral obstruction by the necrotic tissue or blood clots or consecutive obstructive pyelonephritis [5]. Our patient deviated

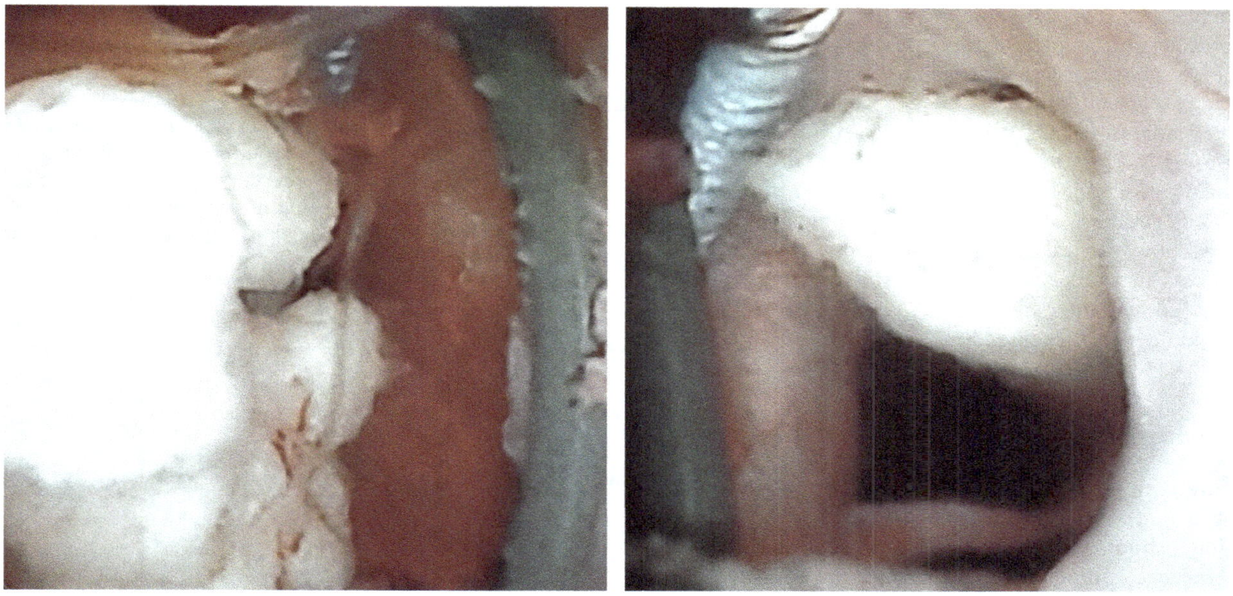

(a) (b)

FIGURE 2: (a) Whitish, fluffy substance representing necrotic, sloughed papilla in inflammatory and hemorrhagic mucosal environment. (b) Sloughing necrotic papilla in the left-mid caliceal system.

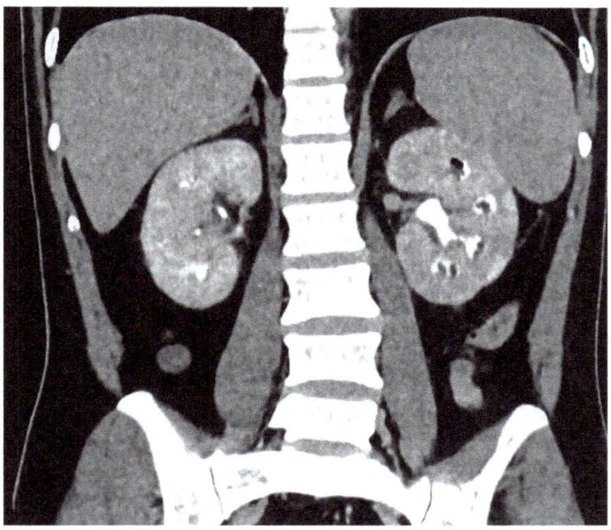

FIGURE 3: Renal papillary necrosis in the left kidney on delayed contrast CT scan on the 5th postoperative day. Coronal reconstruction. Air in the upper caliceal system represents prior instrumentation.

from most of the patients having renal papillary necrosis. He presented with isolated macroscopic hematuria, which progressed to clot urinary retention. No abdominal or flank pain, no fever or chills, and no signs of pyelonephritis could be observed either clinically or biochemically. Due to the continuous bleeding resulting in the significant drop in the hemoglobin level, the patient received blood transfusions and was taken to the operating theater on emergency basis. We expected that the patient had a sort of bladder pathology, because the clinical picture as well as the available preoperative imaging showed abnormality at the upper urinary tract beyond the bladder. Finally, FURS greatly helped us to confirm the diagnosis and completed the missing piece of the puzzle. However, the clinical manifestation, though it was somehow misleading, and laboratory and radiology findings retrospectively were relevant to the diagnosis. Among the well-known risk factors, type II diabetes mellitus was present.

Regarding the surgical process itself, wearing full personal protective equipment is a must in such emergency surgeries in a COVID-19-positive patient. However, due to these pieces of equipment, most of the surgeons have additional intraoperative burdens, negatively affecting their nontechnical skills, such as vision and communication, as well as impacting decision-making processes and also resulting in surgical discomfort and increased fatigue [6].

Another general debate or consideration is whether to perform a laparoscopic/endoscopic emergency surgery during the COVID-19 outbreak or to perform a traditional, appropriate open surgery, instead. Concerning the answer to this question, first of all, nonoperative management should represent the first line in a COVID-19 patient as far as possible. Open surgeries, if needed, might be recommended and should be performed safely in most patients especially in acute care surgery, avoiding the creation of pneumoperitoneum and other smoke-generating and time-consuming maneuvers, which might increase the risk of aerosolization during laparoscopy. Establishing local institutional treatment algorithms or protocols based on international guidelines is essential to manage these patients properly [7, 8]. In our case scenario, if we would have been faced with an uncontrollable bleeding with renal origin, we had also been challenged whether to treat it conservatively or with selective embolization or open surgery, as the last resort, depending mainly on the stability of the patient and the degree of bleeding. In a profuse, life-threating situation, a laparoscopic approach is definitely much less preferable for such patient. Fortunately, ureteroscopy in our patient was safe without increasing the chance of spreading the virus to the staff of the operating theater.

Our patient was COVID-19 positive; however, he was asymptomatic from this point of view and he did not receive any medication for that reason based on the medical COVID-19 protocol of our hospital. Probably, it will remain unknown how his viral infection impacted the basic necrotizing process in the kidneys. We considered his COVID-19 infection coincidental; nonetheless, its negative additional impact could not be excluded.

4. Conclusions

Our case demonstrated that sometimes, papillary necrosis can be a diagnosis of elimination or exclusion. This rare pathology should be suspected after excluding all other, much more common causes of hematuria. At the atypical clinical presentation, the insufficient preoperative imaging modalities can be misleading to and challenging for the urologist in obtaining the right diagnosis.

Based on our case report, we can also conclude that in such a severe pandemic, also with all its negative mental impact, it can be even more challenging for health care providers to stay alert and vigilant and at the same time make the right decision for cases that do not fit in the everyday routine practice.

Consent

No written consent has been obtained from the patient as there is no patient identifiable data included in this case report.

References

[1] E. K. Lang, R. J. Macchia, R. Thomas et al., "Multiphasic helical CT diagnosis of early medullary and papillary necrosis," *Journal of Endourology*, vol. 18, no. 1, pp. 49–56, 2004.

[2] M. D. Griffin, E. J. Bergstralhn, and T. S. Larson, "Renal papillary necrosis-a sixteen-year clinical experience," *Journal of the American Society of Nephrology*, vol. 6, no. 2, pp. 248–256, 1995.

[3] G. Eknoyan, W. Y. Qunibi, R. T. Grissom, S. N. Tuma, and J. C. Ayus, "Renal papillary necrosis: an update," *Medicine (Baltimore)*, vol. 61, no. 2, pp. 55–73, 1982.

[4] D. S. Lima, M. A. F. Riberio, G. Gallo, and S. Di Saverio, "Role of chest CT scan in patient with acute abdomen during the Covid-19 era," *British Journal of Surgery*, vol. 107, no. 7, p. e196, 2020.

[5] J. O. Salo, M. Talja, and T. Lehtonen, "Ureteroscopy in the treatment of ureteral obstruction caused by papillary necrosis," *European Urology*, vol. 13, no. 1-2, pp. 140-141, 1987.

[6] C. Y. Benítez, A. Güemes, J. Aranda et al., "Impact of personal protective equipment on surgical performance during the COVID-19 Pandemic," *World Journal of Surgery*, vol. 44, no. 9, pp. 2842–2847, 2020.

[7] S. Di Saverio, M. Khan, F. Pata et al., "Laparoscopy at all costs? Not now during COVID-19 outbreak and not for acute care surgery and emergency colorectal surgery: a practical algorithm from a hub tertiary teaching hospital in Northern Lombardy, Italy," *Journal of Trauma and Acute Care Surgery*, vol. 88, no. 6, pp. 715–718, 2020.

[8] S. Di Saverio, F. Pata, M. Khan, G. Ietto, E. Zani, and G. Carcano, "Convert to open: the new paradigm for surgery during COVID-19?," *British Journal of Surgery*, vol. 107, no. 7, p. e194, 2020.

20

Concurrent Angiomyolipoma and Clear Cell Renal Cell Carcinoma in the Same Kidney: A Rare Finding in a Patient without Tuberous Sclerosis

Amal Fekkar, Kaoutar Znati, Fouad Zouaidia, Hafsa Elouazzani, Zakia Bernoussi, and Ahmed Jahid

Department of Pathology, Ibn Sina University Hospital Center, Rabat, Morocco

Correspondence should be addressed to Amal Fekkar; amal_fekkar@um5.ac.ma

Academic Editor: Apul Goel

Synchronous renal cell carcinomas (RCC) and angiomyolipomas (AML) occurring in the same kidney are rare. Cases in the setting of tuberous sclerosis (TS) have been reported in the literature. However, the association of these tumors in the same kidney without TS is even more rare. We report here a case of a clear cell renal cell carcinoma (CCRCC) associated with an AML in the same kidney in a 42 years old female lacking the TS diagnostic criteria. The patient underwent a radical nephrectomy. Six months after surgery, the patient is healthy without signs of tumor recurrence or distant metastasis.

1. Introduction

AML are the most common benign tumor of the kidney, however, representing just 1% of surgically removed renal tumors [1]. It belongs to the family of perivascular epithelioid cell tumors (PEComas) and may occur sporadically or in patients with TS. The coexistence of RCC with AML in the same kidney is an uncommon finding, and nearly 80 cases with and without TS have been reported [2]. However, the majority of cases were in patients with TS [3, 4]. TS is an autosomal genetic disorder characterized by an increased risk of developing AML, renal cysts, and RCN. The clinical manifestations are broad, affecting not just the kidneys but also the brain, skin, lungs, and heart [5]. The clinical diagnosis of TS is based on the revised Gomez criteria. Rarely, RCN and AML can occur in the same kidney, sporadically, without TS, as synchronous or metachronous tumors.

2. Case Report

A 42-year-old female, who underwent 18 years ago, extracorporeal shockwave lithotripsy for right kidney stones, presented with six months history of right lumbar region pain associated with dysuria without hematuria. Physical exam showed right-sided abdominal tenderness.

Computed tomography (CT) urography (Figure 1) showed two masses in the midportion of the right kidney with distinct radiologic appearances. The external mass measuring 24 × 23 mm was a fat containing tumor suggesting AML. The internal tumor was fleshy and large measuring 49 × 40 mm. It deformed the renal contour and demonstrated a predominantly heterogeneous enhancement pattern. There was no evidence of lymph node metastases.

The other laboratory findings were within normal limits.

A right radical nephrectomy was done.

The patient had an uneventful postoperative recovery, and no neoadjuvant treatment has been administered. Six months after surgery, the patient is healthy without signs of tumor recurrence or distant metastasis.

On gross examination (Figure 2), the kidney was slightly enlarged weighing 280 g and measuring 130 × 70 × 65 mm. The cut surface revealed 2 masses in the midportion. The largest mass of 47 × 40 mm was encapsulated and firm with a heterogeneous appearance, composed of golden yellow soft

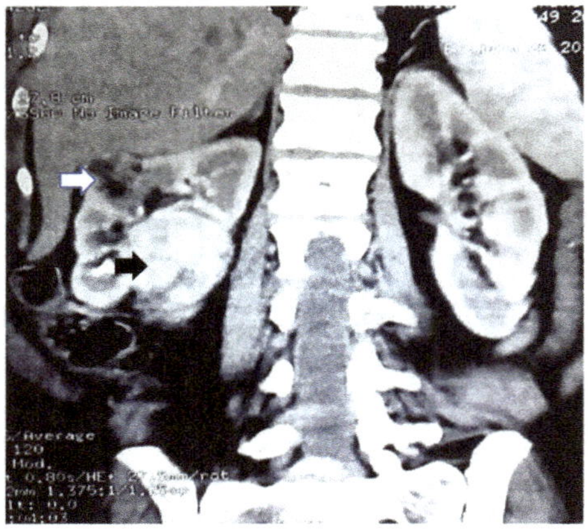

Figure 1: Computerized tomography urography scan showing two tumors in the midportion of the right kidney with distinct radiologic appearances: the external mass (white arrow) is a fat-containing tumor suggesting AML. The internal tumor (black arrow) is solid demonstrating a heterogeneous enhancement pattern.

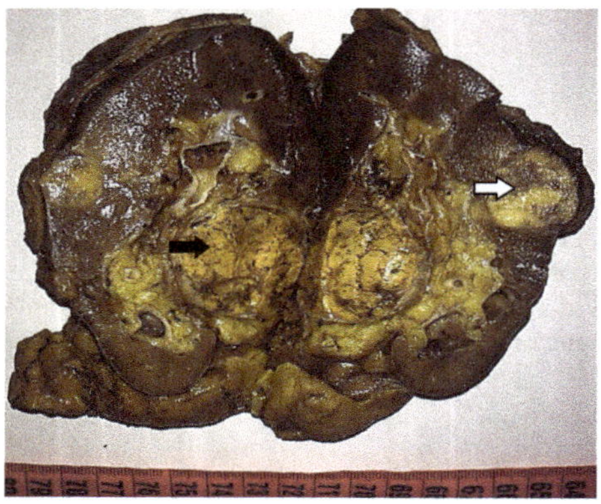

Figure 2: Gross examination revealing two different renal masses: the largest mass (black arrow) was encapsulated and firm composed of golden yellow soft areas with hemorrhagic changes. The smaller mass (white arrow) was well defined and had yellowish, glistening cut surface.

areas with hemorrhagic changes. The smaller mass measuring 25 × 20 mm was well defined and had yellowish, glistening cut surface. It was located at 3 cm from the first lesion.

Microscopic examination of the largest mass showed a malignant proliferation composed of cells with distinct cell membranes, optically clear cytoplasm, and rounded nuclei slightly larger than a red cell with inconspicuous nucleoli (consistent with Fuhrman grade 1). The cells were mainly arranged in sheets and compact nests surrounded by a regular network of thin-walled blood vessels (Figure 3). These features were consistent with the diagnosis of CCRCC.

The smaller lesion corresponded histologically to an AML composed of aggregates of thick-walled blood vessels, admixed with large mature fat cells and smooth muscle cells (Figure 3).

In the immunohistochemical study, AML showed positive immunostaining for melanocytic markers (HMB-45 and Melan-A) and for smooth muscle markers (smooth muscle actin and H-caldesmon) (Figure 4).

3. Discussion

The simultaneous occurrence of two different renal tumors in the same kidney is rare. The combination of these neoplasms can take different aspects. We distinguish separate tumors, collision tumors, and composite tumors. A collision tumor is a meeting of two tumors arising in independent topographical sites. A composite (hybrid) tumor consists of two different neoplasms associated in the same renal nodule. Separate tumors are simultaneous neoplasms of different types occurring in two distinct settings, in association with hereditary disorders or sporadically [3]. In our case, the tumors had a sporadic occurrence and were separated by normal renal tissue.

There have been rare reports of the simultaneous occurrence of RCC and a variety of benign and malignant renal neoplasms within the same kidney. AML with concomitant CCRCC is seen commonly in patients with TS and rarely in patients without this syndrome [3, 4].

In our case, we used the clinical criteria (the revised Gomez Criteria) to rule out the diagnosis of TS; therefore, the patient underwent various clinical and paraclinical examinations from several medical specialists notably in dermatology, cardiology, ophthalmology, neurology, radiology, and dental medicine, and no major or minor clinical feature of TS was determined. In the 2012 International Tuberous Sclerosis Complex Consensus Group, comprising 79 specialists from 14 countries, organized into 12 subcommittees, each led by a clinician with advanced expertise in TS complex and the relevant medical subspecialty, special attention was given to evaluate the sensitivity and specificity of clinical findings with respect to TS diagnosis, and they concluded that clinical features of TS complex continue to be a principal means of diagnosis. The identification of either a TSC1 or TSC2 pathogenic mutation in DNA from the normal tissue is sufficient to make a definite diagnosis of TS but a significant fraction 10% to 25% of TS patients has no mutation identified by conventional genetic testing, and a normal result does not exclude TS or has any effect on the use of clinical diagnostic criteria to diagnose TS [6] (Table 1).

TS is an autosomal dominant disorder caused by the pathogenic mutation of TSC1 or TSC2 genes. It is characterized by mental retardation, seizures, and the development of cellular proliferations involving various organs, such as AML, subependymal giant cell tumors, cutaneous angiofibromas, cardiac rhabdomyomas, lymphangioleiomyomatosis, and pulmonary multifocal micronodular hyperplasia. Renal pathology is encountered in about 60% of TS patients, including renal cysts, AML, and epithelial neoplasms such as RCC and oncocytomas [4].

CCRCC are the most common type of RCC accounting for 65-70% of all renal cancers [1]. They are mostly sporadic and typically solitary cortical tumors. Like other renal

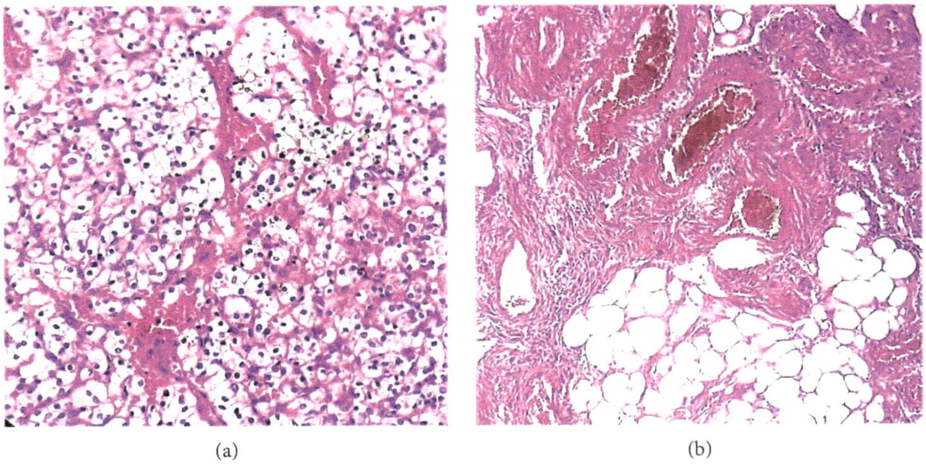

FIGURE 3: Hematoxylin and eosin staining demonstrating as follows. (a) CCRCC composed of nests of cells with clear cytoplasm, surrounded by a network of abundant thin-walled blood vessels. (b) AML composed of aggregates of thick-walled blood vessels, admixed with mature adipose tissue and smooth muscle cells.

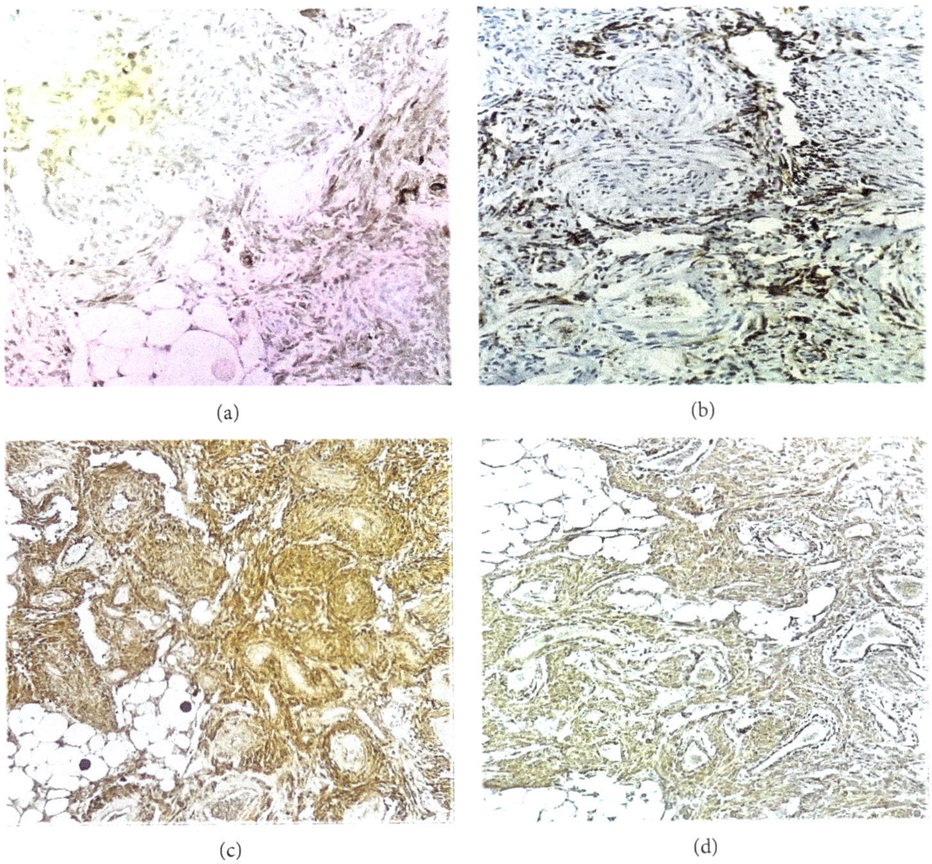

FIGURE 4: Immunohistochemical study of the AML showing the positivity of (a) Melan A, (b) HMB45, (c) H-Caldesmon, and (d) smooth muscle actin.

neoplasms, they could be found incidentally or manifested by nonspecific symptoms such as hematuria or lumbar pain. Radiologically, there is a large overlap of imaging features between benign and malignant renal masses that often makes difficult a correct characterization of these tumors [7]. CCRCC typically shows a heterogeneous consistency, demonstrates a high signal intensity on T2-weighted magnetic resonance imaging (MRI), and is hypervascular on dynamic contrast-enhanced CT or MRI examinations [8]. The diagnosis is made by pathological features. They are

Table 1: Updated diagnostic criteria for tuberous sclerosis complex 2012 (reproduced from Northrup and Krueger 2013).

A. Genetic diagnostic criteria
The identification of either a TSC1 or TSC2 pathogenic mutation in DNA from normal tissue is sufficient to make a definite diagnosis of TS. (note that 10% to 25% of TS patients have no mutation identified by conventional genetic testing, and a normal result does not exclude TS or has any effect on the use of clinical diagnostic criteria to diagnose TS).

B. Clinical diagnostic criteria
Major features
1. Hypomelanotic macules (≥3, at least 5 mm diameter)
2. Angiofibromas (≥3) or fibrous cephalic plaque
3. Ungual fibromas (≥2)
4. Shagreen patch
5. Multiple retinal hamartomas
6. Cortical dysplasias
7. Subependymal nodules
8. Subependymal giant cell astrocytoma
9. Cardiac rhabdomyoma
10. Lymphangioleiomyomatosis*
11. Angiomyolipomas (≥2)*
Minor features
1. "Confetti" skin lesions
2. Dental enamel pits (>3)
3. Intraoral fibromas (≥2)
4. Retinal achromic patch
5. Multiple renal cysts
6. Nonrenal hamartomas
Definite diagnosis: two major features or one major feature with ≥2 minor features
Possible diagnosis: either one major feature or ≥2 minor features
*A combination of the two major clinical features (LAM and angiomyolipomas) without other features does not meet criteria for a definite diagnosis.

morphologically composed of cells with clear or eosinophilic cytoplasm arranged most commonly in solid alveolar and acinar pattern and contain a regular network of small thin-walled blood vessels. The tumor cells express epithelial markers, PAX8, and CD10. Carbonic anhydrase IX had characteristically a diffuse membranous overexpression in 75-100% of CCRCC. In most of these tumors, there is a deletion or an unbalanced chromosomal translocation (3;6, 3;8, or 3;11) that is due to either somatic mutations or hypermethylation-induced inactivation in patients harboring the VHL gene [9].

AML are the most common mesenchymal tumors of the kidney, known for their variable morphology and benign clinical course. They are part of the PEComas family. Most cases of AML are sporadic with higher incidence in women (1/4) and a mean age of 38 years. In patients with TS, AML occur in younger age, and they are usually small, bilateral, and multiple, whereas sporadic AML are usually unilateral and solitary [10]. The clinical features depend on the presence or not of TS. In TS, AML are usually asymptomatic, whereas sporadic AML are more likely larger manifested by flank pain, heamaturia, palpable mass, or revealed by a massive retroperitoneal hemorrhage due to rupture, representing the most dangerous complication. Radiologically, classic AML is the only benign solid renal mass that can be characterized with confidence by imaging through the identification of fat without calcifications on CT or MRI; however, approximately 5% of AMLs are "fat poor," and there are rare cases of renal malignancies that contain fat, mimicking AML [7]. Morphologically, AML are composed of varying quantities of myoid spindle cells, adipose cells, and dysmorphic blood vessels. It is believed that these diverse tissue elements arise from the same cell of origin, the perivascular epithelioid cell, with its potential to differentiate into adipocytes, smooth muscle cells, endothelial cells, and HMB45 immunoreactive cells [11]. Immunohistochemically AML are characterized by the coexpression of melanocytic (HMB-45, Melan-A) and smooth muscle markers. Epithelial markers are always negative. There are several variants of renal AML, distinguished by histological features. The most important to recognize is the epithelioid AML, because of his malignant potential. It is also the subtype that raises the most the problem of differential diagnosis [12]. It can mimic a high-grade sarcomatoid renal cell carcinoma [9]. Histologically, the TS-associated AML are more likely to have an epithelioid component compared with the sporadic AML, which are typically triphasic [12, 13], like in our case.

Both sporadic and TS-associated AML frequently show a loss of heterozygosity at the TSC2-containing region on chromosome 16p and occasionally at the TSC1 region on chromosome 9p34 [9].

In a study, all patients with concomitant sporadic AML and RCN were female. The age range was 49 to 87 years with a mean age of 63.3 years [12]. The patient in our case was a 42-year-old female. Jimenez et al. studied 36 cases of coexistent RCN and AML and found that the majority of tumors associated with AML were CCRCC (62.5%), whereas the second most frequently associated tumor was oncocytoma [14]. Authors recommend the consideration of the possible coexistence of RCC with AML in cases with or without TS in the management of radiologically diagnosed AML accompanied by other renal masses of indeterminate nature [2].

The association of RCC and AML in the same kidney may be coincidental, or there could be a pathogenetic relationship [11]. The theory of cancer stem cells (CSCs) suggests that two or three dissimilar renal tumors could arise from CSCs. Another hypothesis explaining the pathogenesis of the coexistence of different renal tumors might be the evolution of one subtype to another [5]. Some studies claim that the RCN can develop from a preexistent AML [12].

The rarity of the reported cases and the limited follow-up data do not allow an accurate analysis of the prognosis of this combination of neoplasms; although, it seems that the prognosis depends mainly on the pathological stage of the RCC [14].

4. Conclusion

The coexistence of RCC with AML in the same kidney is rare, even more in patients without TS. Such cases should be accumulated and studied, to better understand the relationship among different types of renal tumors and to improve their management. In addition, this case is an opportunity to remind physicians to think of TS in front of this kind of tumor association which is most often seen in the context of this complex and to be aware of the various clinical and genetic diagnostic criteria to confirm or eliminate this diagnosis because the management will not be limited in these cases to the treatment of tumors.

Abbreviations

RCN: Renal cell neoplasm
AML: Angiomyolipomas
TS: Tuberous sclerosis
RCC: Renal cell carcinomas
CCRCC: Clear cell renal cell carcinoma
PEComas: Perivascular epithelioid cell tumors
CSCs: Cancer stem cells
CT: Computed tomography
MRI: Magnetic resonance imaging.

Consent

The patient in the article has given consent for the case report to be published.

References

[1] H. Moch, P. A. Humphrey, T. M. Ulbright, and V. E. Reuter, *WHO Classification of tumours of the urinary system and male genital organs*, vol. 8, 2016lyon, 2016.

[2] A. A. Petrolla and G. T. MacLennan, "Renal cell carcinoma and other concurrent renal neoplasms," *Journal of Urology*, vol. 178, no. 5, pp. 2163–2163, 2007.

[3] J. F. Val-Bernal, F. Villoria, and M. A. Pérez-Expósito, "Concurrent angiomyolipomas and renal cell carcinoma harboring metastatic foci of mammary carcinoma in the same kidney: an incidental autopsy finding in a patient with a follow-up of thirty years," *Annals of Diagnostic Pathology*, vol. 5, no. 5, pp. 293–299, 2001.

[4] A. Kakkar, A. G. Vallonthaiel, M. C. Sharma, G. Bora, A. Panda, and S. Amlesh, "Composite renal cell carcinoma and angiomyolipoma in a patient with tuberous sclerosis: a diagnostic dilemma," *Canadian Urological Association Journal*, vol. 9, no. 7-8, pp. E507–E510, 2015.

[5] J. Guo, M. S. Tretiakova, M. L. Troxell et al., "Tuberous sclerosis-associated renal cell Carcinoma," *American Journal of Surgical Pathology*, vol. 38, no. 11, pp. 1457–1467, 2014.

[6] H. Northrup, D. A. Krueger, H. Northrup et al., "Tuberous Sclerosis Complex Diagnostic Criteria Update: Recommendations of the 2012 International Tuberous Sclerosis Complex Consensus Conference," *Pediatric Neurology*, vol. 49, no. 4, pp. 243–254, 2013.

[7] M. Galia, D. Albano, A. Bruno et al., "Imaging features of solid renal masses," *The British Journal of Radiology*, vol. 90, no. 1077, p. 20170077, 2017.

[8] G. Low, G. Huang, W. Fu, Z. Moloo, and S. Girgis, "Review of renal cell carcinoma and its common subtypes in radiology," *World Journal of Radiology*, vol. 8, no. 5, pp. 484–500, 2016.

[9] S.-Y. Jun, K.-J. Cho, C.-S. Kim, A. G. Ayala, and J. Y. Ro, "Triple synchronous neoplasms in one kidney: report of a case and review of the literature,' *Annals of Diagnostic Pathology*, vol. 7, no. 6, pp. 374–380, 2003.

[10] S. Korula, A. Ekbote, N. Kumar, S. Danda, I. Agarwal, and S. Chaturvedi, "Renal manifestations of tuberous sclerosis among children: an Indian experience and review of the literature," *Clinical Kidney Journal*, vol. 7, no. 2, pp. 134–137, 2014.

[11] K. T. Mai, D. G. Perkins, S. Robertson, J. Thomas, C. Morrash, and J. P. Collins, "Composite renal cell carcinoma and angiomyolipoma: a study of the histogenetic relationship of the two lesions," *Pathology International*, vol. 49, no. 1, pp. 1–8, 1999.

[12] M. Mei, L. E. Rosen, V. Reddy, D. J. Cimbaluk, and P. Gattuso, "Concurrent angiomyolipomas and renal cell neoplasms in patients without tuberous sclerosis: a retrospective study," *International Journal of Surgical Pathology*, vol. 23, no. 4, pp. 265–270, 2015.

[13] T. Hatano and S. Egawa, "Renal angiomyolipoma with tuberous sclerosis complex: how it differs from sporadic angiomyolipoma in both management and care," *Asian Journal of Surgery*, vol. 43, no. 10, pp. 967–972, 2020.

[14] R. E. Jimenez, J. N. Eble, V. E. Reuter et al., "Concurrent angiomyolipoma and renal cell neoplasia: a study of 36 cases," *Modern Pathology*, vol. 14, no. 3, pp. 157–163, 2001.

21

Metastatic Renal Cell Carcinoma with Level IV Thrombus: Contemporary Management with Complete Response to Neoadjuvant Targeted Therapy

Abhishek Bhat,[1] Bruno Nahar,[1] Vivek Venkatramani,[1] Indraneel Banerjee,[1] Oleksandr N. Kryvenko,[1,2,3] and Dipen J. Parekh[1,3]

[1] *Department of Urology, University of Miami Miller School of Medicine, Miami, FL, USA*
[2] *Department of Pathology and Laboratory Medicine, University of Miami Miller School of Medicine, Miami, FL, USA*
[3] *Sylvester Comprehensive Cancer Center, University of Miami Miller School of Medicine, Miami, FL, USA*

Correspondence should be addressed to Abhishek Bhat; axb1722@med.miami.edu

Academic Editor: Fumitaka Koga

Renal cell carcinoma, particularly the most common clear cell type, is one of the most aggressive of urological cancers with significant risk of metastatic spread. It also has a propensity for venotropism with a proportion of tumors developing thrombi up to the right atrium. The response with newly adopted targeted therapy has been considered to be in the evolutionary stage with no clear role with respect to debulking or reducing the size of the inferior vena cava (IVC) thrombus. We describe a case of a right-sided metastatic RCC with Level IV thrombus initially managed with Pazopanib followed by Nivolumab and Adalimumab followed by cytoreductive nephrectomy and IVC thrombectomy in the post-targeted therapy setting with complete curative response.

1. Introduction

Renal cell cancers (RCC) comprise 3.8% of all new cancers in the United States with 90% of renal tumors being RCC and about 80% being clear cell type [1, 2]. The management of clinical Stage II and III renal cancers with inferior vena cava (IVC) extension includes radical nephrectomy [3]. Targeted therapy for advanced and metastatic RCC is widely used in first and second line treatments. We describe a case of advanced stage RCC with extension of thrombus into the right atrium and widespread visceral metastases who was initially treated with targeted therapy and then underwent posttherapy cytoreductive nephrectomy with IVC thrombectomy and metastasectomy with complete cure after downstaging had been achieved.

2. Case Report

A 57-year-old woman with good performance status was detected to have a large right renal mass with adrenal extension and tumor thrombus extending to the right atrium (Figures 1 and 3). She was also noted to have enhancing liver lesions (Figure 2), suggestive of metastatic disease (cT4N1M1). Pulmonary embolus and retroperitoneal lymphadenopathy were also noted. Biopsy of the mass revealed clear cell renal cell carcinoma, WHO ISUP nucleolar grade 3. She received Apixaban 10mg/day for management of pulmonary embolus.

She was started on Pazopanib 800 mg orally once daily which was later switched to Nivolumab after she developed upper gastrointestinal bleeding secondary to a duodenal ulcer.

Interval imaging 6 months after targeted therapy revealed a decrease in the size of the primary renal mass, although the thrombus extension into the IVC still persisted with development of new hilar lymphadenopathy and segmental pulmonary embolism. Nivolumab was continued and 3-month PET/CT showed further reduction in the size of the renal mass with thrombus extension now to the level of liver. There were new enhancing masses in the liver suspicious

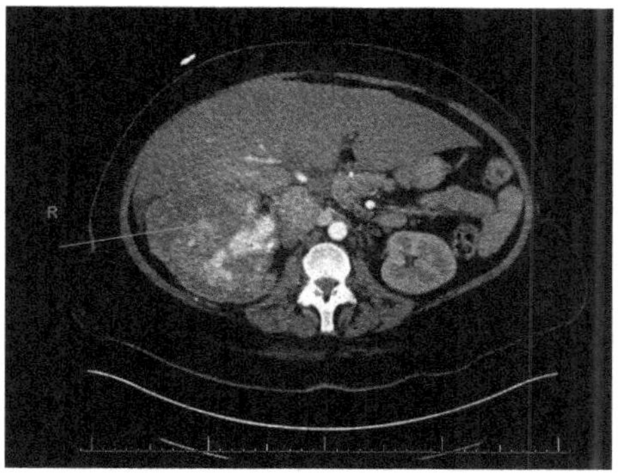

FIGURE 1: Right renal tumor with IVC thrombus.

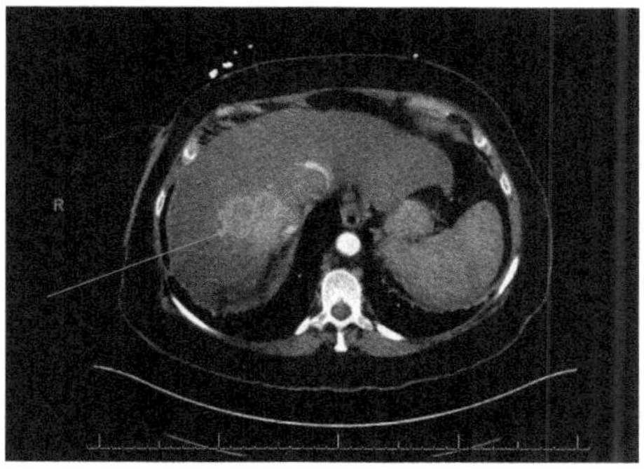

FIGURE 2: Liver metastases.

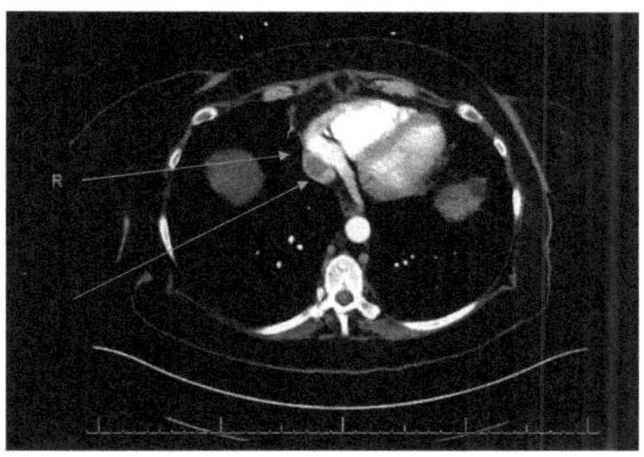

FIGURE 3: Extension of IVC thrombus to the right atrium.

for metastases with subcarinal, precarinal, and bilateral hilar mediastinal lymphadenopathy.

She was initiated on Cabozantinib in addition to the Nivolumab in view of new lymphadenopathy. She tolerated the new regimen very well and was completely symptom-free with this therapeutic combination (Figure 4). New imaging with PET/CT showed no FDG avid lesions anywhere in the body including the IVC thrombus with significant reduction in the size of the renal mass. MRI Angiogram of the abdomen showed the IVC thrombus invading the IVC lateral wall and situated below the hepatic veins (Figure 5).

Based on the imaging, it was decided to proceed with posttherapy right cytoreductive nephrectomy with IVC thrombectomy. The anticoagulant was stopped and bridging was done with Heparin prior to the surgery. Intraoperative findings were that of a large renal mass with an infiltrating IVC thrombus in the retrohepatic location (using TEE assistance) with no gross evidence of metastases. Open radical nephrectomy with IVC thrombectomy and caval reconstruction was carried out with complete tumor thrombus resection (Figure 6). The patient did well postoperatively and was discharged on 6th postoperative day symptom-free.

Radical nephrectomy specimen examination showed a necrotic nonviable carcinoma consistent with an RCC with complete response measuring 7 cm in size with perinephric extension. The tumor was extensively sampled and no viable carcinoma was detected (Figure 7). The necrotic tumor was surrounded by a thick fibromuscular pseudocapsule typically see in clear cell renal cell carcinoma which maintains its structure and did not have necrosis [4]. IVC specimen

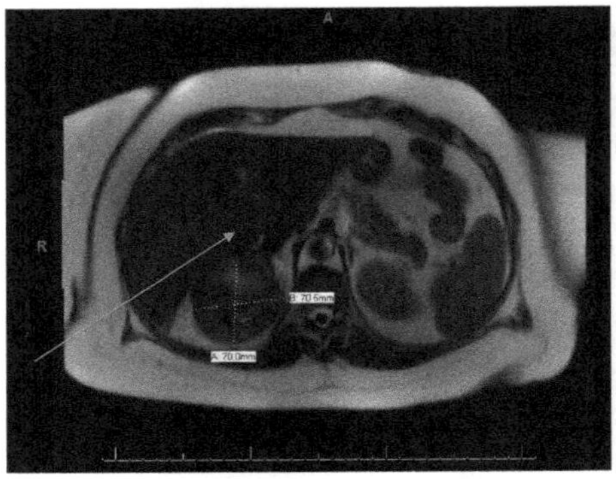

FIGURE 4: Resolution of liver metastases following neoadjuvant therapy.

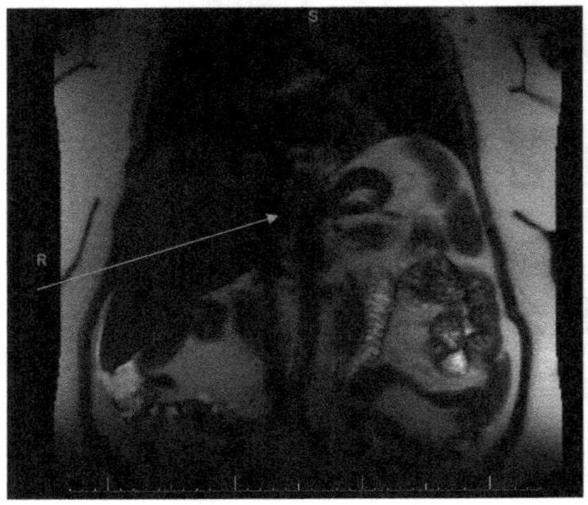

FIGURE 5: Presence of IVC thrombus at the infrahepatic level after neoadjuvant therapy.

showed a necrotic nonviable carcinoma in the lumen of renal vein as well (Figure 8). The AJCC 8th edition pathological stage was ypT0Nx Mn/a.

She was fully back to her activities of daily living with no complaints at the time of her first follow-up visit to the clinic at the postoperative visit at 3 weeks. She will continue to follow up with both the Urological Oncology and Medical Oncology teams. She has not been planned for adjuvant targeted therapy at this stage in view of no evidence of residual disease.

3. Discussion

The management of metastatic RCC with Level IV IVC thrombus is complex and requires multimodality treatments. Current available literature supports the potential increasing role of targeted therapy in the neoadjuvant setting for the management of metastatic RCC and advanced RCC. The therapy does seem safe and feasible with no significant complications. The priority in this case from our standpoint was to achieve substantial downgrading of the tumor and to ensure control of metastatic disease. When this had been accomplished, the next step was posttherapy cytoreductive nephrectomy with IVC thrombectomy.

Pazopanib is a preferred Category 1 option for first line treatment of patients with relapsed or medically unresectable Stage IV clear cell RCC. This is supported by the results of the COMPARZ and the PISCES trial which showed a comparable oncological control with fewer side effects reported [5–7].

The data for first line Nivolumab in combination with Ipilimumab for favorable risk patients has been mixed. The Checkmate 214 trial showed that the combination of Nivolumab and Ipilimumab produced a higher objective response rate (42% vs 27%, $p<0.001$) and a higher complete response rate (9% vs 1%, $p<0.001$) compared to Sunitinib monotherapy [7]. This has led to the combination being recommended as a Category 1, preferred treatment option for first line treatment for intermediate and poor risk patients with previously untreated, relapsed or medically unresectable predominantly Stage IV clear cell renal cell carcinoma.

Patients treated with Cabozantinib as a primary treatment modality showed a significantly increased median progression free survival (PFS) compared to those treated with Sunitinib. They also showed a significantly higher objective response rate (ORR) compared to Sunitinib (46% vs 18%) [8].

One of the benefits of preoperative systemic treatment is the possible reduction in the size of the primary tumor to make it resectable. This has received variable reporting in literature with wide variation in the treatment protocols and adoption. Despite this, there does seem to be some evidence to achieve downstaging in truly unresectable tumors. Thomas et al. reported a series of 19 patients with unresectable

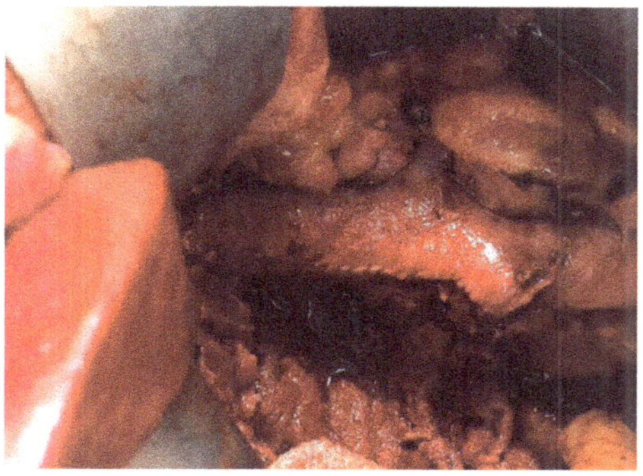

FIGURE 6: Radical Nephrectomy with complete IVC thrombectomy and caval reconstruction.

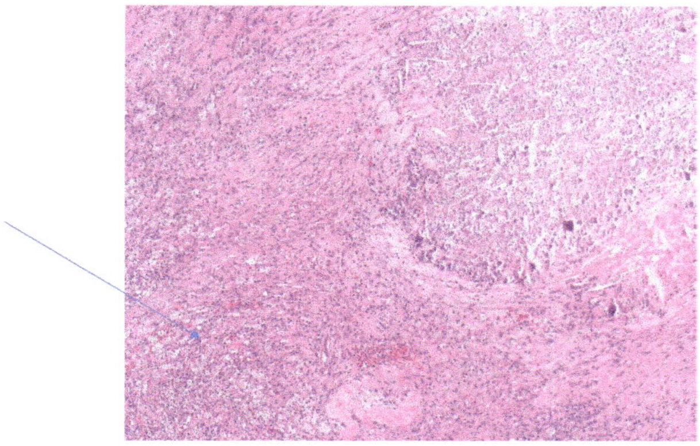

FIGURE 7: Necrotic tumor with calcifications surrounded by foamy histiocyte reaction.

or bilateral tumors who received neoadjuvant Sunitinib. 15 patients were able to undergo radical nephrectomy thereafter with mean reduction in tumor size by 16% and significant reduction in tumor burden [9]. In another case series, there was significant tumor size reduction by 14%. Three of 10 patients underwent radical nephrectomy after 4 weeks of Sunitinib with significant tumor necrosis being reported on pathology due to the antiangiogenic action of the targeted therapy [10].

The commonly used RECIST criteria to look for response to standardized treatment may not be effective as antiangiogenic therapy may not affect the size of the tumor but effectively produces intratumoral necrosis which is not assessed at all [11]. Further, it has been demonstrated in studies that loss of intratumoral enhancement and density may be more reliable indicators of preoperative tumor therapy than tumor size alone [12].

Preoperative therapy to produce a reduction in the level of IVC thrombus has remained ineffective with IVC thrombectomy alone remaining the standard of care. Much of the existing literature on the use of preoperative therapy in the setting of an IVC thrombus comes from single center studies. The study by Cost et al. demonstrated there was minimal clinical effect on RCC thrombi with only one case of thrombus level regression from Level IV to Level II [13].

There have been data in the form of randomized controlled trials to demonstrate that overall survival does not increase with a cytoreductive nephrectomy in intermediate and poor risk patients. However this data is not robust for favorable risk patients [14]. Our patient was in the intermediate risk category in view of synchronous metastatic disease and targeted therapy along with posttherapy cytoreductive nephrectomy showed dramatic response, with downstaging of the tumor thrombus as well. This aspect of targeted therapy needs more studies and trials and could prove to be an effective management of select patients with advanced disease.

4. Conclusion

Downstaging the advanced primary tumor, tumor thrombus, and metastases provides an option of radical nephrectomy. Although current literature does not advocate neoadjuvant therapy for downstaging the level of IVC thrombus, we found a significant downstaging in the level of the thrombus from Level IV to Level II. Although the standards for neoadjuvant therapy have still not been established due to paucity of literature, more research is required to shed light on management of such tumors.

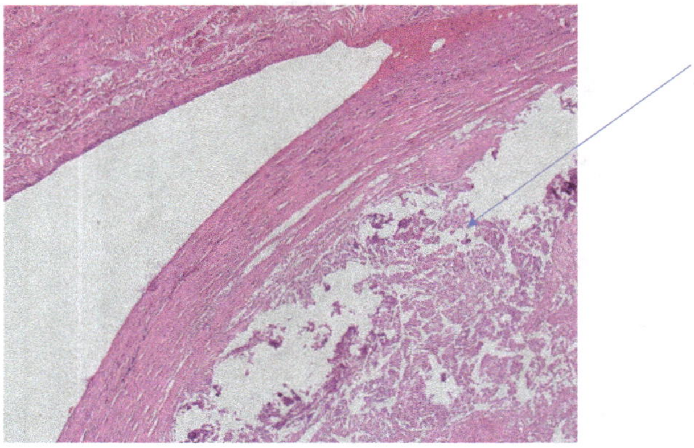

FIGURE 8: Necrotic tumor in renal vein.

References

[1] B. C. Leibovich, C. M. Lohse, P. L. Crispen et al., "Histological subtype is an independent predictor of outcome for patients with renal cell carcinoma," *The Journal of Urology*, vol. 183, no. 4, pp. 1309–1316, 2010.

[2] H. Moch, T. Gasser, M. B. Amin, J. Torhorst, G. Sauter, and M. J. Mihatsch, "Prognostic utility of the recently recommended histologic classification and revised TNM staging system of renal cell carcinoma: a swiss experience with 588 tumors," *Cancer*, vol. 89, no. 3, pp. 604–614, 2000.

[3] J.-H. Luo, F.-J. Zhou, D. Xie et al., "Analysis of long-term survival in patients with localized renal cell carcinoma: laparoscopic versus open radical nephrectomy," *World Journal of Urology*, vol. 28, no. 3, pp. 289–293, 2010.

[4] L. Roquero, O. N. Kryvenko, N. S. Gupta, and M. W. Lee, "Characterization of fibromuscular pseudocapsule in renal cell carcinoma," *International Journal of Surgical Pathology*, vol. 23, no. 5, pp. 359–363, 2015.

[5] R. J. Motzer, N. B. Haas, F. Donskov et al., "Randomized phase III trial of adjuvant pazopanib versus placebo after nephrectomy in patients with localized or locally advanced renal cell carcinoma," *Journal of Clinical Oncology*, vol. 35, no. 35, pp. 3916–3923, 2017.

[6] R. J. Motzer, T. E. Hutson, D. Cella et al., "Pazopanib versus sunitinib in metastatic renal-cell carcinoma," *The New England Journal of Medicine*, vol. 369, no. 8, pp. 722–731, 2013.

[7] R. J. Motzer, N. M. Tannir, D. F. McDermott, O. Arén Frontera, B. Melichar, T. K. Choueiri et al., "Nivolumab plus ipilimumab versus sunitinib in advanced renal-cell carcinoma," *The New England Journal of Medicine*, vol. 378, no. 14, pp. 1277–1290, 2018.

[8] T. K. Choueiri, S. Halabi, B. L. Sanford et al., "Cabozantinib versus sunitinib as initial targeted therapy for patients with metastatic renal cell carcinoma of poor or intermediate risk: the alliance A031203 CABOSUN trial," *Journal of Clinical Oncology: Official Journal of the American Society of Clinical Oncology*, vol. 35, no. 6, pp. 591–597, 2017.

[9] A. A. Thomas, B. I. Rini, B. R. Lane et al., "Response of the primary tumor to neoadjuvant sunitinib in patients with advanced renal cell carcinoma," *The Journal of Urology*, vol. 181, no. 2, pp. 518–523, 2009.

[10] A. Bex, A. A. M. van der Veldt, C. Blank et al., "Neoadjuvant sunitinib for surgically complex advanced renal cell cancer of doubtful resectability: Initial experience with downsizing to reconsider cytoreductive surgery," *World Journal of Urology*, vol. 27, no. 4, pp. 533–539, 2009.

[11] N. J. Hellenthal, W. Underwood, R. Penetrante et al., "Prospective clinical trial of preoperative sunitinib in patients with renal cell carcinoma," *The Journal of Urology*, vol. 184, no. 3, pp. 859–864, 2010.

[12] C. L. Cowey, J. R. Fielding, and W. Kimryn Rathmell, "The loss of radiographic enhancement in primary renal cell carcinoma tumors following multitargeted receptor tyrosine kinase therapy is an additional indicator of response," *Urology*, vol. 75, no. 5, pp. 1108–1113.el, 2010.

[13] N. Cost, S. Delacroix, J. Sleeper et al., "The impact of targeted molecular therapies on the level of renal cell carcinoma vena caval tumor thrombus," *European Urology*, vol. 59, no. 6, pp. 912–918, 2011.

[14] A. Méjean, A. Ravaud, S. Thezenas, S. Colas, J-B. Beauval, K. Bensalah et al., "Sunitinib alone or after nephrectomy in metastatic renal-cell carcinoma," *The New England Journal of Medicine*, vol. 3, no. 0, 2018.

22

Robotic-Assisted Partial Nephrectomy and Adrenalectomy: Case of a Pheochromocytoma Invading into Renal Parenchyma

Zeynep G. Gul, Christine W. Liaw, Avinash Reddy, and Reza Mehrazin

Department of Urology, Icahn School of Medicine at Mount Sinai, New York, NY, USA

Correspondence should be addressed to Christine W. Liaw; christineliaw6@gmail.com

Academic Editor: David Duchene

Although upper pole renal masses and adrenal masses can usually be distinguished on cross-sectional imaging, large masses can obscure the boundaries between the kidney and adrenal gland. We describe a unique case of an adrenal pheochromocytoma in a 42-year-old female who was referred for robotic partial nephrectomy. During the procedure, the patient developed severe hypertension. The case was aborted, and the workup revealed pheochromocytoma. After appropriate pretreatment, the patient underwent a successful robotic adrenalectomy and partial nephrectomy. Therefore, we recommend screening patients with hypertension and large upper pole masses for pheochromocytoma to better direct preoperative management.

1. Introduction

Pheochromocytomas are catecholamine-secreting tumors that arise from the chromaffin cells of the adrenal medulla or the paraganglia. Pheochromocytomas represent about 5% of all adrenal masses [1]. Although they are both located within Gerota's fascia, adrenal and renal masses are usually easily distinguished on imaging. Here, we describe a unique case of an adrenal pheochromocytoma in a 42-year-old African American female who was referred for robotic partial nephrectomy.

2. Case Presentation

The patient presented to an outside hospital with chest pain, shortness of breath, and diaphoresis. She was found to be hypertensive and have an elevated troponin with ST depressions on EKG. During the hospital admission, the patient required intubation secondary to hypertensive emergency and flash pulmonary edema. Workup included a left heart catheterization, which showed normal coronaries, and a CT angiogram, which revealed a large right renal mass. The patient was diagnosed with congestive heart failure and discharged after a 6-day admission on lisinopril, metoprolol, furosemide, and aspirin.

The patient was then referred to our center for robotic partial nephrectomy. In the office, the patient was well appearing and normotensive. An MRI renal mass protocol was ordered to further evaluate the renal lesion and revealed a 5.7 cm, heterogeneous, exophytic right upper pole renal mass (Figure 1). On the day of the surgery, the case began uneventfully; the robotic ports were placed and the abdomen was insufflated without any issues. The da Vinci Xi® robot was docked, but during the initial mobilization of the bowel, the patient developed severe hypertension up to 270/110 mmHg. Insufflation was immediately discontinued, and subsequently, her systolic blood pressure dropped to the 180s. Anesthesia started clevidipine and esmolol drips, and her blood pressure normalized to 110/80. The case was aborted, and the patient was admitted for workup of a possible pheochromocytoma.

Endocrinology was consulted and performed a complete evaluation. Significant findings included elevated plasma normetanephrine and metanephrine levels, which were 4533 pg/ml (normal 0-145 pg/mL) and 1410 (normal 0-62 pg/mL), respectively. She was diagnosed with a

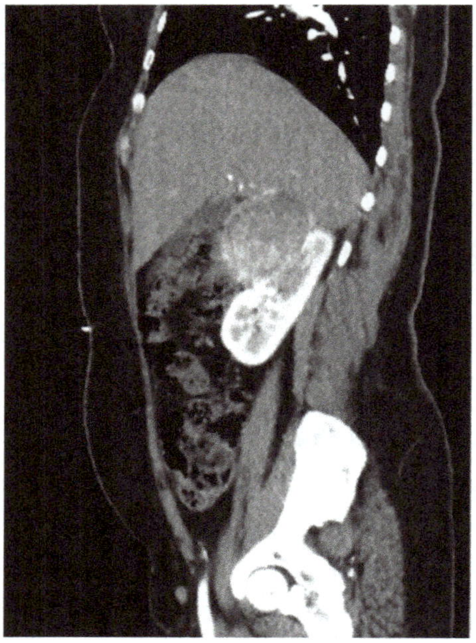

Figure 1: A 5.7 cm mass that appears to arise from the right kidney.

pheochromocytoma and started on phenoxybenzamine 10 mg twice a day and nifedipine 60 mg. Metoprolol was continued and lisinopril was stopped. She was discharged home.

One month later, she returned to the operating room for robotic right adrenalectomy and partial nephrectomy. Initially, the medial attachments and vasculature feeding the tumor were controlled using clips and electrocautery. Next, the main adrenal vein was controlled and the mass was circumferentially dissected. The mass appeared to penetrate into the upper pole of the kidney, and the upper pole renal parenchyma had to be excised in order to resect the entire tumor. The renal parenchymal bed was then repaired using a barbed suture. The procedure was uneventful and the patient was discharged on postoperative day one. Final pathology revealed an 8.3 cm pheochromocytoma involving the adrenal gland and adjacent to the renal parenchyma (Figure 2).

3. Discussion

In general, upper pole renal masses and adrenal masses can be distinguished by cross-sectional imaging. However, with large masses, it can be more difficult to identify boundaries between the kidney and adrenal gland. There have been a limited number of case reports in which adrenal masses were thought to be renal masses or vice versa [2–4]. In the case of our patient, the appearance of the mass on imaging was suggestive of a renal origin. First, MRI demonstrated the characteristic "claw" sign, which describes when the normal parenchyma of the organ of origin wraps around the developing mass (Figure 3(a)). Second, the adrenal gland was identified on imaging and thought to be displaced by the renal mass (Figure 3(b)).

Of note, one interesting point is that the patient was started on a beta blocker for the initial diagnosis of congestive heart failure. With her true diagnosis of pheochromocytoma, we would expect rebound hypertension. Singular beta blockade with the unopposed vasoconstriction leads to rebound hypertension; alpha blockade is more critical during the medical management of pheochromocytomas [5].

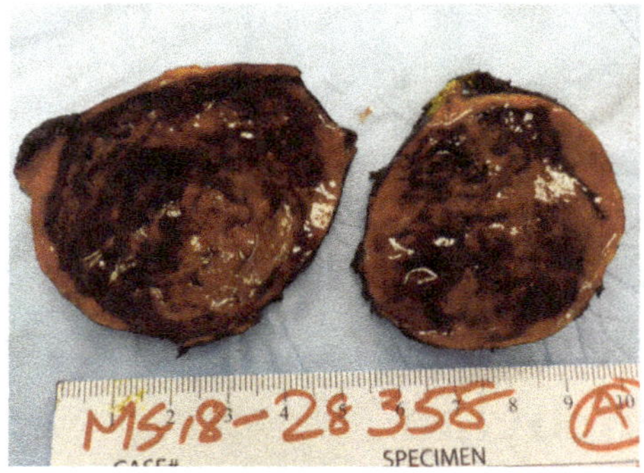

Figure 2: Final gross pathology specimen.

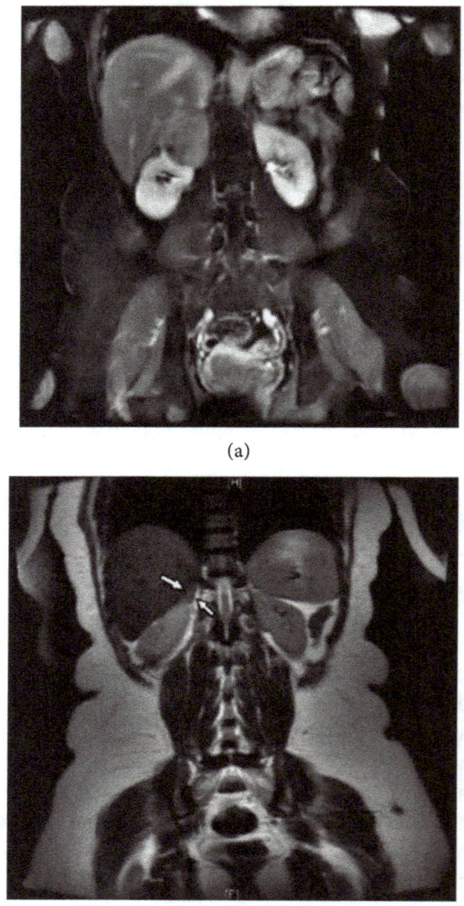

(a)

(b)

Figure 3: (a) The renal parenchyma can be seen creeping alongside the mass, a finding known as the "claw" sign, and is consistent with a mass of renal origin. (b) The right adrenal gland was identified on MRI and noted to be distinct from the renal mass.

4. Conclusion

Current guidelines state that all incidentally diagnosed adrenal masses should undergo a metabolic workup to exclude pheochromocytoma [1]. However, no guidelines exist on the indications for metabolic workup when the mass is not clearly adrenal in origin. Considering that the incidence of pheochromocytomas is 0.2-0.6% among all patients with a new diagnosis of hypertension [1], we suspect that among patients with hypertension and a large upper pole renal mass the incidence of pheochromocytomas is much higher. Therefore, we recommend screening patients with hypertension and large upper pole masses for pheochromocytomas in order to better direct preoperative management.

Consent

Informed consent was obtained from the patient regarding this publication.

References

[1] J. W. M. Lenders, Q. Y. Duh, G. Eisenhofer et al., "Pheochromocytoma and paraganglioma: an endocrine society clinical practice guideline," *The Journal of Clinical Endocrinology and Metabolism*, vol. 99, no. 6, pp. 1915–1942, 2014.

[2] M. K. Moslemi, S. Al-Mousawi, and M. H. Dehghani Firoozabadi, "Renal cell carcinoma mimicking adrenal tumor," *Journal of Oncology*, vol. 2010, Article ID 987128, 3 pages, 2010.

[3] S. T. Laroia, V. Jain, and A. Rastogi, "Beyond the boundaries: enigma of distinguishing exophytic upper pole renal cell carcinoma from an adrenal mass," *World Journal of Nephrology and Urology*, vol. 4, no. 2, pp. 222–225, 2015.

[4] M. Adas, B. Koc, G. Adas, O. Yalcin, S. Celik, and Ö. Kemik, "Pitfalls in the diagnosis of pheochromocytoma: a case series and review of the literature," *Journal of Epidemiological Research*, vol. 2, no. 2, pp. 49–55, 2015.

[5] R. Darr, J. W. M. Lenders, L. C. Hofbauer, B. Naumann, S. R. Bornstein, and G. Eisenhofer, "Pheochromocytoma - update on disease management," *Therapeutic Advances in Endocrinology and Metabolism*, vol. 3, no. 1, pp. 11–26, 2012.

23

Novel Technique for Hand-Assisted Laparoscopic Nephrectomy for Advanced Renal Cell Carcinoma with Renal Vein and Inferior Vena Cava Thrombi: Three Case Reports

Yuichi Machida,[1] Hiroki Yoshiuchi,[2] Yuko Kitano,[2] Yoshikazu Kuroki,[2] Masato Kamizuru,[2] and Junji Uchida[1]

[1]*Department of Urology, Osaka Metropolitan University Graduate School of Medicine, 1-4-3 Asahi-machi, Abeno-ku, Osaka 545-8585, Japan*
[2]*Department of Urology, Yao Municipal Hospital, 1-3-1, Ryuge-cho, Yao-City, Osaka 581-0069, Japan*

Correspondence should be addressed to Yuichi Machida; ymachida0719@gmail.com

Academic Editor: Tun-Chieh Chen

Introduction. The treatment of thrombi in the renal vein (RV) and inferior vena cava (IVC) requires advanced laparoscopic experience. We present three cases of hand-assisted laparoscopic nephrectomy (HALN) using a novel technique for treating advanced renal cell carcinoma (RCC) with thrombi in the RV and IVC. *Case Presentation.* Three patients with RCC with RV or IVC thrombus below level I underwent HALN. Two patients had right RCC with RV and IVC thrombi. One patient had left RCC with an RV thrombus. We hooked a vessel loop to the end of the thrombus and pulled it up manually to make space for vascular processing. The RV was narrowed and dissected using Hem-o-lok clips or an Endo GIA stapler. *Conclusion.* In carefully selected cases, renal vascular processing could be easily and safely performed using a vessel loop in HALN with thrombectomy.

1. Introduction

In 2000, Savage and Gill reported the first laparoscopic radical nephrectomy (LRN) for a case of renal cell carcinoma (RCC) with thrombus extending into the renal vein (RV) [1]. To date, multiple case reports and case series have been presented on the successful use of pure laparoscopic, laparoscopic-assisted, or hand-assisted LRN and thrombectomy. These studies used the Satinsky vascular clamp or laparoscopic bulldog clamp to control the inferior vena cava (IVC), which requires experience in laparoscopic vascular suturing.

Reports have shown that hand-assisted laparoscopic nephrectomy (HALN) has the advantages of shorter operative time and fewer complications than LRN [2–4]. However, if the RV does not have enough space for vascular clips or endoscopic stapling devices, laparoscopic IVC suturing must be performed by placing a laparoscopic clamp or an open conversion, which reduces the advantages of HALN.

Here, we report the results of a case series of the modified HALN technique with vascular loops in patients with advanced RCC with RV and IVC thrombi below level I.

2. Case Presentation

Three patients with RCC with RV or IVC thrombus below level I underwent HALN at Yao Municipal Hospital between January 2016 and December 2020. Tumor thrombus level was defined according to the Mayo classification of macroscopic venous invasion in RCC, with level I defined as a thrombus either at the entry of the RV or within the IVC less than 2 cm from the confluence of the RV and IVC. The same surgeon performed all surgeries.

The patient was placed in the lateral decubitus position. The port layout is shown in Figure 1. An 8 cm incision was

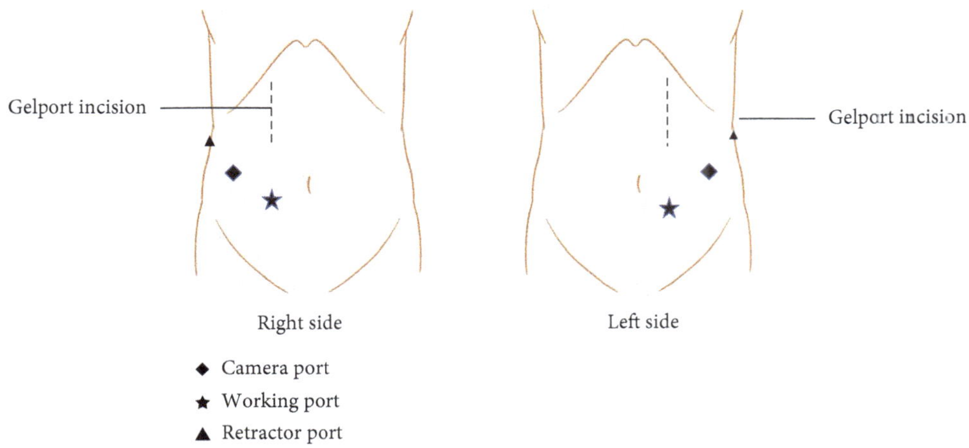

FIGURE 1: Placement of the hand port and trocars.

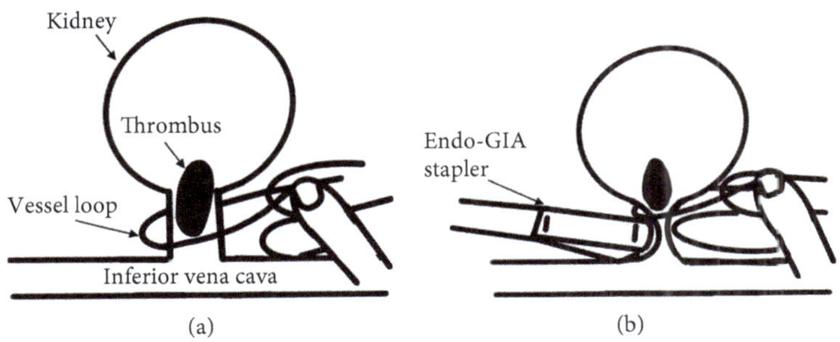

FIGURE 2: Schema of vascular processing in hand-assisted laparoscopic nephrectomy. (a) Thrombus tip is hooked using a vessel loop. (b) Thrombus is pulled up using the vessel loop, creating space for it to be processed using the Endo GIA stapler.

made from below the costal arch along the outer edge of the rectus abdominis muscle through which the GelPort® was inserted. The incision position of the hand port was higher than that in conventional HALN [5]. This modification allowed the intra-abdominal hand to be closer to the renal hilum for easier handling.

The schema of vessel processing using a vessel loop is shown in Figure 2. A laparoscopic retractor was used to elevate the kidney from the caudal side, and the renal artery was ligated using Hem-o-lok® clips before approaching the RV. Doppler ultrasound was performed to identify the end of the tumor thrombus. We hooked a vessel loop to the end of the thrombus and pulled it up manually to make space for vascular processing. The RV was narrowed and dissected using an Endo GIA stapler or Hem-o-lok clips. The specimen was removed from the hand port incision.

Figure 3 shows computed tomography (CT) or magnetic resonance imaging and intraoperative findings of the cases with right RCC (cases 1 and 2), and Figure 4 shows those of the case with left RCC (case 3). In case 1, CT demonstrated a tumor thrombus extending 0.5 cm into the IVC. In case 3, the thrombus extended 2 mm beyond the right aortic border to within 1.5 cm of the left border of the IVC. In all cases, the thrombi could be pulled up proximally using a vessel loop, facilitating subsequent vascular ligation with an Endo GIA stapler or Hem-o-lok clips. The procedure was successful in all patients without open conversion or complications. All patients had negative resection margins.

3. Discussion

In this study, we demonstrated our modified HALN technique using a vessel loop in patients with RCC with RV and IVC thrombi below level I. The greatest advantage of this novel technique may be that the end of the thrombus can be hooked onto the vessel loop and pulled up while elevating the renal hilus via delicate manipulation of the fingertips. An intra-abdominal hand improves tactile feedback to the surgeon, thereby lowering the threshold for laparoscopic surgery [5]. Since adhesions around the renal hilus are expected in such an invasive cancer, inadvertent manipulation using forceps may lead to bleeding, so that manipulation by blunt dissection of the fingertips might be the optimal technique to avoid surgical complications. This novel technique may allow simpler and less invasive vascular treatment of the RV with thrombus. Furthermore, if the tumor thrombus is inadequately resected by our method, or if there is bleeding due to inadequate vascular control,

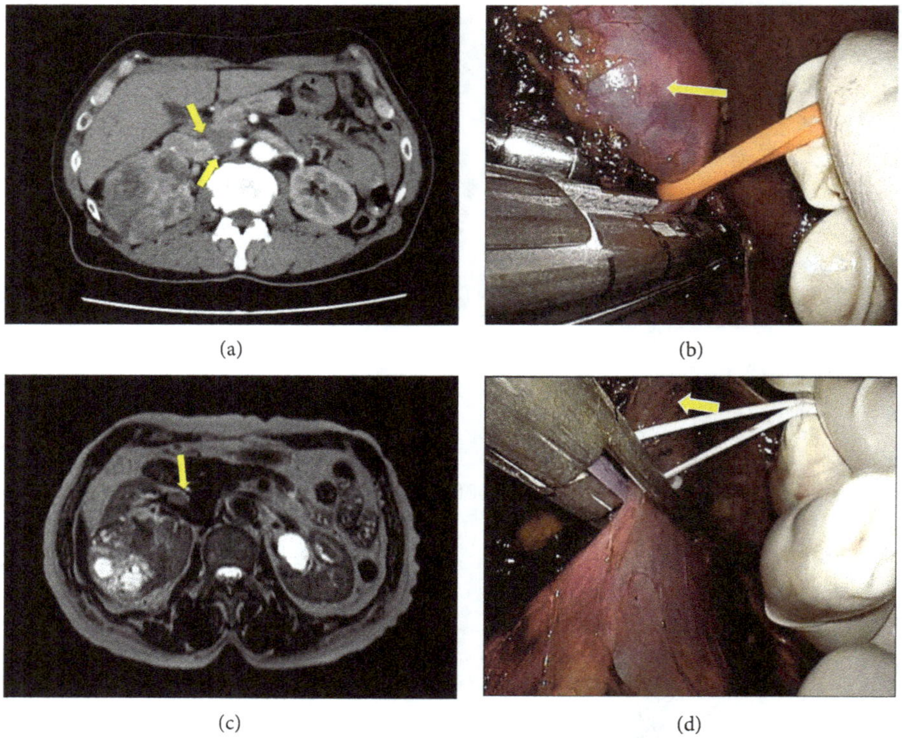

FIGURE 3: Imaging and intraoperative findings of the cases of right renal cell carcinoma (RCC) with thrombus ((a, b) case 1 and (c, d) case 2). (a) Computed tomography demonstrated a renal tumor thrombus extending 0.5 cm into the inferior vena cava. (b) The tumor was pulled up within the renal vein using the vessel loop, and the renal vein was divided using the Endo GIA stapler. (c) Magnetic resonance imaging demonstrated a renal tumor thrombus within the renal vein. (d) The tumor was pulled up using the vessel loop, and the renal vein was divided using the Endo GIA stapler. Arrowheads indicate the tip of the tumor thrombus.

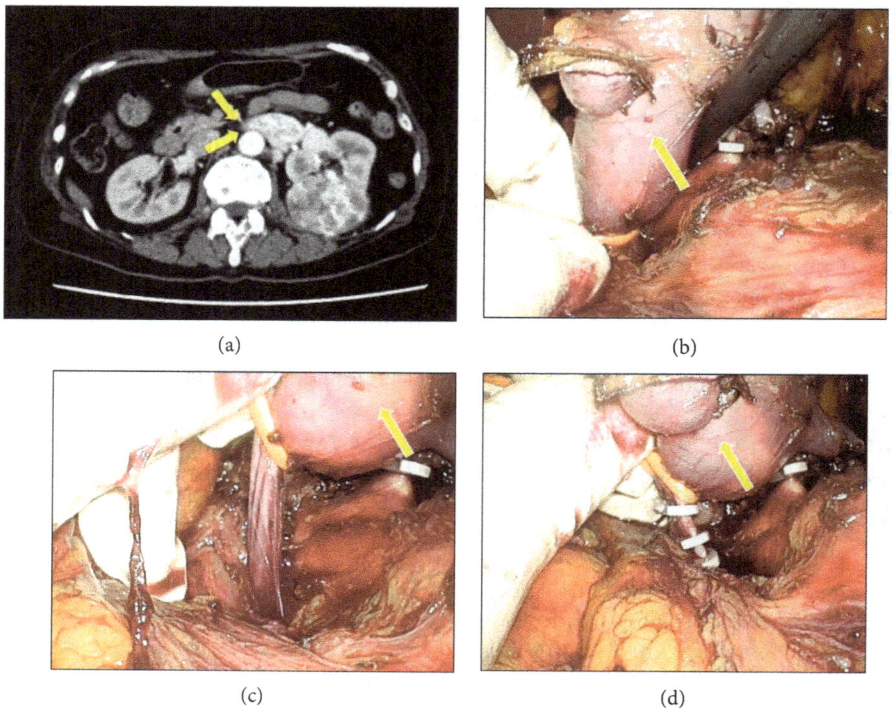

FIGURE 4: Imaging and intraoperative findings of the cases with left renal cell carcinoma with thrombus (case 3). (a) Computed tomography demonstrated a thrombus extending 2 mm beyond the right aortic border. (b) A vessel loop hooked to the thrombus tip. (c) The thrombus was pulled up using a vessel loop. (d) The left renal vein was dissected using Hem-o-lok clips. Arrowheads indicate the tip of the tumor thrombus.

the position of our hand port allows easy access to the renal vessels, making it easy to treat the vessels under direct vision through the hand port incision even when laparoscopic techniques are difficult to perform.

Although the dissection of the RV with thrombus has been reported to be possible in pure laparoscopic surgery by forceps manipulation, milking the thrombus and clipping the RV are difficult, and securing the field of view in the renal hilum is more difficult than that in HALN. Moreover, HALN has been reported to have advantages when the tumor is massive or the patient's medical complications require a prompt response; HALN may avoid unnecessary conversion to open surgery [6].

However, there might be significant limitations in the use of this novel HALN technique. It can only be used for treating RCC with thrombus that has little progression to the IVC. If a vessel loop cannot be hooked to the edge of the thrombus because of thrombus development, vascular dissection using this procedure is impossible. In such cases, the IVC can be clamped laparoscopically using a bulldog or Satinsky clamp and closed by running a 3-0 polypropylene suture after tumor removal, requiring a more complex technique [7, 8]. Kovac and Luke reported that for a case of right RCC with a 1 cm thrombus extending into the IVC undergoing HALN, lateral traction by hand was applied to the right kidney, allowing the thrombus to be pulled into the RV and away from the IVC [9]. In this study, a laparoscopic retractor was used to elevate the kidney from the caudal side, allowing the thrombus to return into the RV. However, in cases where the thrombus does not return to the RV after such a procedure, the aforementioned suture technique is required, and the surgeon must be proficient in laparoscopic suture techniques.

4. Conclusions

We demonstrated that HALN is technically safe and effective for renal tumors with thrombus below level I. The use of a vessel loop in dissecting the RV with thrombus is easier to divide with an endovascular stapler or Hem-o-lok clips than previously reported techniques.

Ethical Approval

The patient provided informed consent to publish images and details in the study.

Acknowledgments

We express our appreciation to the operation room personnel of Yao Municipal Hospital.

References

[1] S. J. Savage and I. S. Gill, "Laparoscopic radical nephrectomy for renal cell carcinoma in a patient with level I renal vein tumor thrombus," *The Journal of Urology*, vol. 163, no. 4, pp. 1243-1244, 2000.

[2] C. P. Nelson and J. S. Wolf Jr., "Comparison of hand assisted versus standard laparoscopic radical nephrectomy for suspected renal cell carcinoma," *The Journal of Urology*, vol. 167, no. 5, pp. 1989–1994, 2002.

[3] S. P. Hedican, T. D. Moon, P. S. Lowry, and S. Y. Nakada, "Hand-assisted laparoscopic renal surgery in the morbidly and profoundly obese," *Journal of Endourology*, vol. 18, no. 3, pp. 241–244, 2004.

[4] F. Hernandez, K. H. Rha, P. A. Pinto et al., "Laparoscopic nephrectomy: assessment of morcellation versus intact specimen extraction on postoperative status," *The Journal of Urology*, vol. 170, no. 2, pp. 412–415, 2003.

[5] S. P. Sterrett and S. Y. Nakada, "Hand-assisted radical laparoscopic nephrectomy," *BJU International*, vol. 102, no. 3, pp. 404–415, 2008.

[6] X. Guo, H. Wang, Y. Xiang, X. Jin, and S. Jiang, "Safety and oncological outcomes for large (stage >/=T2b) and locally advanced renal cell carcinoma: comparison between laparoscopic and modified hand-assisted laparoscopic radical nephrectomy," *The Journal of International Medical Research*, vol. 48, no. 10, p. 300060520961238, 2020.

[7] W. Wang, L. Wang, J. Xu, T. S. Adams, Y. Tian, and W. Lv, "Pure retroperitoneal laparoscopic radical nephrectomy for right renal masses with renal vein and inferior vena cava thrombus," *Journal of Endourology*, vol. 28, no. 7, pp. 819–824, 2014.

[8] O. Cinar, K. O. Gunseren, C. Cicek, B. A. Vuruskan, and H. Vuruskan, "Laparoscopic transperitoneal radical nephrectomy for renal masses with level I and II thrombus," *Journal of Laparoendoscopic & Advanced Surgical Techniques. Part A*, vol. 29, no. 1, pp. 35–39, 2019.

[9] J. R. Kovac and P. P. Luke, "Hand-assisted laparoscopic radical nephrectomy in the treatment of a renal cell carcinoma with a level II vena cava thrombus," *International Braz J Urol*, vol. 36, no. 3, pp. 327–331, 2010.

24

Renal Carcinoma and Kartagener Syndrome: An Unusual Association

Hamza Dergamoun, Abdelilah El Alaoui, Imad Boualaoui, Hachem Sayegh, Lounis Benslimane, and Yassine Nouini

Department of Urology A, Ibn Sina Hospital, Mohammed V University, Rabat, Morocco

Correspondence should be addressed to Hamza Dergamoun; hamza.dergamoun@gmail.com

Academic Editor: Giorgio Carmignani

Background. The association of renal cell carcinoma and Kartagener's syndrome is unusual, and only eleven cases have been reported in the literature. The purpose of this work is to analyze this unusual association of Kartagener's syndrome and renal cell tumor and to study the main diagnostic and therapeutic aspects through our observation and review of the literature. *Case Presentation.* We report the case of a 50-year-old patient, with a history of recurrent respiratory infections, in whom a renal tumor was simultaneously diagnosed with Kartagener's syndrome, represented by situs inversus, bronchiectasia, and chronic sinusitis. The patient was treated by partial nephrectomy, and the histological examination showed a clear cell carcinoma. Through this observation and a review of the literature, we try to analyze this association as well as the main diagnostic and therapeutic aspects. *Conclusion.* The association of situs inversus and renal cell carcinoma is very rare—preoperative assessment and anatomy knowledge are crucial for a better adaptation of the surgical technique.

1. Background

Kartagener's syndrome is rare. Bronchiectasis, chronic sinusitis, and situs inversus are the classic three abnormalities. This syndrome is a part of primary ciliary dyskinesias (PCD), a rare genetic group of diseases that involve a constitutional abnormality of the cilia leading to respiratory damages [1, 2]. More rarely, PCD may be associated with cardiac, renal, or sensory defects, resulting in complex phenotypes. There is no known evidence that situs inversus increases the risk of malignancy [3]. The association of renal cell carcinoma and Kartagener's syndrome is unusual, and only 11 cases have been reported in the literature.

We report a case of renal cell carcinoma (RCC) discovered in a patient with Kartagener's syndrome. According to our knowledge, this case is the first reported in our country, and the 2nd case in the world treated with partial nephrectomy.

Through this observation and a review of the literature, we try to analyze this association as well as the main diagnostic and therapeutic aspects.

2. Case Presentation

We report the case of 50-year-old patient, married for 12 years, without children, a regular chronic smoker (30 pack years), who suffered from recurrent pulmonary infections. He consulted for right lumbago beginning 8 months earlier, nonrelieved by analgesic treatment. The patient's overall condition was preserved and no hematuria has been noticed.

An abdominal ultrasound showed cystic lesions of the right kidney containing multiple thick septa, without vegetation, measured 73×72 mm. The liver is found in the left hypochondriac region and the spleen on the right one, confirming the situs inversus. A chest X-ray revealed dextrocardia (Figure 1).

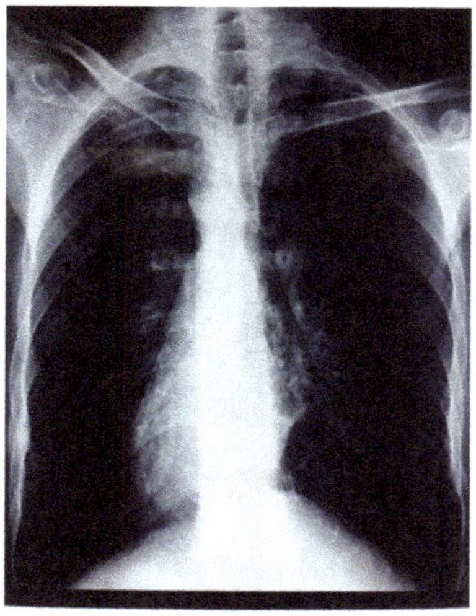

Figure 1: Chest X-ray showing dextrocardia.

Enhanced abdominal computed tomography (CT) has confirmed the situs inversus and showed a bulky mass in the right kidney, measuring 7 cm × 8 cm (anterolateral and craniocaudal) with cystic patches and multiple images of thickened septa (Figure 2). There were no tumor thrombus in the renal vein or the inferior vena cava.

Functional respiratory tests were also performed and revealed an irreversible obstructive airway disorder and pulmonary hyperinflation. Azoospermia was found in the sperm test, preoperative renal function was normal, and the rest of biological assessment showed no other abnormalities.

We diagnosed our patient as having a T2bN0M0 renal tumor. The favorable RENAL nephrometry score (6a) allow us to put forward a partial nephrectomy with open approach, by a flank incision along the eleventh intercostal space (Figure 3). The histologic examination of the surgical specimen revealed a renal cell carcinoma—the margins were not affected.

In immediate postoperative, the patient has presented with a hematuria but the renal function was still be normal. The patient was discharged at postoperative on day 5. *In the absence of standardized data*, we plan to carry out a follow-up according to the recommendations of the *French Association of Urology* of a renal tumor with low risk, either the realization of a scanner at 6 months followed by every year for 3 years, a final control at 5 years and a monitoring of the renal function by assaying plasma creatinine at the same time as the scanner [4].

One year later, the patient is still alive, without any metastases and with a normal renal function.

3. Discussion

A review of the literature unveils the rarity of this association. Only eleven cases have been published. Bertini and Boileau described firstly the same case in a 54-year-old woman [5]. Oake and Drachenberg studied the operative considerations for the treatment of renal carcinoma in a 65-year-old man with situs inversus [6]. The age of patients varies between 43 and 83 years with only one woman and ten men. Six patients had the tumor in the left side when five in the right one. Nine patients had a curative treatment by radical nephrectomy, while only one palliative treatment and another treated by partial nephrectomy. Five cases of clear cell carcinoma had been reported (Table 1).

Surgery in these patients with situs inversus is particular. The modifications in surgical anatomy for the reversed abdominal organs complicates the surgical attitudes. Surgical treatment presents many technical issues; moreover, several surgical techniques have been described including laparoscopic techniques. To reduce these surgical difficulties, Makiyama et al. described the first case of a laparoscopic nephroureterectomy in a patient with situs inversus; the team developed a laparoscopic simulator specially dedicated to the reversed anatomy to allow preoperative training [7].

Patient's preoperative evaluation with CT scan and magnetic resonance imaging can be helpful to explore anatomical variations and determine surgical approach. Literature reports increased the frequency of vascular anomalies associated to the situs inversus; in addition to the transposed position of the aorta and vena cava, Makiyama et al. [7] in their case report found 2 renal arteries to the right kidney and a right renal vein passing over the aorta and ramifying an adrenal vein, a lumbar vein, and a gonadal vein. Oake and Drachenberg [6] report a case of patient with two renal veins and a number of extrarenal arteries travelling both anterior and posterior to the inferior vena cava.

The second case of renal cell carcinoma reported in a patient with situs inversus in the world mentioned a lower than normal origin of the left renal vein [8].

The management of renal vessels should be carefully performed because of the transposed position of the aorta and the inferior vena cava and the elevated incidence of associated vascular abnormalities.

Radiological image, such as 3D-constructed CT, may specify the different variations and facilitate the management of the surgical procedure. The use of magnetic resonance scanning preoperatively allows detailed planning of the approach as required.

The surgical approach is not standardized, and an exhaustive preoperative assessment (CT, MRS) seems to be the best way to orient towards the safest technique.

We did not use the laparoscopic approach in our case because of the rarity of that and lack of facility due to anatomical variations. We suppose that partial nephrectomy will be very difficult in laparoscopic approach.

Preoperative evaluation and postoperative follow-up are very important in these patients that have cardiac, pulmonary, and renal anomalies [8].

4. Conclusion

The association of situs inversus and renal cell carcinoma is very rare. To our knowledge, this is the first reported case in Morocco. Preoperative assessment and knowledge

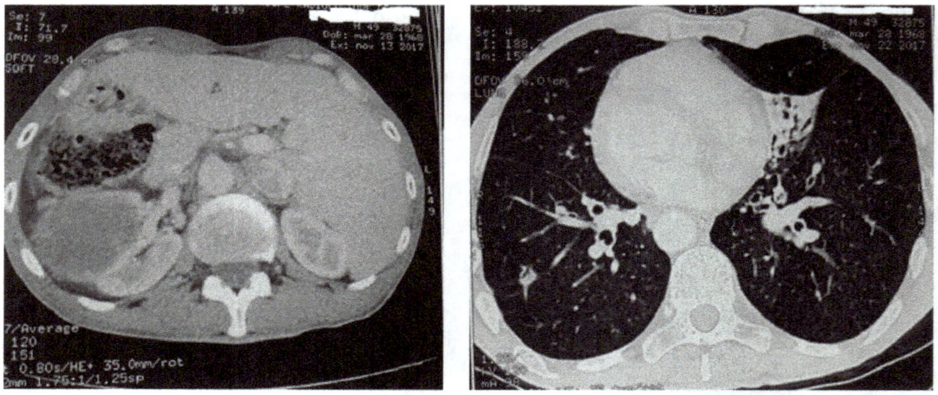

(a) (b)

FIGURE 2: Computed tomography demonstrated a mass in the right kidney and mirror-image organs with left-to-right reversal (a) and bronchiectasia with situs inversus (b).

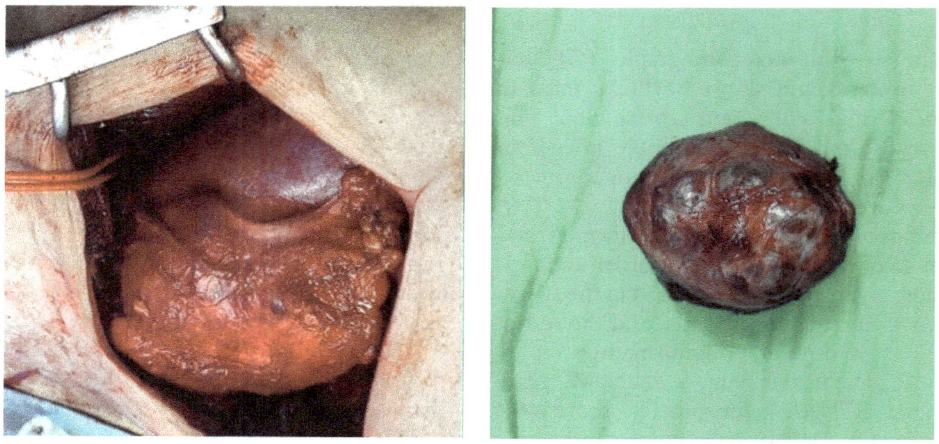

(a) (b)

FIGURE 3: Intraoperative image showing the kidney and the tumor lesion (a) and specimen of partial nephrectomy (b).

TABLE 1: Literature review: clinical cases published of situs inversus and renal carcinoma.

No.	Case report	Age/sex	Location	Open/Lap nephrectomy	Radical/partial nephrectomy	Histology
1	Bertini and Boileau 1987 [5]	54/F	Right	Open	Radical	–
2	Treiger et al. 1993 [8]	82/M	Left	Open	Radical	–
3	Adler and Lerner 1998 [3]	58/M	Left	Open	Radical	–
4	Jimenez Verdejo et al. 2000 [9]	43/M	Right	Open	Radical	–
5	Jewell and Bowa 2001 [10]	43/M	Left	Open	Radical	Clear cell
6	Takagi et al. 2008 [11]	50/M	Left	Open	Radical	–
7	Makiyama et al. 2012 [7]	61/M	Right	Lap	Radical	–
8	Rangarajan et al. 2013 [12]	65/M	Right	Nonsurgical	–	Clear cell
9	Terakawa et al. 2014 [13]	81/M	Left	Lap	Radical	Clear cell
10	Sağlam et al. 2015 [14]	52/M	Right	Open	Partial	Clear cell
11	Oake and Drachenberg 2017 [6]	65/M	Left	Open	Radical	Clear cell
12	Our study	50/M	Right	Open	Partial	Clear cell

F: female; Lap: laparoscopic; M: male.

of anatomy are crucial and allow for better adaptation of the surgical technique.

Abbreviations

PCD: Primary ciliary dyskinesias
VHL: von Hippel-Lindau disease
CT: Computed tomography
RCC: Renal cell carcinoma
MRS: Magnetic resonance scanning.

References

[1] B. A. Afzelius, "A human syndrome caused by immotile cilia," *Science*, vol. 193, no. 4250, pp. 317–319, 1976.

[2] M. Kartagener, "Zur pathogenese der Bronchiektasien," *Beiträge zur Klinik der Tuberkulose und spezifischen Tuberkulose-Forschung*, vol. 83, no. 4, pp. 489–501, 1933.

[3] H. L. Adler and S. P. Lerner, "Renal cell carcinoma and situs inversus viscerum," *The Journal of Urology*, vol. 160, 6 Part 1, pp. 2141-2142, 1998.

[4] K. Bensalah, L. Albiges, J. C. Bernhard et al., "RETRACTED: Recommandations françaises du Comité de Cancérologie de l'AFU – Actualisation 2018–2020 : prise en charge du cancer du reinFrench ccAFU guidelines – Update 2018–2020: Management of kidney cancer: management of kidney cancer," *Progrès en Urologie*, vol. 28, no. 12S, pp. S3–S31, 2018.

[5] J. E. Bertini Jr. and M. A. Boileau, "Renal cell carcinoma in a patient with situs inversus totalis," *Journal of Surgical Oncology*, vol. 34, no. 1, pp. 29–31, 1987.

[6] J. Oake and D. Drachenberg, "A case of renal cell carcinoma in a patient with situs inversus: operative considerations and a review of the literature," *Canadian Urological Association Journal*, vol. 11, no. 5, pp. 233–236, 2017.

[7] K. Makiyama, R. Sakata, H. Yamanaka, T. Tatenuma, F. Sano, and Y. Kubota, "Laparoscopic nephroureterectomy in renal pelvic urothelial carcinoma with situs inversus totalis: preoperative training using a patient-specific simulator," *Urology*, vol. 80, no. 6, pp. 1375–1378, 2012.

[8] B. F. Treiger, R. Khazan, S. M. Goldman, and F. F. Marshall, "Renal cell carcinoma with situs inversus totalis," *Urology*, vol. 41, no. 5, pp. 455–457, 1993.

[9] A. Jimenez Verdejo, J. L. Martinez Torres, F. Palao Yago et al., "Carcinoma de células renales en paciente con situs inversus y síndrome de kartagener," *Actas Urologicas Españolas*, vol. 24, no. 2, pp. 169–172, 2000.

[10] J. Jewell and K. Bowa, "Situs inversus with renal neoplasm: a case report," *East and Central African Journal of Surgery*, vol. 6, pp. 95–97, 2001.

[11] Y. Takagi, M. Narushima, and T. Shimoji, "A case of renal cell carcinoma with situs inversus totalis," *Japanese Journal of Clinical Urology*, vol. 62, pp. 315–317, 2008.

[12] S. Rangarajan, B. Sunil, and A. S. Shet, "Situs inversus and metastatic renal cell carcinoma: a case report," *International Journal of Case Reports and Images*, vol. 3, pp. 1–5, 2013.

[13] T. Terakawa, H. Miyake, H Tanaka, T. Inoue, and M. Fujisawa, "Feasibility of a retroperitoneal approach as a surgical strategy for patients with situs inversus totalis: presentation of a patient undergoing laparoscopic radical nephrectomy for renal cell carcinoma," *International Cancer Conference Journal*, vol. 3, no. 1, pp. 8–10, 2014.

[14] E. Sağlam, A. Türk, A. Selimoğlu, M. K. Demirkol, N. P. Sağlam, and A. Özgül, "Renal cell carcinoma in a patient with Kartagener syndrome: first case report in English language," *Journal of Urological Surgery*, vol. 1, no. 1, pp. 33–35, 2015.

25

Renal Angiomyolipoma Mimicking a Well-Differentiated Retroperitoneal Liposarcoma

Honoka Fuse,[1] Masaya Ito,[1] Kosuke Takemura,[1] Shuzo Ikuta,[2] Toru Motoi,[3] Tomotake Okuma,[4] Madoka Kataoka,[1] and Fumitaka Koga[1]

[1]*Department of Urology, Tokyo Metropolitan Cancer and Infectious Diseases Center Komagome Hospital, Tokyo, Japan*
[2]*Department of Radiology, Tokyo Metropolitan Cancer and Infectious Diseases Center Komagome Hospital, Tokyo, Japan*
[3]*Department of Pathology, Tokyo Metropolitan Cancer and Infectious Diseases Center Komagome Hospital, Tokyo, Japan*
[4]*Department of Musculoskeletal Oncology, Tokyo Metropolitan Cancer and Infectious Diseases Center Komagome Hospital, Tokyo, Japan*

Correspondence should be addressed to Masaya Ito; ito.uro@cick.jp and Fumitaka Koga; f-koga@cick.jp

Academic Editor: Bharat Rekhi

A 37-year-old Burmese woman presented with an incidentally found retroperitoneal fat-containing tumor. The tumor was 9 cm in the longest diameter, surrounding the right kidney, and composed of homogenous adipose tissue with thickened septum-like structures and spotty nonadipose structures, which were enhanced on contrast-enhanced computed tomography and magnetic resonance imaging. The tumor did not show either a beak sign or synchronous angiomyolipoma-like lesion in the kidneys. The tumor had irregular septa, thin blood vessels, and spotty small soft-tissue nodules. The tumor did not contain any heterogeneously enhanced solid lesions suspicious for dedifferentiated liposarcomas. Based on these imaging findings, a clinical diagnosis of a well-differentiated liposarcoma was made. Under the consensus of a multidisciplinary cancer board, she was recommended to undergo core-needle biopsy to confirm the clinical diagnosis. However, she declined to undergo biopsy for financial reasons. She underwent kidney-sparing retroperitoneal tumor resection. Histopathologically, the tumor was an angiomyolipoma with positive immunostaining for HMB45 and Melan A. The present case suggests the importance of core-needle biopsy prior to surgical intervention for retroperitoneal fat-containing tumors.

1. Introduction

Several types of fat-containing tumors arise in the retroperitoneum. Of these, the differential diagnosis between well-differentiated liposarcomas (WDLs) and large renal angiomyolipomas (AMLs) is sometimes challenging [1, 2]. Although large AMLs are generally exophytic and extend into the perinephric space, both WDLs and large renal AMLs might present as large fat-containing tumors attached to the kidneys. Despite the radiographic similarities, treatment options for these tumors are quite different. The standard of care for WDLs is surgical resection because of the possible acquisition of an enhanced aggressive phenotype such as that of dedifferentiated liposarcomas (DDLs) [3], whereas patients with AMLs have several treatment options including active surveillance, selective arterial embolization, ablative therapies, surgical treatment, and the administration of mammalian target of rapamycin (mTOR) inhibitors [4]. Thus, it is important to establish accurate diagnoses for the appropriate management of retroperitoneal fat-containing tumors. Here, we report a case of a renal AML mimicking a retroperitoneal WDL.

2. Case Presentation

A 37-year-old Burmese woman presented with an incidental retroperitoneal tumor. Contrast-enhanced computed tomography (CT) revealed a tumor measuring 9 cm in the longest diameter surrounding the right kidney (Figure 1). The tumor consisted of adipose tissue and thickened irregular septum-like structures showing early enhancement on CT. The tumor did not demonstrate a “beak sign,” a sharp beak shape

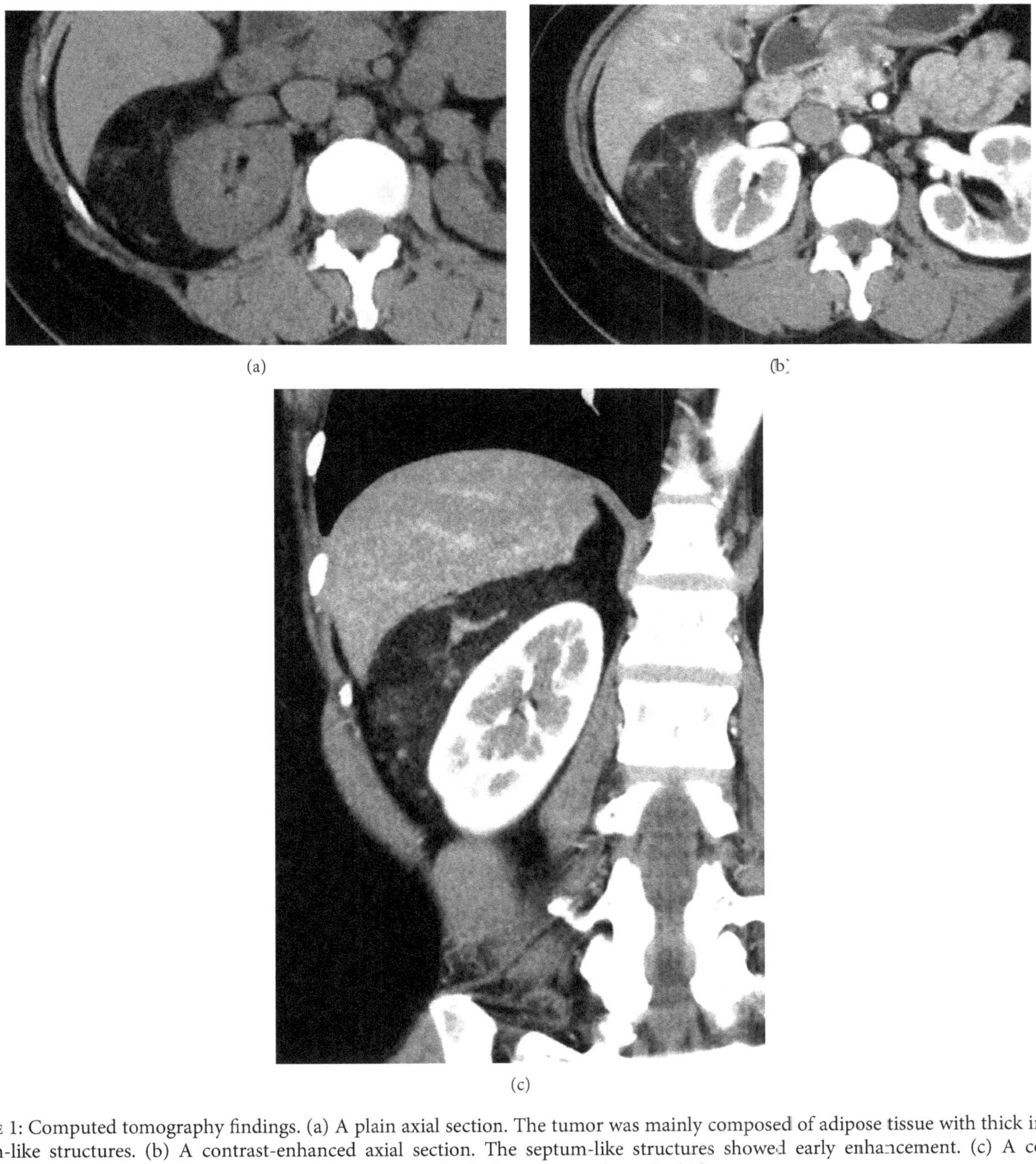

FIGURE 1: Computed tomography findings. (a) A plain axial section. The tumor was mainly composed of adipose tissue with thick irregular septum-like structures. (b) A contrast-enhanced axial section. The septum-like structures showed early enhancement. (c) A contrast-enhanced coronal section. There was no beak sign or sharp beak shape arising from the kidneys.

arising from the kidneys, nor an "embedded organ sign," encasement of the organ of origin in the tumor, both of which are often observed in cases of renal AMLs [5]. The tumor had thin blood vessels and spotty small soft-tissue nodules. On the other hand, the tumor did not present with hemorrhage, aneurysm, or intratumoral calcification. There were no other synchronous AML-like lesions in the ipsilateral or contralateral kidney, nor did tumor vessels extend through the renal parenchyma. The tumor contained no solid lesions suspicious for DDLs. On fat-suppressed T1-weighted magnetic resonance imaging (MRI), the tumor had a homogenously low-intensity area containing a weakly high-intensity area with a thick irregular septum-like structure (Figure 2(a)) exhibiting strong enhancement (Figure 2(b)). Her case was evaluated in a cancer board composed of urologists, soft-tissue oncologists, radiation oncologists, radiologists, and pathologists, wherein the consensus of a clinical diagnosis of a retroperitoneal WDL was reached. Even though we strongly recommended core-needle biopsy before surgery, she declined this and desired upfront surgical resection of the tumor for financial reasons. She subsequently underwent kidney-sparing retroperitoneal

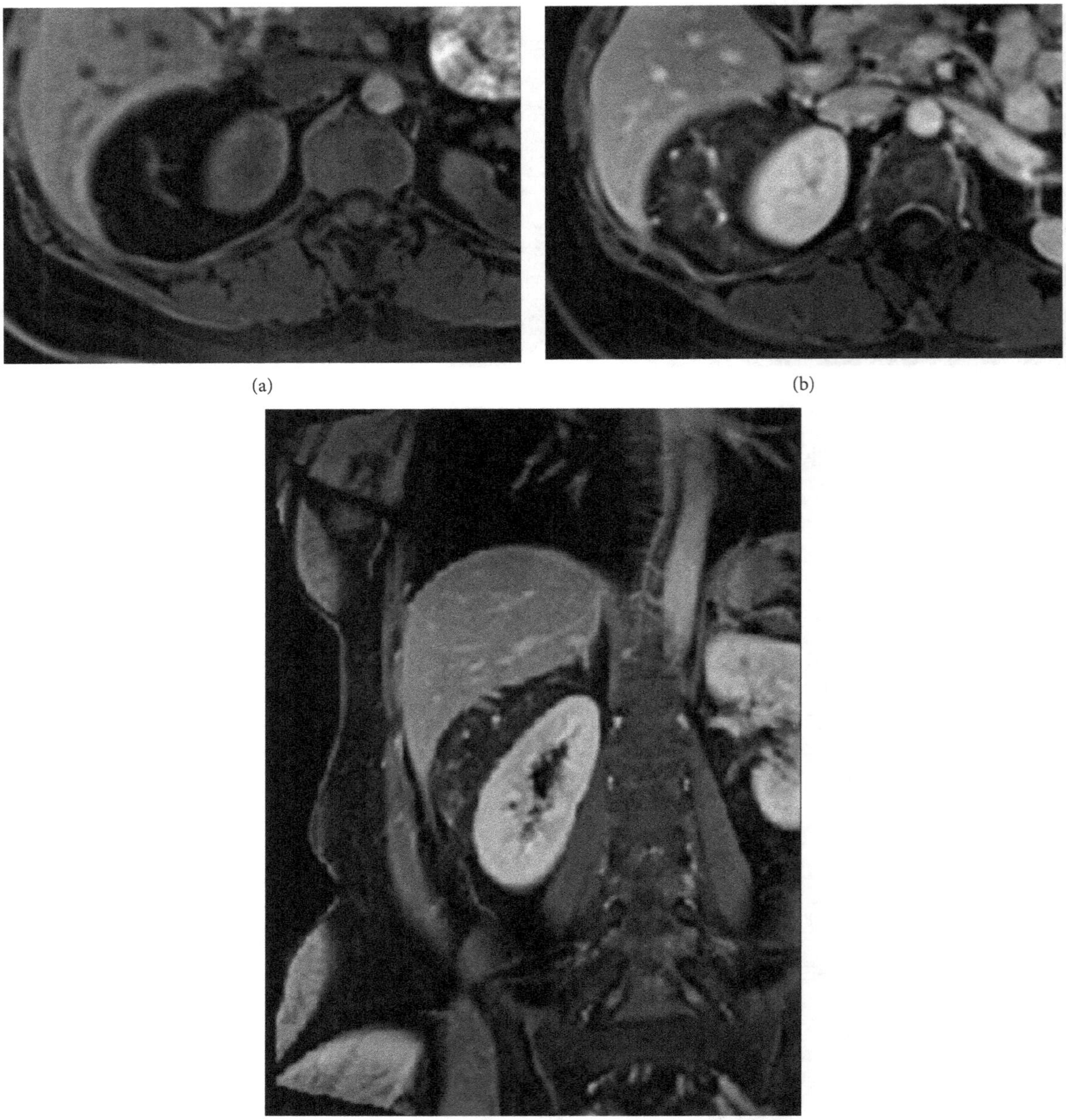

FIGURE 2: Magnetic resonance imaging findings. (a) Fat-suppressed T1-weighted scans. The tumor was mainly composed of a homogenously low-intensity area, including a weakly high-intensity area with thick irregular septum-like structures. (b) Dynamic contrast-enhanced image. The septum-like structures showed strong enhancement. There was no beak sign or sharp beak shape arising from the kidneys. (c) Coronal section of dynamic contrast-enhanced image. The tumor surrounded the right kidney with no beak sign.

tumor resection through a minimum-incision endoscopic surgery [6], and she was discharged without complications. Histopathological examination revealed a heterogeneous tumor consisting of mature adipose tissue, spindle and epithelioid smooth muscle cells, and abnormal thick-walled blood vessels (Figure 3(a)). There were no atypical cells corresponding to the diagnosis of malignancy. Immunohistochemically, the tumor cells tested strongly and diffusely positive for HMB45 (Figure 3(b)). The tumor cells also tested positive for Melan A, smooth muscle actin, and S-100. Consequently, a definite diagnosis of AML was established.

3. Discussion

We encountered a case of a renal AML mimicking a WDL. It is occasionally challenging to differentiate AMLs from WDLs because both tumors might appear as similar large fat-containing perinephric masses. To distinguish them radiologically, it has been reported that renal AMLs often exhibit characteristic findings of a "beak sign" and "embedded organ sign" on CT and MRI [5]. Additionally, AMLs have been reported to possess identical features of the presence of synchronous AML-like lesions in other areas and the presence

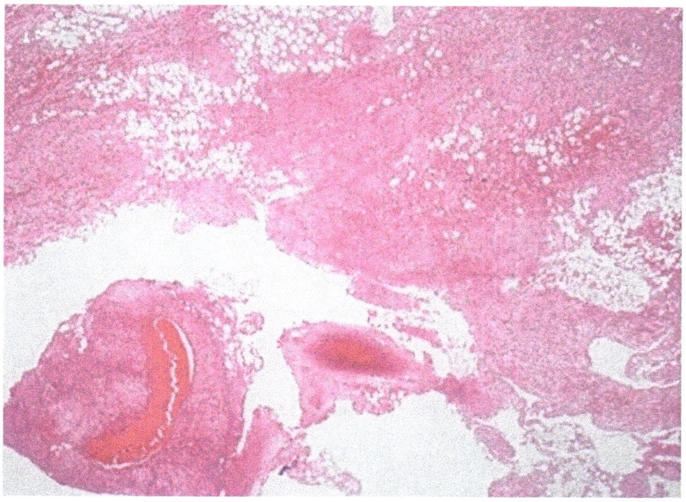

(a)

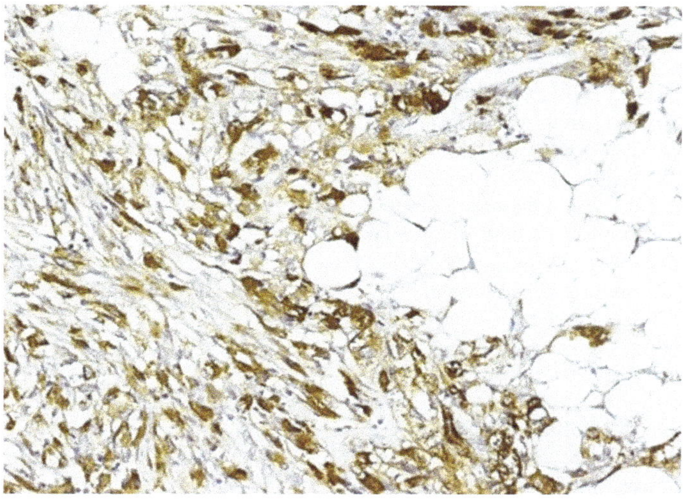

(b)

FIGURE 3: Histopathological findings. (a) Hematoxylin–eosin stain (×40). The tumor consisted of mature adipose tissue, smooth muscle cells, and thick-walled abnormal vessels. (b) Immunostaining for HMB45, a marker of angiomyolipoma, was positive in the tumor cells (×200).

of hemorrhage, aneurysm, and tumor vessels extending through the renal parenchyma [7]. In the present case, none of these features of AMLs were observed.

WDLs and DDLs are known to originate from retroperitoneal soft tissue and harbor adipose tissue and thickened irregular septum-like structures exhibiting strong enhancement [5, 8]. Although WDLs and DDLs have several common features, including irregular septa, thin blood vessels, and intratumoral calcification [7], distinct differences lie in that DDLs are frequently accompanied by solid nodules that are strongly enhanced on contrast-enhanced CT and are completely independent from fatty elements [7, 9], while WDLs exhibit features of soft-tissue nodules with weaker contrast enhancement [10]. In the present case, a clinical diagnosis of a retroperitoneal WDL was established because most features of WDLs were observed apart from intratumoral calcification, whereas none of the features of DDLs were observed. Hence, we considered that a WDL was the most probable diagnosis and that core-needle biopsy would provide additional information before surgical intervention. If a tumor biopsy had been performed and an AML had been suggested before the surgery, she could have chosen a less invasive treatment option, including selective arterial embolization, ablative therapies, and the administration of mTOR inhibitors [4]. Active surveillance could also have been an option, although large AMLs harbor the risk of spontaneous rupture [11, 12].

4. Conclusions

We encountered a case of a renal AML mimicking a WDL on imaging examinations. The important role of core-needle biopsy is suggested for accurate clinical diagnosis and proper management of retroperitoneal fat-containing tumors.

Acknowledgments

We would like to thank Editage (https://www.editage.com) for the English language editing.

References

[1] G. Sharma, A. Jain, P. Sharma, S. Sharma, V. Rathi, and P. K. Garg, "Giant exophytic renal angiomyolipoma masquerading as a retroperitoneal liposarcoma: a case report and review of literature," *World Journal of Clinical Oncology*, vol. 9, no. 7, pp. 162–1666, 2018.

[2] M. Nishino, K. Hayakawa, M. Minami, A. Yamamoto, H. Ueda, and K. Takasu, "Primary retroperitoneal neoplasms: CT and MR imaging findings with anatomic and pathologic diagnostic clues," *RadioGraphics*, vol. 23, no. 1, pp. 45–57, 2003.

[3] A. M. Crago and M. A. Dickson, "Liposarcoma: multimodality management and future targeted therapies," *Surgical Oncology Clinics of North America*, vol. 25, no. 4, pp. 761–773, 2016.

[4] A. S. Flum, N. Hamoui, M. A. Said et al., "Update on the diagnosis and management of renal angiomyolipoma," *The Journal of Urology*, vol. 195, 4 Part 1, pp. 834–846, 2016.

[5] A. M. Shaaban, M. Rezvani, M. Tubay, K. M. Elsayes, P. J. Woodward, and C. O. Menias, "Fat-containing retroperitoneal lesions: imaging characteristics, localization, and differential diagnosis," *RadioGraphics*, vol. 36, no. 3, pp. 710–734, 2016.

[6] H. Suzuki, K. Takemura, K. Sakamoto et al., "A case of renal pelvic cancer complicated by horseshoe kidney treated with RoboSurgeon gasless single-port retroperitoneoscopic nephroureterectomy," *Case Reports in Urology*, vol. 2018, Article ID 3231480, 4 pages, 2018.

[7] Q. Wang, Y. H. Juan, Y. Li et al., "Multidetector computed tomography features in differentiating exophytic renal angiomyolipoma from retroperitoneal liposarcoma: a strobe-compliant observational study," *Medicine*, vol. 94, no. 37, article e1521, 2015.

[8] M. J. Kransdorf, L. W. Bancroft, J. J. Peterson, M. D. Murphey, W. C. Foster, and H. T. Temple, "Imaging of fatty tumors: distinction of lipoma and well-differentiated liposarcoma," *Radiology*, vol. 224, no. 1, pp. 99–104, 2002.

[9] A. D. Levy, M. A. Manning, W. B. Al-Refaie, and M. M. Miettinen, "Soft-tissue sarcomas of the abdomen and pelvis: radiologic-pathologic features, part 1-common sarcomas: from the radiologic pathology archives," *RadioGraphics*, vol. 37, no. 2, pp. 462–483, 2017.

[10] P. Bhosale, J. Wang, D. Varma et al., "Can abdominal computed tomography imaging help accurately identify a dedifferentiated component in a well-differentiated liposarcoma?," *Journal of Computer Assisted Tomography*, vol. 40, no. 6, pp. 872–879, 2016.

[11] K. Yamakado, N. Tanaka, T. Nakagawa, S. Kobayashi, M. Yanagawa, and K. Takeda, "Renal angiomyolipoma: relationships between tumor size, aneurysm formation, and rupture," *Radiology*, vol. 225, no. 1, pp. 78–82, 2002.

[12] X. F. Xu, X. H. Hu, Q. M. Zuo, J. Zhang, H. Y. Xu, and Y. Zhang, "A scoring system based on clinical features for the prediction of sporadic renal angiomyolipoma rupture and hemorrhage," *Medicine*, vol. 99, no. 20, article e20167, 2020.

26

Jackstone in the Kidney: An Unusual Calculus

Serozsha Goonewardena, Umesh Jayarajah, Sanka Nalinda Kuruppu, and Manoj Hilary Fernando

Department of Urology, National Hospital of Sri Lanka, Colombo, Sri Lanka

Correspondence should be addressed to Umesh Jayarajah; umeshe.jaya@gmail.com

Academic Editor: Claudio Simeone

Jackstones are stones in the urinary tract that have the characteristic appearance resembling six-pointed toy jacks. They are nearly always reported to occur in the urinary bladder, and the occurrence in less capacious renal pelvis is unusual. We report a solitary, typical jackstone in the renal pelvis without significant outflow obstruction that was successfully treated with retrograde intrarenal surgery followed by extracorporeal shockwave lithotripsy. This highlights the complex pathophysiological mechanisms in stone formation which needs to be further studied. It is important to recognize the characteristic shape of the renal calculi on the radiological investigation in the diagnosis of the jackstones.

1. Introduction

Jackstones are stones in the urinary tract that have the characteristic appearance resembling six-pointed toy jacks. They are nearly always reported to occur in the urinary bladder [1, 2]. Interestingly, the first probable case of jackstone in the kidney was reported in 1906. Fowler in his paper described a similar stone and stated that "They occur in the renal pelvis, cysts of the kidney, or, as freely movable calculi, in the bladder" [3]. Fowler used words almost identical to those of Ord and Shattock way back in 1895 [4]. However, there is very limited literature about this rare type of calculus. Therefore, we report an unusual case of a jackstone in the kidney.

2. Case Presentation

A 63-year-old woman presented with painless intermittent visible haematuria of 4 months duration with no history of flank pain, fever, or vomiting. She had type 2 diabetes mellitus for 18 years. Clinical examination was unremarkable. X-ray KUB showed a typical jackstone in the right kidney (Figure 1(a)). Noncontrast computerized tomography KUB (NCCT-KUB) confirmed the presence of jackstone in the renal pelvis of the right kidney with mild hydronephrosis and no proximal hydroureter (Figures 1(b) and 1(c)). The stone size was 2.4 cm × 2.3 cm, and the stone density was 1355 Hounsfield units. A 99m Technetium-DTPA (Diethylenetriamine Penta-acetic Acid) diuretic renography ruled out significant obstruction with a differential function of 45% in the right kidney. She underwent cystoscopy which excluded bladder pathology accounting for visible haematuria. Right retrograde intrarenal surgery using a 7.5 Fr semirigid ureteroscope and Holmium : YAG lasertripsy completely fragmented the jackstone in the kidney (Figure 1(d)). A retrograde JJ stent was placed, and subsequent extracorporeal shockwave lithotripsy rendered her stone-free before the stent was removed. She had an unremarkable recovery. Facilities were not available for stone analysis.

3. Discussion

Jackstone in the kidney is exceedingly rare, and our review of the literature revealed only few previous reports [3, 5]. Grases et al. reported a 33-year-old man with two stones in the kidney of which the smaller stone (15 mm) was a jackstone. It had a nucleus of organic matter on which calcium oxalate monohydrate (COM) crystals have grown in a columnar

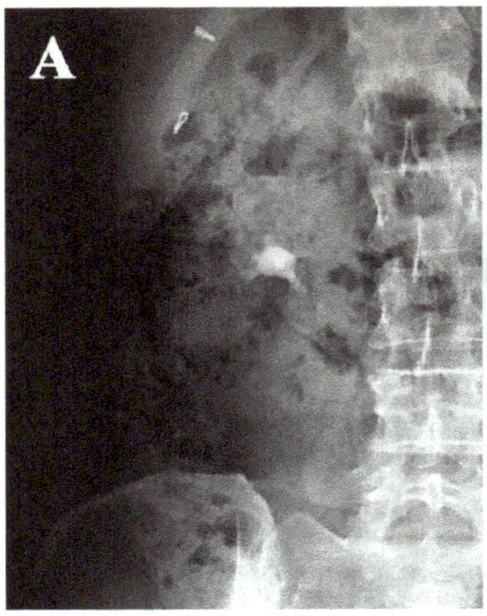

(a)

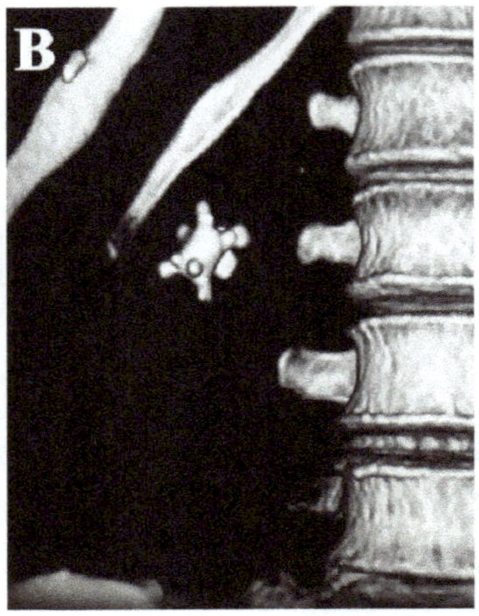

(b)

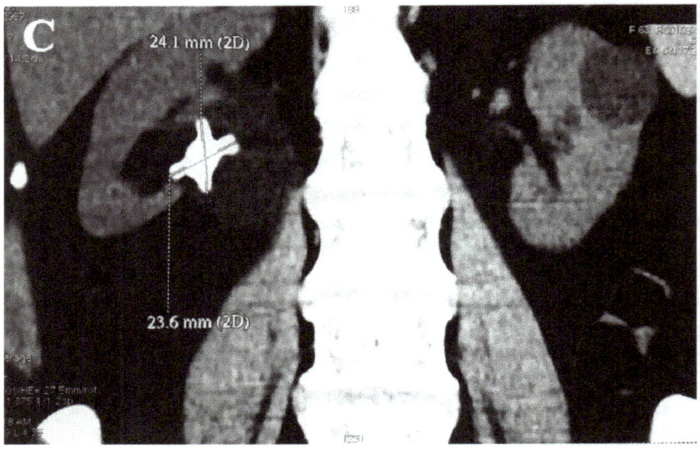

(c)

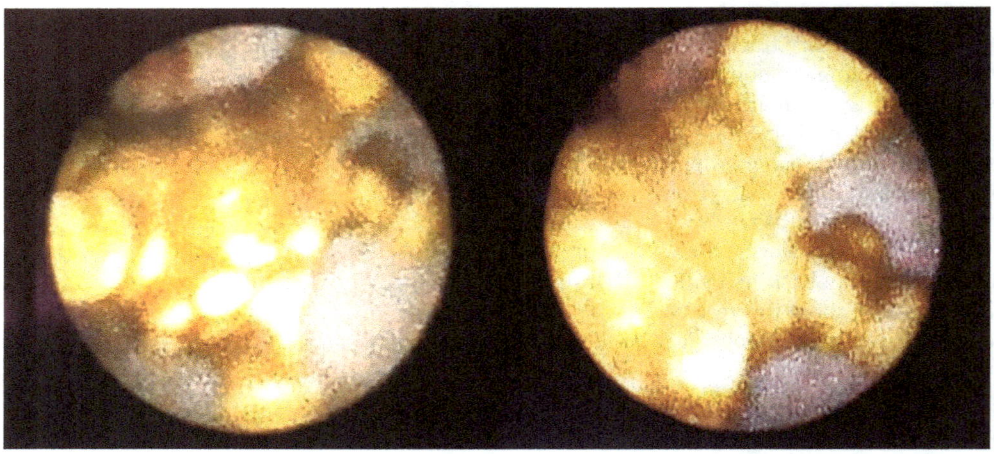

(d)

FIGURE 1: (a) X-ray: typical jackstone in the right kidney. (b) Reconstructed image of noncontrast computerized tomography (NCCT) confirming the presence of jackstone. (c) NCCT showing the right renal jackstone with mild hydronephrosis and no proximal hydroureter. (d) Endoscopic images showing a jackstone.

concentric structure. The presence of organic matter in the urine acting as a nidus was postulated as a possible reason for the formation of the jackstone found in this patient. However, jackstones in the bladder may be composed of COM or calcium oxalate dihydrate (COD). COM (whewhellite) stones are usually smooth, whereas those composed of COD (Weddellite) tend to be irregular and yellow [2, 6].

Our case is unique as the patient presented with a solitary large jackstone (2.3 × 2.4 cm) that had a typical appearance as that of jackstones found in the bladder. In the previous case report by Grases et al., the typical appearance as seen with bladder jackstones was absent. The possible reason for the typical appearance in our patient may be the capacious renal pelvis that may have facilitated the formation of the jackstone. The composition of the jackstone in our patient is most likely COM. This is because the stone density was rather high (1355 HU), and its surface was relatively smooth (Figure 1(d)). In such a jackstone, Rao et al. found that COM is the main constituent [6]. Unfortunately, facilities were not available for stone analysis.

The exact pathophysiology of development of jackstone is poorly understood. Outflow obstruction remains the most common cause of bladder calculi in adults which was also seen with jackstones in the bladder [2]. However, interestingly in our patient, there was no significant obstruction at the pelviureteric junction demonstrated in the renogram curve.

We report a solitary, large, typical jackstone in the renal pelvis without significant outflow obstruction. This highlights the complex pathophysiological mechanisms in stone formation within the urinary system which needs to be further studied. It is important to recognize the characteristic shape of the renal calculi on the radiological investigation in the diagnosis of the jackstones.

Abbreviations

KUB: Kidney-ureter-bladder
NCCT: Noncontrast computed tomography
DTPA: Diethylenetriamine pentaacetic acid
COM: Calcium oxalate monohydrate
COD: Calcium oxalate dihydrate.

Consent

Informed written consent was obtained from the patient for publication of this manuscript, including images or other personal or clinical details of the patient.

Disclosure

The case report was presented as an abstract in the annual conference of the Sri Lanka Medical Association, "133rd Anniversary International Medical Congress in 2020", https://slma.lk/wp-content/uploads/2020/08/SLMA-Abstract-Book-2020.pdf.

Authors' Contributions

SASG and UJ conceived and designed the report and collected and organized the data. UJ, MHF, SASG, and SNK wrote the initial and final draft of the article and provided logistic support. All authors have critically reviewed and approved the final draft and are responsible for the content and similarity index of the manuscript. Serozsha Goonewardena and Umesh Jayaraja have equal contribution.

References

[1] D. Subasinghe, S. Goonewardena, and V. Kathiragamathamby, "Jack stone in the bladder: case report of a rare entity," *BMC Urology*, vol. 17, no. 1, p. 40, 2017.

[2] K. J. Singh, A. Tiwari, and A. Goyal, "Jackstone: A rare entity of vesical calculus," *Indian Journal of Urology*, vol. 27, no. 4, p. 543, 2011.

[3] H. A. Fowler, "The microscopic structure of urinary calculi of oxalate of lime, with special reference to the spiculated variety," *Johns Hopkins Hospital Reports*, vol. 13, pp. 507–556, 1906.

[4] W. M. Ord and S. G. Shattock, *On the microscopic structure of urinary calculi of oxalate of lime*, Adlar and Son, Bartholomew Close, 1895.

[5] F. Grases, A. Costa-Bauza, R. M. Prieto et al., "Rare calcium oxalate monohydrate calculus attached to the wall of the renal pelvis," *International Journal of Urology*, vol. 18, no. 4, pp. 323–325, 2011.

[6] M. V. Rao, J. S. Agarwal, and N. Chhotray, "Scanning electron microscopic studies of the ultrastructure of Jack stone calculi," *The Indian Journal of Medical Research*, vol. 77, pp. 288–294, 1983.

27

Ureterocalyceal Fistula: A Rare Complication of Laparoscopic Partial Nephrectomy

Fayez T. Hammad

College of Medicine and Health Sciences, United Arab Emirates University and Mediclinic Al Ain, Al Ain, UAE

Correspondence should be addressed to Fayez T. Hammad; fayezhammad@hotmail.com

Academic Editor: Giorgio Carmignani

Background. Postoperative urinary leak is a well-documented complication following partial nephrectomy. It usually presents as persistent discharge from the retroperitoneal drain, nephrocutaneous fistula, urinary collection, systemic manifestations, or abdominal symptoms. Herein, we report for the first time on a case of urinary leak postlaparoscopic partial nephrectomy which did not heal and led to the formation of ureterocalyceal fistula. *Case Presentation.* A 41-year-old male presented with a coincidental renal mass at the inferiomedial aspect of the right kidney. He underwent laparoscopic partial nephrectomy. On the third postoperative day, he developed fever. CT scan showed minimal urine leak from the tumor site and a JJ stent was inserted. Due to severe bladder symptoms, the stent was removed and a perirenal drain was inserted and removed in few days. He did well initially but in two weeks, he started to develop urinary tract infections. Repeat CT scan showed ongoing urinary leak from the site of the previous surgery. Retrograde pyelography demonstrated a complete UPJ stenosis with an ureterocalyceal fistula. Trial for reanastomosis failed due to severe adhesions and small intrarenal pelvis. An ureterocalyceal anastomosis has to be performed to another calyx. *Conclusion.* We report for the first time on an ureterocalyceal fistula following laparoscopic partial nephrectomy. This complication might be prevented by a careful dissection of the area close to the ureter or by an insertion of a JJ stent for an adequate time if a ureteric injury is suspected.

1. Background

Nephron-sparing surgery has become the standard of care for clinical stage T1a and selected clinical stage T1b renal tumors [1–3]. This is due to the superior functional outcomes and equivalent oncologic results compared with radical nephrectomy. Despite the advancement in technology, it remains a challenging procedure associated with several postoperative complications [4, 5].

Postoperative urinary leak following partial nephrectomy is a well-documented complication with an incidence ranging from 18% in some series to less than 2% in the most recent ones [4–6]. It usually presents as persistent discharge from the retroperitoneal drain, nephrocutaneous fistula, urinary collection, systemic manifestations, or abdominal symptoms [6–8].

Herein, we report for the first time on a case of urinary leak postlaparoscopic partial nephrectomy which led to the formation of a ureterocalyceal fistula.

2. Case Presentation

A 41-year-old male presented with a coincidental right renal mass. He gave a history suggestive of chronic prostatitis and had mild urinary frequency and occasional mild urgency. He also had a history of previous open appendectomy. Preoperative CT scan showed a heterogeneously enhancing mass at the inferior pole of the right kidney suggestive of neoplastic lesion (PADUA score 8) (Figure 1(a)) for which he underwent transperitoneal laparoscopic partial nephrectomy with 25 minutes warm ischemia time and the surgery was uneventful. During surgery, the right colon was reflected medially, followed by dissection of the renal hilum, and identification of the artery and vein. The tumor was identified and the resection margins were identified and marked with cautery. After clamping the renal artery, the tumor was resected with an approximately 3-5 mm rim of normal renal parenchyma. We could not identify any urinary leak and the resection bed was sutured using polyglactin in a

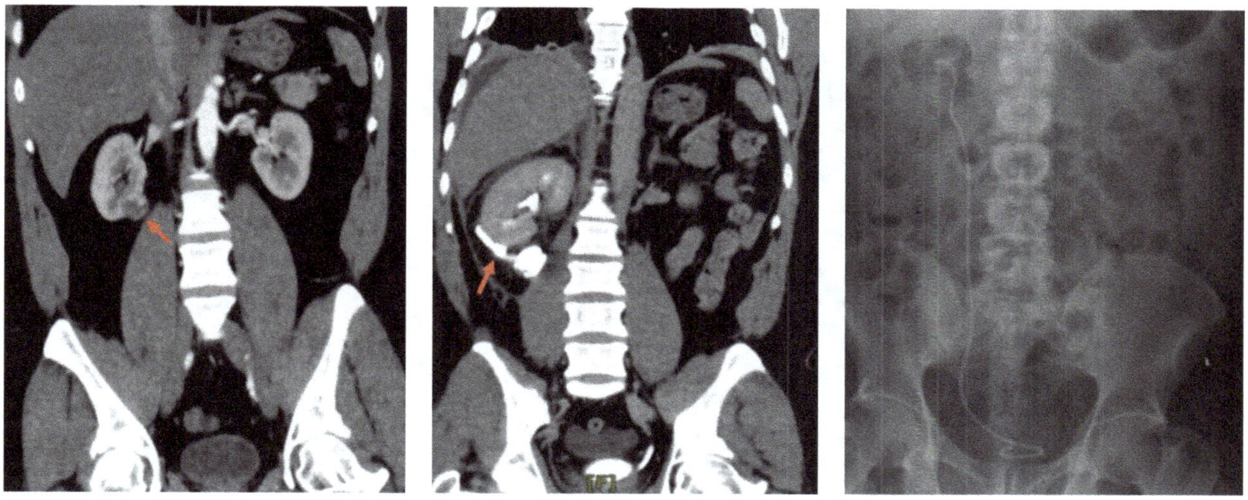

(a) (b) (c)

Figure 1: (a) Preoperative CT scan showing the lesion at the inferiomedial aspect of the right kidney. (b) Delayed phase CT scan demonstrating the urine leak from the site of partial nephrectomy. (c) Postoperative plain X-ray showing the JJ stent in position.

running fashion. The renal capsule was approximated over a small piece of *Surgicel* using polyglactin as well. Histopathology demonstrated a 2.9 × 3.8 × 3.4 cm Fuhrman grade II clear cell carcinoma which was confined to the capsule (T1a N0 M0).

Postoperatively, he did well and the drain was removed after 48 hours as it was bringing only 45 cc of serosanguinous fluid as suggested by potassium and creatinine levels, which were similar to the serum values. One day later, he developed high-grade fever, and CT scan showed minimal urine leak from the site of the partial nephrectomy (Figure 1(b)). He refused nephrostomy tube insertion, so he underwent cystoscopy and JJ stent insertion on the 6th postop day. During the procedure, retrograde pyelography showed no abnormality in the upper ureter or kidney apart from the leak from the site of surgery. Therefore, 26 cm, 6 FR stent was inserted easily (Figure 1(c)) and a Foley's catheter was fixed. The patient was discharged on the eighth postop day.

Three days postdischarge, he presented with severe bladder spasms and insisted on catheter removal which was reinserted 24 hours later. He then developed fever with minimal abdominal pain for which he was admitted on the 9th postdischarge day. CT scan showed extravasation of urine at the site of the previous surgery with fluid collection (3.8 × 1.8 cm) associated with few gas bubble and mild right pleural reaction. He was offered a nephrostomy tube but he totally refused again, so he was convinced to have a perirenal drain, which was inserted in the presence of the JJ stent and urethral catheter. Subsequently, he continued to have severe bladder spasms despite the antimuscarinic agents. Indeed, he tried several times to pull the catheter which got blocked and all the urine from both kidneys was coming out from the perirenal drain. In view of this and the agony that he had, we decided to remove the JJ stent and urethral catheter and leave only the perirenal drain.

Subsequently, almost half of urine output was coming out from the perirenal drain. Another CT scan showed the pigtail drain tube to be adjacent to the site of partial nephrectomy and no contrast was going down the ureter. So, the drain was pulled out 2 cm under CT guidance. CT scan then showed free drainage of urine along the ureter. The drain was left in place for two days during which it did not drain any urine. The patient felt well with no fever, so the drain was removed three days later. During all this time, the kidney did not show any significant dilation on either ultrasound or CT scan.

Postdischarge, he did well initially, but in few days, he started to develop urinary tract infections that were occasionally associated with low-grade fever but no abdominal pain. Ultrasound again did not show any abnormality. One month later, he was readmitted with high-grade fever. CT scan showed an ongoing leak which was, this time, more medial with minimal dilation of the collecting system. A trial to insert a JJ stent failed and retrograde pyelography showed normal ureter up to approximately 3 cm below the ureteropelvic junction which had a blind end and there was a fistula between the upper ureter and lower calyceal system (ureterocalyceal fistula) (Figures 2(a) and 2(b)). Using an ureteroscope, a trial to negotiate the way to the UPJ was not successful. A nephrostomy tube was inserted and a trial to pass a JJ stent and guidewire, antegradely, also failed. Six weeks later, he had another trial to pass the stent antegradely which also failed. He then underwent an open surgical exploration through an anterior midline incision. A trial to bridge the gap between the upper ureter and renal pelvis failed due to the intrarenal nature of the pelvis and the severe adhesion, and indeed, there was a small injury of the IVC during dissection. So, with huge difficulty, a ureterocalyceal anastomosis was finally performed to another calyx (one of the anterior calyces) despite the nondilated nature of the calyces, previous surgery in the area, and the reasonably thick renal parenchyma as he totally refused the idea of nephrectomy. This required resection of a small wedge of renal tissues to prevent future anastomotic stenosis.

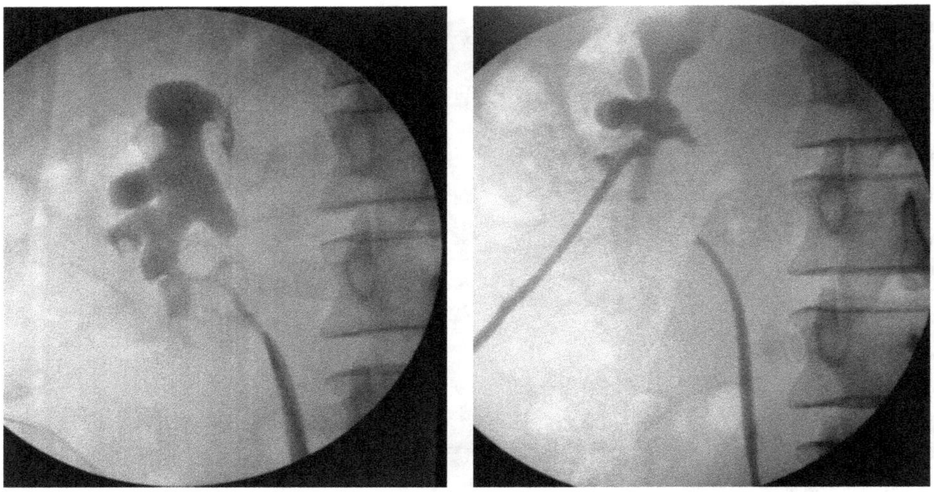

(a) (b)

FIGURE 2: (a) Retrograde pyelography showing a fistulous tract between the upper ureter and the inferior calyceal system. The blind end of the renal pelvis is also seen. (b) Simultaneous retrograde and antegrade pyelography following the insertion of the nephrostomy tube.

Postoperatively, he did well and was discharged on the 7th postoperative day.

3. Discussion

Postoperative urinary leak following partial nephrectomy is a well-documented complication [6, 8]. The majority of these cases present as persistent discharge from the retroperitoneal drain, nephrocutaneous fistula, urinary collection, abdominal symptoms, or systemic manifestation [6–8]. The management of urinary leak depends on the presentation, extent of leak, and the status of the patient and includes spontaneous resolution, retrograde ureteral stents insertion, insertion of a nephrostomy tube, or percutaneous drainage of the perirenal urinoma or even nephrectomy [6, 7]. This is the first case of urinary leak postlaparoscopic partial nephrectomy which did not heal despite several attempts of drainage and led to the formation of a ureterocalyceal fistula.

In the current case, it is difficult to ascertain the cause of the stenosis of the upper ureter but it appears that a combination of urinary leak at the site of partial nephrectomy and a possible ureteric injury had resulted in the formation of the ureterocalyceal fistula. The most likely cause for the expected ureteric injury was an inadvertent diathermy injury to the vascular supply of the ureter or even a direct but unnoticed ureteric injury as the tumor was relatively close to the ureter. The fact that no direct injury was obvious during laparoscopic dissection and the fact that the retrograde pyelography and the insertion of JJ stent were totally uneventful when performed almost a week after surgery indicate that the injury was a mild one which took some time to cause a break in the ureteric wall and fistula formation. One of the factors that could have caused or at least contributed to the ureteric injury is the infections and collections, which formed postoperatively in the adjacent area. Other remote possibility was the inadvertent injury by the percutaneous needle during drainage of the perirenal collection which was located at the lower pole and upper ureter.

In this case, no glue was used during the procedure. In this regard, there was a report of urine leak associated with fibrin glue which led to almost complete occlusion and stricture formation of the upper ureter which was associated with enfolding of the ureter by fibrin glue causing marked stiffness and adhesions [9].

The early removal of the JJ stent due to severe bladder spasms and intolerance despite the use of anticholinergics must have also contributed to the formation of the fistula. If the stent was kept in for longer time, this probably would have ended in ureteric stricture but prevented this complication.

In conclusion, herein we report on the first case of a ureterocalyceal fistula following laparoscopic partial nephrectomy of an inferiomedial renal tumor. Careful dissection of the tissues in the medical aspect adjacent to the ureter and leaving a JJ stent for an adequate period in case of suspicion of ureteric injury might prevent such complication.

Abbreviations

JJ stent: Double J stent.

Ethical Approval

The patient had consented for publications and the report met the local ethics committee regulations (Mediclinic Ethical Committee).

Consent

The patient had consented for publications in a written format.

Authors' Contributions

FH performed the procedures and for the two cases, did the literature review, consented patents, collected data, and wrote the manuscript.

References

[1] A. Finelli, N. Ismaila, B. Bro et al., "Management of small renal masses: American Society of Clinical Oncology clinical practice guideline," *Journal of Clinical Oncology*, vol. 35, no. 6, pp. 668–680, 2017.

[2] Z. Kirkali, "The motion: open partial nephrectomy is the standard of care for small resectable solid renal masses," *European Urology*, vol. 51, no. 2, pp. 561–2; discussion 564, 2007, discussion 564.

[3] J. J. Meeks and C. M. Gonzalez, "Standard of care for small renal masses in the 21st century," *JAMA Surgery*, vol. 150, no. 7, pp. 672-673, 2015.

[4] U. Boylu, C. Basatac, U. Yildirim, F. F. Onol, and E. Gumus, "Comparison of surgical, functional, and oncological outcomes of open and robot-assisted partial nephrectomy," *Journal of Minimal Access Surgery*, vol. 11, no. 1, pp. 72–77, 2015.

[5] A. Masson-Lecomte, D. R. Yates, V. Hupertan et al., "A prospective comparison of the pathologic and surgical outcomes obtained after elective treatment of renal cell carcinoma by open or robot-assisted partial nephrectomy," *Urologic Oncology*, vol. 31, no. 6, pp. 924–929, 2013.

[6] T. Erlich, Y. Abu-Ghanem, J. Ramon, Y. Mor, B. Rosenzweig, and Z. Dotan, "Postoperative urinary leakage following partial nephrectomy for renal mass: risk factors and a proposed algorithm for the diagnosis and management," *Scandinavian Journal of Surgery*, vol. 106, no. 2, pp. 139–144, 2016.

[7] S. D. Kundu, R. H. Thompson, G. J. Kallingal, G. Cambareri, and P. Russo, "Urinary fistulae after partial nephrectomy," *BJU International*, vol. 106, no. 7, pp. 1042–1044, 2010.

[8] J. J. Meeks, L. C. Zhao, N. Navai, K. T. Perry, R. B. Nadler, and N. D. Smith, "Risk factors and management of urine leaks after partial nephrectomy," *The Journal of Urology*, vol. 180, no. 6, pp. 2375–2378, 2008.

[9] C. J. Wang, D. B. Kong, B. H. Shen et al., "Ureteral obstruction and urinary fistula due to fibrin glue after partial nephrectomy: a case report and review of the literature," *Oncology Letters*, vol. 5, no. 3, pp. 825–828, 2013.

28

Late-Onset Bilateral Choroidal Metastases from Clear Cell Renal Cell Carcinoma

Constantinos D. Georgakopoulos, Athina Pallikari, Panagiotis Plotas, and Olga E. Makri

Department of Ophthalmology, Medical School, University of Patras, Rio, 265 04 Patras, Greece

Correspondence should be addressed to Olga E. Makri; makriolga@upatras.gr

Academic Editor: Tun-Chieh Chen

Aim. To present a case of clear cell renal cell carcinoma with late-onset bilateral choroidal metastases. *Case Report.* A 57-year-old male patient in the Oncology Clinic complained of reduced vision in the right eye (OD) for 7 days. The patient, who was under immunotherapy with nivolumab, had been diagnosed with clear cell renal cell carcinoma in the left kidney 15 years ago that recurred in the right kidney before 2 years. Metastases in the brain, lungs, and bones had also been diagnosed. On ophthalmological examination, the visual acuity was 20/50 OD and 20/20 in the left eye (OS). Dilated fundus examination in OD revealed a single raised oval-shaped yellowish choroidal nodule infratemporally with macular involvement. A similar lesion, sparing the macula, was observed in OS. Fundus autofluorescence revealed diffuse punctate hyperautofluorescence on the lesions. Serous macular detachment was also observed in OD. A standardized A-scan ultrasound demonstrated an irregular structure of the lesions with moderate to high internal reflectivity. Based on the history and clinical and echographic characteristics, the diagnosis of bilateral choroidal metastases from renal cell carcinoma was set. *Conclusion.* Choroidal metastases from the primary renal tumor are extremely rare. The time interval between primary malignancy and choroidal metastasis is reported to be 12-96 months. Bilateral choroidal metastases have been described in 9 cases. We describe a rare case where bilateral choroidal metastases were diagnosed 15 years after the initial diagnosis of clear cell renal cell carcinoma.

1. Introduction

Renal cell carcinoma (RCC) is a rare but potentially fatal malignancy among adults, as it is characterized by a strong tendency to metastasize unpredictably to any organ, even decades after surgical removal of the primary tumor [1]. Approximately one-third of patients with RCC will eventually develop a distant metastatic tumor, a fact that results in a guarded prognosis [2]. The most common metastatic locations are the lungs, bones, liver, and brain, whereas the uveal tract is an extremely rare site of kidney tumor spread as it represents about 4% of all uveal metastatic malignancies [3].

The choroid is one of the most highly vascularized tissues of the body and comprises a common site of uveal metastatic disease. A large retrospective chart review reported choroidal involvement in 88% of the 950 cases with uveal metastases studied [4]. Breast and lung cancer are the most common primary tumor sites in cases of choroidal metastases, while metastases originating from kidneys are rare [3, 4].

We present a case of bilateral choroidal metastases originating from RCC that occurred 15 years after the diagnosis of the primary tumor.

2. Case Presentation

A 57-year-old hospitalized male patient presented with decreased vision in the right eye (OD) during the last week. His medical history was significant with left radical nephrectomy before 15 years due to a histologically proven clear cell renal carcinoma (Fuhrman grade II [5]). Tumor recurrence was detected 2 years ago, and the patient underwent right

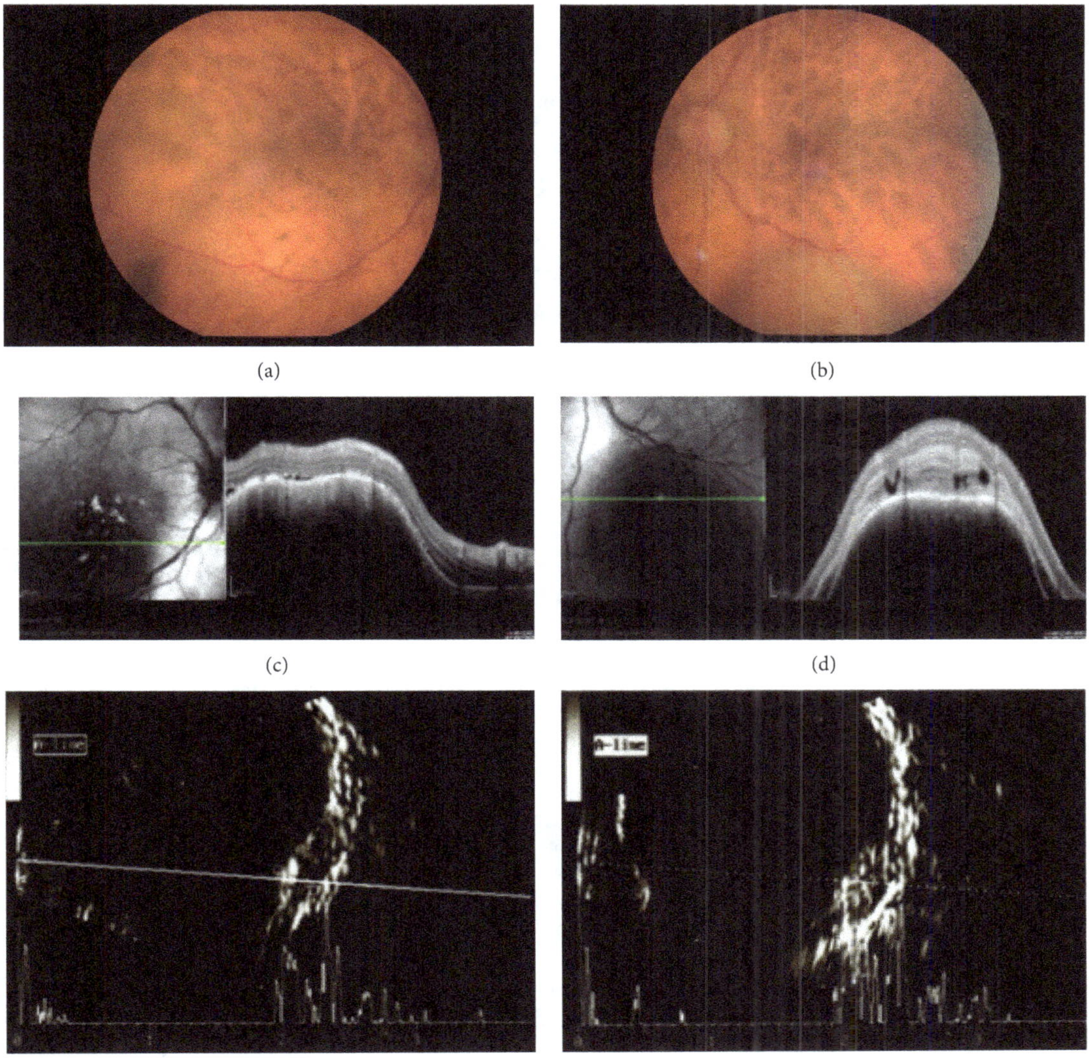

Figure 1: Color fundus image of the right eye (a) revealed an elevated, oval-shaped, lightly pigmented, orange, subretinal lesion in the inferotemporal quadrant with secondary serous retinal detachment extending to the macula. In the left eye (b), a nonpigmented, reddish-white, subretinal lesion below the inferior temporal arcade was observed. Examination with optical coherence tomography in the right eye (c) revealed eradication of the choriocapillaries and irregular choroidal surface overlying the lesion and in the left eye (d) showed a dome-shaped choroidal morphology, compression of the overlying choriocapillaris, and intraretinal fluid at the site of the lesion. Ultrasound examination showed dome-shaped choroidal lesions in the right (e) and left (f) eyes with a medium-to-high internal reflectivity and a dense acoustic sign.

heminephrectomy (stage pT1bNx according to the 8th edition of the AJCC Cancer Staging Form). Secondary brain, pulmonary, and bone metastases had also been developed. The patient was under immunotherapy with nivolumab.

On ophthalmologic examination, his best-corrected visual acuity was 20/50 in (OD) and 20/20 in the left eye (OS). The slit-lamp biomicroscopy of the anterior segment was unremarkable in both eyes. Funduscopic examination of OD showed an elevated, oval-shaped, lightly pigmented, orange, subretinal lesion at the inferotemporal quadrant with secondary serous retinal detachment that extended to the macula (Figure 1(a)). A flat pigmented naevus temporal to the lesion was also present. The fundoscopy of OS revealed a nonpigmented, reddish-white, subretinal lesion below the inferior temporal arcade (Figure 1(b)).

Optical coherence tomography (OCT) in OD demonstrated eradication of the choriocapillaries and irregular choroidal surface overlying the lesion associated with a serous retinal detachment that extended to the macula (Figure 1(c)). In OS, OCT showed a dome-shaped choroidal morphology, compression of the overlying choriocapillaries, and intraretinal fluid at the site of the lesion (Figure 1(d)). Fundus autofluorescence revealed scattered hyperfluorescent clumps of the lesion in OD, whereas the lesion in OS was hypofluorescent. Fluorescence angiography was contraindicated.

Table 1: Cases of renal cell carcinoma with metastases to the choroid. In nine cases, the choroidal metastases were bilateral.

Study	Number of cases	Mean age at diagnosis (years)	Sex		Laterality		Diagnosis of metastasis before primary tumor	Interval between diagnosis of primary tumor and metastasis (years)
			Male	Female	Unilateral	Bilateral		
Shields et al. [3]	46	66	34	12	39	7	2	N/A
Sountoulides et al. [6]	4	49.6	3		N/A	N/A	0	1-8
Haimovici et al. [7]	5	61.4	4	1	4	1	2	6-18
Bellerive et al. [8]	1	73	1			1	0	25

Ultrasound examination showed bilateral dome-shaped choroidal lesions measuring 8.2 mm base and 3.0 mm height in OD and 7.2 mm base and 3.4 mm height in OS (Figure 1 (e), (f)). The lesions had medium-to-high internal reflectivity with a dense acoustic sign.

Based on the medical history and the clinical and multimodal imaging findings, the patient was diagnosed with bilateral choroidal metastases originating from a RCC that occurred 15 years ago. Due to the patient's low life expectancy and poor systemic status, it was decided not to proceed to biopsy of the metastatic sites and any local therapeutic regimen while systemic immunotherapy was continued. The patient expired 3 months after the occurrence of choroidal metastases.

3. Discussion

Ocular metastases comprise an extremely uncommon site of distant spread from RCC and may be the initial manifestation of a previously undiagnosed RCC. The uveal tract is the most frequent site of ocular metastatic disease from RCC [6] (Table 1). Haimovici et al. presented 5 cases with RCC-related choroidal metastases that occurred 6-18 years after nephrectomy [7]. In a retrospective review, Sountoulides et al. documented 19 cases with RCC suffered from ocular metastatic disease. Interestingly, the choroid was implicated in 4 out of 19 cases, and the time interval between the diagnosis of RCC and metastasis varied from 1 to 8 years [6]. There is one rare case of unilateral choroidal metastasis that developed 25 years after nephrectomy due to RCC [8].

A review of the literature revealed a small number of cases with bilateral kidney-related choroidal metastases. More precisely, in a retrospective review of 1111 patients with uveal metastases, bilateral kidney cancer-related choroidal metastases were found in 7 out of 46 cases with metastatic kidney tumor [3]. The orangish appearance of the uveal mass may indicate renal origin, but may also be found in metastases originating from a thyroid carcinoma or a carcinoid tumor [7]. Additionally, RCC choroidal metastases are usually characterized by a slightly higher height-to-base ratio in A-scan ultrasonography compared to those originating from other metastatic cancers, whilst the mean thickness of the mass has been reported to be approximately 4 mm [4].

The diagnosis of a choroidal metastasis is based on medical history and ophthalmoscopic and echographic characteristics, whereas uncertain cases require fine needle aspiration biopsy [4, 7]. Differential diagnosis of choroidal metastases includes choroidal melanomas, haemangiomas, granulomas, and choroidal osteomas [9]. The treatment depends on the systemic status of the patient and the number and location of choroidal tumors. In cases with poor systemic status, observation is preferred. Other treatment modalities include systemic chemotherapy with drugs used for the primary cancer, immunotherapy, hormone therapy, or radiotherapy in multifocal and bilateral metastases. Proton beam radiotherapy, plaque radiotherapy, transpupillary radiotherapy, or photodynamic therapy is the preferred treatment strategy for solitary metastasis while enucleation is suggested for blind painful eyes [9].

In conclusion, we describe an extremely rare case where bilateral choroidal metastases were diagnosed 15 years after the initial diagnosis of a clear cell RCC. Choroidal metastases from RCC represent a rare condition that should not be overlooked. Therefore, a high index of suspicion is required with sufficient investigation of patients with a history of RCC who complain of visual symptoms, even decades after the RCC diagnosis.

Consent

Informed consent was obtained from the patient regarding this publication.

Authors' Contributions

All authors have read and approved the final version of the manuscript.

References

[1] R. J. Motzer, N. H. Bander, and D. M. Nanus, "Renal-cell carcinoma," *The New England Journal of Medicine*, vol. 335, no. 12, pp. 865–875, 1996.

[2] A. Jemal, R. Siegel, E. Ward, T. Murray, J. Xu, and M. J. Thun, "Cancer statistics, 2007," *CA: a Cancer Journal for Clinicians*, vol. 57, no. 1, pp. 43–66, 2007.

[3] C. L. Shields, R. J. Welch, K. Malik et al., "Uveal metastasis: clinical features and survival outcome of 2214 tumors in 1111

patients based on primary tumor origin," *Middle East African Journal of Ophthalmology*, vol. 25, no. 2, pp. 81–90, 2018.

[4] C. L. Shields, J. A. Shields, N. E. Gross, G. P. Schwartz, and S. E. Lally, "Survey of 520 eyes with uveal metastases," *Ophthalmology*, vol. 104, no. 8, pp. 1265–1276, 1997.

[5] S. A. Fuhrman, L. C. Lasky, and C. Limas, "Prognostic significance of morphologic parameters in renal cell carcinoma," *The American Journal of Surgical Pathology*, vol. 6, no. 7, pp. 655–664, 1982.

[6] P. Sountoulides, L. Metaxa, and L. Cindolo, "Atypical presentations and rare metastatic sites of renal cell carcinoma: a review of case reports," *Journal of Medical Case Reports*, vol. 5, no. 1, p. 429, 2011.

[7] R. Haimovici, E. S. Gragoudas, Z. Gregor, R. D. Pesavento, W. F. Mieler, and J. S. Duker, "Choroidal metastases from renal cell carcinoma," *Ophthalmology*, vol. 104, no. 7, pp. 1152–1158, 1997.

[8] C. Bellerive, G. Allaire, and S. Callejo, "A late onset of choroidal metastasis from renal cell carcinoma simulating melanoma," *Canadian Journal of Ophthalmology*, vol. 52, no. 3, pp. e108–e110, 2017.

[9] S. Arepalli, S. Kaliki, and C. L. Shields, "Choroidal metastases: origin, features, and therapy," *Indian Journal of Ophthalmology*, vol. 63, no. 2, pp. 122–127, 2015.

An Intratumoral Aneurysm and an Extrarenal Synchronous Cystic Tumour in a Case of a Renal Cell Carcinoma

Supun De Silva[1] **Lalani De Silva**[1] **Susantha De Silva**,[2] **and Priyani Amarathunga**[3]

[1]*Postgraduate Institute of Medicine, University of Colombo, Sri Lanka*
[2]*Urology Unit 02, National Hospital of Sri Lanka, Colombo, Sri Lanka*
[3]*Department of Pathology, Faculty of Medicine, University of Colombo, Sri Lanka*

Correspondence should be addressed to Supun De Silva; supun85@gmail.com

Academic Editor: Tun-Chieh Chen

Background. Renal cell carcinoma is a heterogeneous group of malignant tumors originating from the kidney. We report a case of a renal cell carcinoma with two very rare associates, i.e., a large intratumoral aneurysm and a synchronous extrarenal cystic tumor outside the main tumor. *Case Presentation.* A 31-year-old woman, who presented with painless hematuria and loin pain, was diagnosed to have a large renal mass measuring $15 \times 9 \times 8.5$ cm with an intralesional arterial aneurysm measuring 4.5×3.5 cm on radiological examination. During surgery, a separate cystic tumor measuring $5 \times 4.5 \times 4$ cm with distinct vascular supply was noted anteromedial to the kidney, in addition to the renal mass. The histology of the main tumor was compatible with t(6:11) type microphthalmia-associated transcription factor (MiT) family translocation RCC. The aneurysm was of venous origin histologically, and a radiologically demonstrable arteriovenous fistula was recognized retrospectively. The extrarenal cyst has also showed similar histology to that of main tumor and had no evidence of a degenerated lymph node. *Discussion.* Although few cases were reported with various vascular anomalies associated with a renal tumor, this is the first ever case to find an arteriovenous fistula with a secondary venous aneurysm located inside a malignant renal mass. Similarly, no solid RCC is reported to present with an extrarenal malignant cystic nodule. The prognostic and oncological significance of the extrarenal malignant cyst is unclear. Both of these extraordinary features of this case were not properly identified on preoperative imaging. Reviewing the preoperative imaging when pathology reports are available helps to overcome difficulties in making the final diagnosis of complex cases. *Conclusion.* RCCs can house vascular anomalies like arteriovenous fistula and venous aneurysms and can exist with concomitant extrarenal malignant cystic nodules.

1. Introduction

Renal cell carcinoma (RCC) is a heterogeneous group of malignant tumors originating from the kidney. It is known to be associated with a variety of vascular anomalies. Several types of vascular anomalies like renal artery aneurysms (RAAs), venous aneurysms (VAs), and arteriovenous fistulas (AVF) were found to coexist with RCC. However, all of those vascular anomalies reported so far were located outside the tumor mass or in most cases, outside the kidney. Multifocality and coexistence of both solid and cystic components in one tumor are also known phenomena with RCC. In most instances, both of these special features were found inside the ipsilateral kidney. A well-demonstrable extrarenal malignant cystic nodule is never reported to coexist with any type of solid RCC. Here, we report the first ever case to have an intratumoral AVF and a VA together with an extrarenal synchronous malignant cyst in an adult microphthalmia-associated transcription factor (MiT) family translocation RCC. The discovery of two extraordinary features in an extremely rare type of RCC makes this case unique.

2. Case Presentation

A 31-year-old lactating mother was investigated for painless hematuria and vague loin pain. She has given birth to her first baby 10 months before, and by that time, she did not have any symptoms related to the genitourinary system. Her

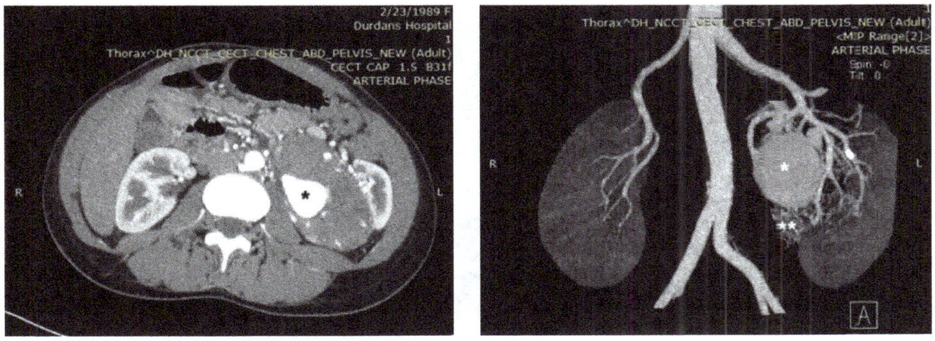

(a) (b)

FIGURE 1: Contrast enhanced CT images of the tumour. (a) An axial section showing the left renal tumour showing the aneurysm (asterisk). The tumour involves the entire kidney except a thin rim of normally enhancing renal tissue at the upper outer region. (b) CT renal angiogram showing multiple feeding arteries and the aneurysm (asterisk). The vasculature of the extrarenal cystic nodule (double asterisks) is also seen inferior to the aneurysm.

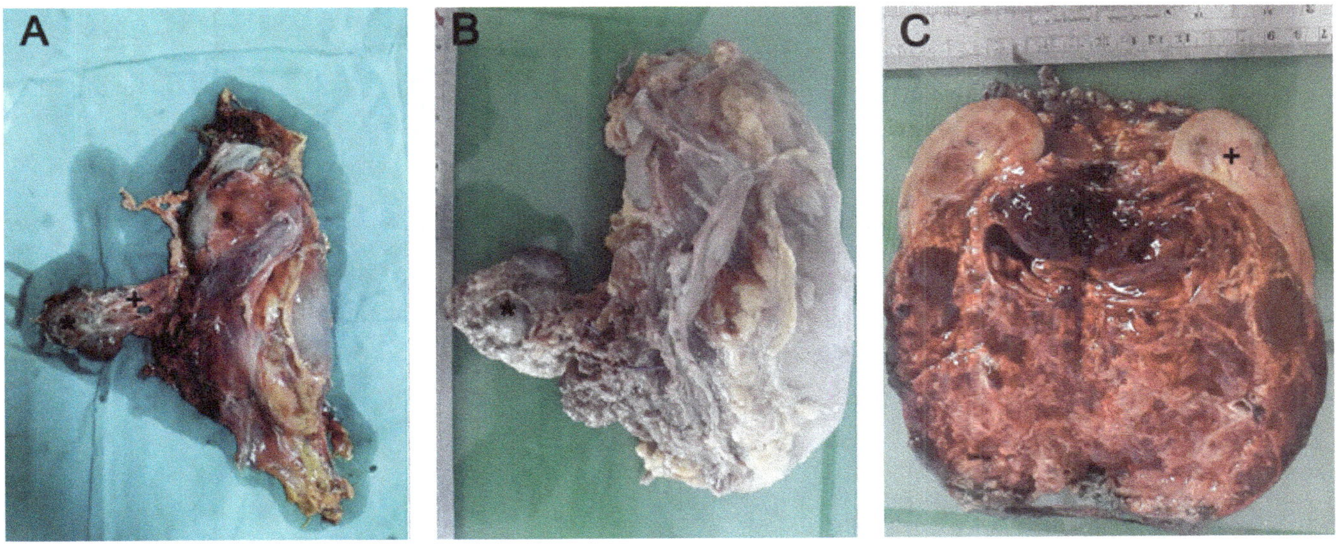

(a) (b) (c)

FIGURE 2: Macroscopic appearance of the tumour. (a) An immediate postoperative image of the specimen showing the left kidney, extrarenal tumor nodule (asterisk) and the vessels supplying it (+). (b) The external appearance of the specimen after formalin fixation demonstrating the separate tumor nodule (asterisk). (c) Cut surface showing the tumour involving the entire kidney sparing a thin rim of normal kidney tissue (+) and the aneurysm filled with a blood clot (asterisk).

antenatal ultrasound scans also had not detected any evidence of a maternal renal mass. There was no history of any familial cancer syndromes. There was a large, nontender, ballotable mass in the left loin. Apart from that, her physical examination was unremarkable. An ultrasound scan of the abdomen has found a large mass lesion involving the left kidney. A contrast-enhanced computerized tomogram (CECT) further detailed the lesion. It was a large, lobulated, well-demarcated, solid, and cystic tumor measuring $15 \times 9 \times 8.5$ cm arising from the mid to upper zones of the left kidney. Additionally, there was an aneurysm of 4.5×3.5 cm inside the tumor, the feeding artery of which could also be identified (Figure 1). There were few suspicious hilar and para-aortic lymph nodes. There was no evidence of distant metastasis and the other kidney was normal. Her serum creatinine was 0.78 mmol/l.

She was offered open radicle nephrectomy. During surgery, it was noted that there was another separate soft, cystic lesion anteromedial to the main tumour. It measured $5 \times 4.5 \times 4$ cm and had distinct blood supply (Figure 2). There were multiple hilar and para-aortic lymph nodes, which were sampled. The postoperative period was uneventful, and the patient was discharged on the third postoperative day.

Macroscopically, the main tumor measured $13.5 \times 7.5 \times 5.5$ cm and involved the upper and mid zones of the kidney. It was lobulated and well defined with large cystic and hemorrhagic areas. There was a blood-filled cavity in the posteromedial aspect of the kidney measuring $4.5 \times 3.8 \times 3.5$ cm which is compatible with the radiologically identified aneurysm (Figure 2). The extrarenal cystic lesion was multiloculated with thin septae and was filled with straw color fluid. Microscopically, the tumor was composed of two different

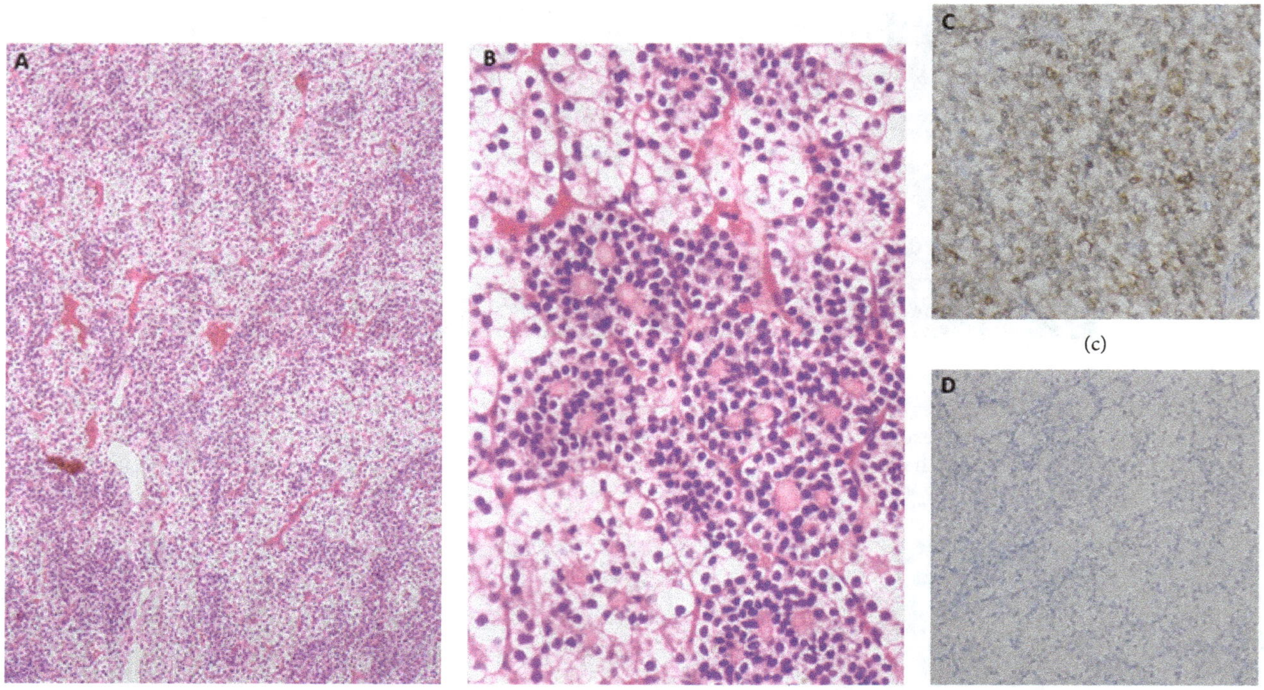

(a) (b) (c) (d)

FIGURE 3: Microscopic appearance of the tumour. (a) Closely packed nests comprising a dual population of cells—H&E 40x. (b) High-power view showing nests of large polygonal cells with clear cytoplasm, surrounded by a thin capillary network. The admixed second population of small cells are forming rosettes around deeply eosinophilic basement membrane like material—H&E 400x. (c) Positive immune-staining for Melan-A. (d) Negative staining for Vimentin.

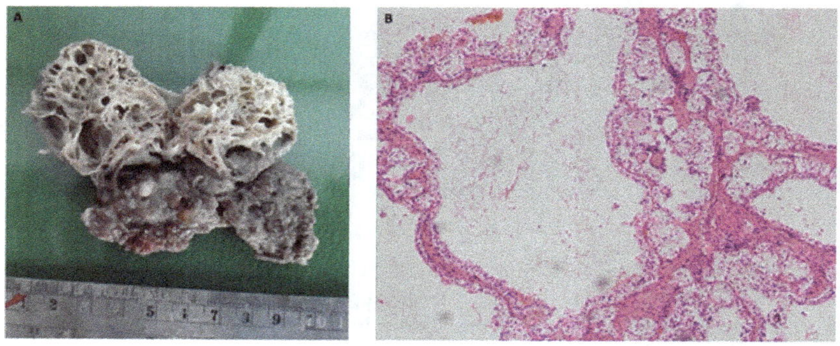

(a) (b)

FIGURE 4: The extrarenal tumor nodule. (a) A cut section showing multilocular cystic structure with thin fibrous septae. (b) Microscopy showing thin-walled cysts lined by a dual population of cells, similar to the main tumour—H&E 200x.

populations of malignant cells arranged in nests. The center of the nests was formed by closely packed small rounded cells with central rounded nuclei and scanty eosinophilic cytoplasm. The periphery of the nests had large polygonal cells with central rounded nuclei and abundant clear cytoplasm (Figure 3). Some areas had sheets of large polygonal cells. Numerous psammoma bodies were also found. Immunohistochemical analysis revealed diffuse cytoplasmic positivity for Melan-A and negative staining for Vimentin, HMB 45, and CD 117. All these features were compatible with MiT family translocation RCC. The tumor had invaded the branches of the renal vein and renal sinus fat, but there was no breach of the renal capsule (pT_{3a}). The intratumoral cystic lesion was lined by thin-walled vascular endothelium compatible with a venous aneurysm. The septae of the extrarenal cystic nodule were lined by multiple layers of large polygonal cells which were morphologically identical to those in the main tumor. The immunohistochemical staining pattern of it was also identical that of the primary tumour, i.e., diffuse cytoplasmic positivity for Melan-A and negative staining for Vimentin, HMB 45, and CD 117 (Figure 4). Thirteen out of 15 lymph nodes were positive for tumor deposits (pN1). Thus, the final pathological stage of the tumor was pT_{3a}, N_1, and M_0. A positron emission tomography (PET) scan carried out three months after the surgery did not detect any residual or metastatic tumor in this patient.

3. Discussion

Vascular anomalies are not uncommon in highly vascular tumors like RCCs with a higher tendency for vascular invasion and hematogenous spread. Proper identification of the location and the origin of a vascular lesion like an AVF or an aneurysm is pivotal for preoperative planning to avoid catastrophes during surgery. In the index case, the intratumoral aneurysm which was readily identified in the early arterial phase of the CECT was reported as an arterial aneurysm of one of the posterior sectoral branches of the renal artery. However, the wall of the aneurysm was composed of venous tissue histologically. Upon further inquiry into the CT angiography of the lesion, a small venous tributary was also identified in relation to the aneurysm. Therefore, the lesion was finally labeled as a venous aneurysm, distal to an arteriovenous fistula (AVF). An identical case of a venous aneurysm secondary to an AVF was reported by *Ferrante* et al. which was also identified as an arterial aneurysm, on preoperative radiology [1]. Five cases of RAA were reported so far to coexist with a RCC [2–5]. In all of the above cases, the aneurysm was found to be located outside the tumour. This is the only reported case so far, to have an aneurysm located inside a tumour mass of a RCC.

The existence of cystic RCC and coexistence of renal cysts with solid RCC are well known. In this patient, a separate cystic lesion was identified with readily identifiable distinct vascular supply. This lesion, which was retrospectively identified in the CECT, was not recognized as a separate mass in the initial report. The radiology team has considered it as a necrotic area of the main tumor, initially. The discovery of the same malignant epithelium with similar immunostaining pattern in the cyst made the case more interesting. The impact of this malignant nodule upon the staging and the prognosis of this patient cannot be determined as no such case is ever reported. It cannot be considered as a different malignancy because it shares the same histological and immunohistochemical features of the main tumor. It can neither be considered as a lymph node invaded by the tumor as no lymphatic tissue was identified inside the cyst. The origin of this malignant nodule remains elusive.

MiT family translocation renal cell carcinomas are a rare form of RCC having either Xp11 or t(6:11) chromosomal translocations. They are predominantly seen in the pediatric age group but extremely rare in adults and indicate poorer prognosis [6–8]. Xp11 subtype is commoner and found to account for 1.6% of adult RCCs in one series [9]. The t(6:11) translocation carcinomas are much rarer than Xp11 subtype and the incidence of which is 0.02% of all RCC [10]. Morphologically, they tend to mimic the various types of RCCs, including clear cell, papillary, and even epitheloid angiomyolipomas [6]. They are characteristically biphasic, with small cells clustered around basement membrane material and large polygonal epithelioid cells in the periphery which is compatible with the histology of this case report. The histopathological features of the two types are known to overlap, which can explain the abundance of psammoma bodies in the index case, which is a feature of Xp11 RCCs. Cytogenetic and specific immunohistochemical studies (TFE3 and TFEB) are necessary for both the confirmation of MiT translocation and for subtyping. We had to resort to surrogate immunohistochemical markers in this case as those studies are not available in Sri Lanka.

Both extraordinary features of this case were not precisely recognized preoperatively. The final diagnosis of both features necessitated several meetings with the pathology, radiology, oncology, and urology teams. Both the AVF/VA and the separate cystic tumor could be identified retrospectively in CECT. This emphasizes the importance of having multidisciplinary team meetings to discuss complex cases like the index case. Moreover, the oncological and prognostic implications of the extrarenal malignant cyst are a matter for further discussion.

4. Conclusion

RCCs can harbor vascular anomalies like AVF and VA which can make surgery challenging. Synchronous malignant cysts can exist even outside the kidney in cases with RCC. Reviewing preoperative imaging when pathology reports are available helps to overcome difficulties in making the final diagnosis in complex cases.

Consent

Informed, written consent was obtained for the publication of this article from the patient involved.

References

[1] A. Ferrante, C. di Stasi, F. Pierconti, and F. Snider, "Incidental finding of right renal venous aneurysm in a patient with symptomatic ipsilateral renal carcinoma: a case report," *Cardiovascular Pathology*, vol. 14, no. 6, pp. 327–330, 2005.

[2] R. A. Casillas, L. Romero, and C. de Virgilio, "Coexisting renal cell carcinoma and renal artery aneurysm," *Annals of Vascular Surgery*, vol. 16, no. 3, pp. 353–357, 2002.

[3] C. Selli, M. Carini, D. Turini, and A. Schifano, "Renal cell carcinoma associated with renal artery aneurysm. Report of two cases," *Urologia Internationalis*, vol. 38, no. 6, pp. 374–377, 1983.

[4] O. Ichiyanagi, M. Ishigooka, Y. Suzuki et al., "Renal cell carcinoma with renal artery aneurysm," *International Urology and Nephrology*, vol. 30, no. 4, pp. 385–390, 1998.

[5] Z. Wang, W. Xiong, C. Pan et al., "Coexisting renal cell carcinoma and renal artery aneurysm: a case report and literature review," *Experimental and Therapeutic Medicine*, vol. 9, no. 6, pp. 2356–2358, 2015.

[6] P. Cutruzzula, D. Cahn, D. Kivlin, C. Tong, D. Edwards, and M. Amster, "A review of translocation T(6;11) renal cell carcinoma Tumors in the adult patient," *Current Urology*, vol. 10, no. 2, pp. 69–71, 2017.

[7] Q. Rao, Q. Y. Xia, L. Cheng, and X. J. Zhou, "Molecular genetics and immunohistochemistry characterization of uncommon and recently described renal cell carcinomas," *Chinese Journal of Cancer Research*, vol. 28, no. 1, pp. 29–49, 2016.

[8] K. Peckova, T. Vanecek, P. Martinek et al., "Aggressive and nonaggressive translocation t(6;11) renal cell carcinoma: comparative study of 6 cases and review of the literature," *Annals of Diagnostic Pathology*, vol. 18, no. 6, pp. 351–357, 2014.

[9] Y. Komai, M. Fujiwara, Y. Fujii et al., "Adult Xp11 translocation renal cell carcinoma diagnosed by cytogenetics and immunohistochemistry," *Clinical Cancer Research*, vol. 15, no. 4, pp. 1170–1176, 2009.

[10] J. I. Geller, P. Argani, A. Adeniran et al., "Translocation renal cell carcinoma: lack of negative impact due to lymph node spread," *Cancer*, vol. 112, no. 7, pp. 1607–1616, 2008.

Metastatic Urothelial Carcinoma from Transplanted Kidney with Complete Response to an Immune Checkpoint Inhibitor

Ryan S. Chiang,[1] Ashton A. Connor,[2] Brant A. Inman,[3] Wen-Chi Foo,[4] David N. Howell,[4] John F. Madden,[4] Matthew J. Ellis,[5] Aparna S. Rege,[2] and Michael R. Harrison[6]

[1]*Department of Medicine, Stanford University Medical Center, Stanford, CA, USA*
[2]*Division of Abdominal Transplant Surgery, Department of Surgery, Duke University School of Medicine, Durham, NC, USA*
[3]*Division of Urology, Department of Surgery, Duke University School of Medicine, Durham, NC, USA*
[4]*Department of Pathology, Duke University School of Medicine, Durham, NC, USA*
[5]*Divisions of Nephrology and Abdominal Transplant, Departments of Medicine and Surgery, Duke University School of Medicine, Durham, NC, USA*
[6]*Division of Medical Oncology, Department of Medicine, Duke University School of Medicine, Durham, NC, USA*

Correspondence should be addressed to Michael R. Harrison; michael.harrison@duke.edu

Academic Editor: Fumitaka Koga

Background. Donor-derived malignancy is a rare complication in patients who undergo organ transplant. Approaches to treatment have largely been individualized based on clinical circumstances given the lack of evidence-based guidelines, with therapeutic options ranging from discontinuation of immunosuppression and transplantectomy to the addition of chemotherapy or radiotherapy. *Case Presentation.* Herein, we describe a 60-year-old woman with metastatic donor-derived upper tract urothelial carcinoma (UTUC) discovered nine years postrenal transplant. Molecular diagnostic studies using polymerase chain reaction amplification of short tandem repeat alleles and HLA tissue typing proved that the urothelial carcinoma originated from donor tissue. She achieved sustained complete remission with transplant nephroureterectomy, retroperitoneal lymphadenectomy, immunosuppression withdrawal, and immunotherapy with pembrolizumab. Routine radiologic surveillance has demonstrated 15-month progression-free survival to date off pembrolizumab, and she is now under consideration for retransplantation. *Conclusions.* Immunotherapy using checkpoint inhibitors can serve as a novel treatment option for patients in the clinical predicament of having a solid organ transplant and simultaneous metastatic malignancy. In this report, we also discuss the oncogenic potential of BK virus, the use of checkpoint inhibitors in urothelial carcinoma, and the feasibility of retransplant for this patient population.

1. Background

Nearly 36,500 transplants were performed in the U.S. in 2018, of which renal transplants comprised the majority at over 21,100 [1]. Solid organ transplant recipients are at higher risk of malignancies, due partly to immunosuppressive medications, decreased immune system surveillance, and risk of oncogenic viral infection [2, 3]. Donor-related malignancy is relatively rare and can be categorized as donor-transmitted if presenting shortly after transplant or donor-derived if many years later [4–6]. There are several reported cases of donor-related malignancies achieving complete remission after transplant organ resection, immunosuppression withdrawal, and occasionally chemotherapy or radiotherapy [7–10]. Features reported in 36 published allograft upper tract urothelial carcinoma (UTUC) cases include long latency (mean 10 years) from transplant to disease presentation, immunosuppression and BK infection as risk factors, and highly aggressive tumor biology [10]. Ortega et al. described a case of donor-derived UTUC discovered nine years postrenal transplant and complicated by BK viremia six years posttransplant successfully managed with transplant nephrectomy and immunosuppression withdrawal [11].

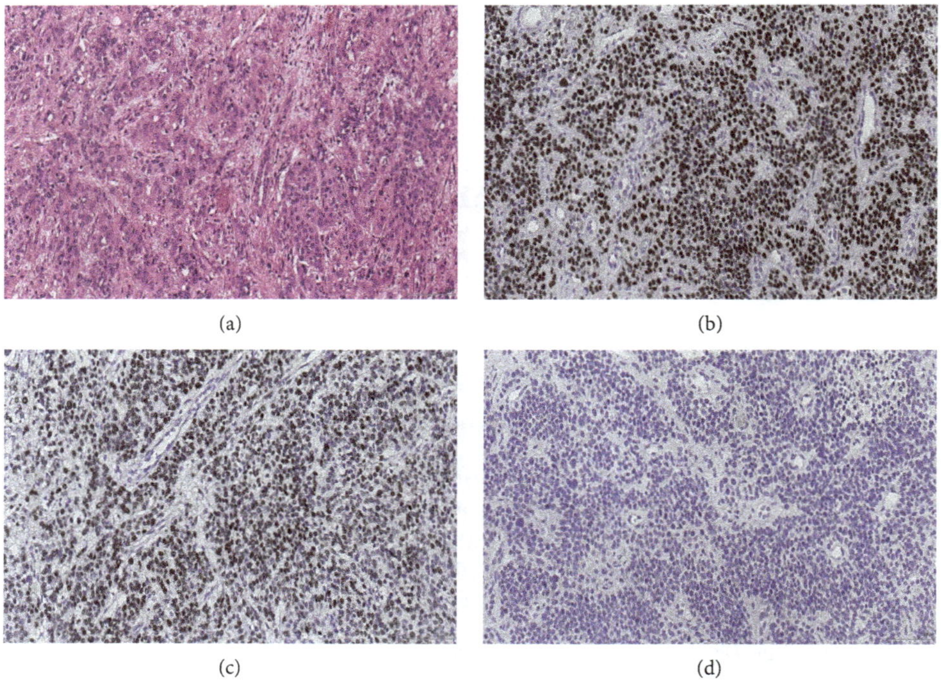

FIGURE 1: (a) The nephrectomy specimen demonstrated infiltrative nests of tumor cells with prominent nucleoli, moderate pleomorphism, and scattered mitoses (H&E). (b) Nuclear expression for p63 in the tumor cells supports the diagnosis of urothelial carcinoma. (c) SV40/BKV stain showing positive staining in the tumor cells. (d) PAX8 is negative in tumor cells, excluding renal cell carcinoma.

Here, we describe a patient who presented with high-grade stage IV UTUC of donor origin ten years after renal allotransplantation. Our patient was treated with transplant nephroureterectomy, retroperitoneal lymphadenectomy, immunosuppression withdrawal, and immunotherapy with pembrolizumab, achieving a sustained complete response.

2. Case Presentation

A 51-year-old Chinese woman with dialysis-dependent end-stage renal disease secondary to IgA nephropathy underwent deceased donor kidney transplant. Donor medical history did not include malignancies. Recipient medical history included vulvar and cervical intraepithelial dysplasia. She had stable creatinine 2.0 mg/dL on tacrolimus, mycophenolate, and prednisone, despite chronic BK viral infection.

Nine years posttransplant, she presented with a several-month history of episodic severe lower abdominal pain. Abdominal computed tomography (CT) revealed a $5.8 \times 5.5 \times 4.6$ cm renal allograft hilar mass, with FDG-avid supraclavicular, mesenteric, retroperitoneal, pulmonary, and hepatic lesions on PET. This imaging, urine cytology, allograft biopsy, and diagnostic laparoscopy were concordant for stage IV UTUC. She underwent transplant nephrectomy and retroperitoneal lymphadenectomy, with final pathology demonstrating pT4N2M0R1 UTUC, with malignant epithelium, high-grade atypia, interstitial fibrosis, tubular atrophy, and extranodal extension, with the largest foci measuring 1.5 cm. There was neither rejection nor IgA nephropathy recurrence. Immunohistochemistry (IHC) stains were negative for C4d and PAX8 and positive for p63, GATA3, CK20, p16, and SV40/BKV (see Figure 1), consistent with UTUC with BK viral protein expression. Next-generation sequencing results were notable for microsatellite-stable, undeterminable tumor mutational burden, EGFR amplification, KDM6A L945fs∗25, and RAF1 amplification. PD-L1 IHC analysis showed a combined positive score of zero (therefore, PD-L1-negative). Chimerism was assessed by PCR amplification of fifteen short tandem repeats and by HLA tissue typing, both showing concordance between donor and malignancy, but not recipient, implying allograft origin.

Despite stopping immunosuppression, disease progression was seen on restaging CT scans two months later. Multidisciplinary cancer conference consensus was for PD-1 blockade with pembrolizumab. She received 28 cycles of pembrolizumab 200 mg IV every three weeks over about 19 months, achieving complete radiological response, with 15-month progression-free survival to date off therapy (see Figure 2). Surveillance imaging continues at 3-month intervals.

3. Discussion

We present a case of post-renal-allotransplantation donor-derived, disseminated UTUC that achieved complete response with transplant nephrectomy, retroperitoneal lymphadenectomy, immunosuppression cessation, and immunotherapy. There have been several cases described in the literature where withdrawal of immunosuppression has been sufficient for treatment of squamous cell carcinomas, undifferentiated epithelioid tumor, and donor-derived urothelial carcinoma in renal transplant patients [11–14]. To our knowledge, this is the first reported case where a patient who developed donor-

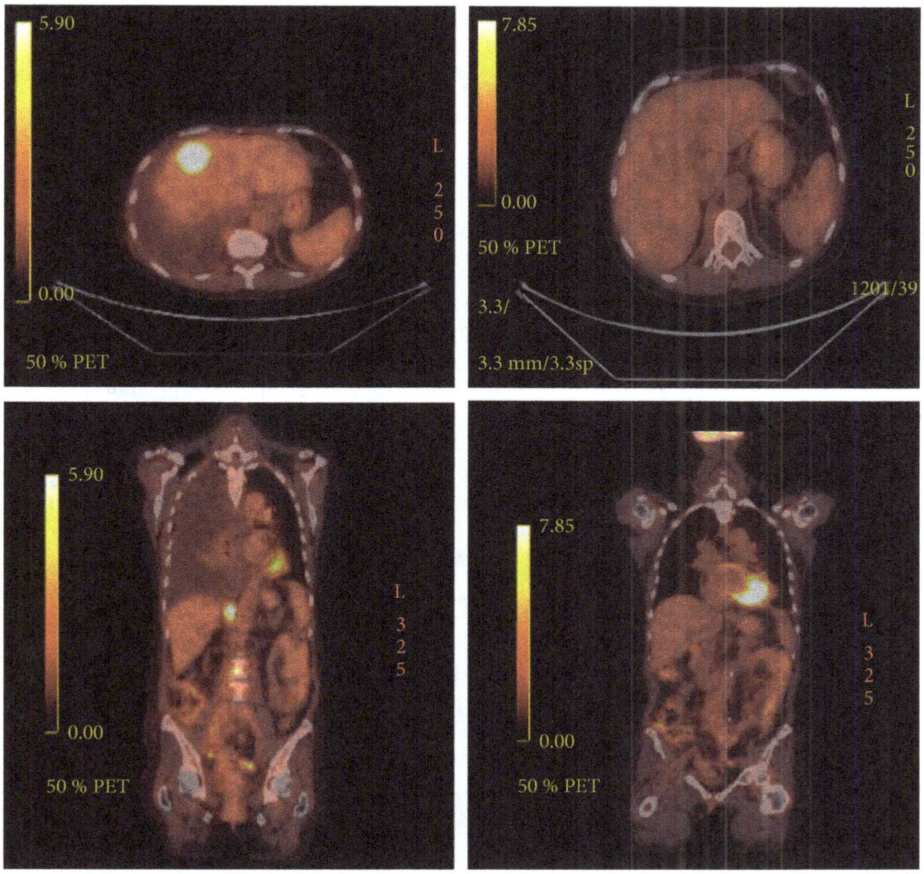

FIGURE 2: PET/CT scans showing improvement in metastatic disease with reduction in hepatic mass and decreased retroperitoneal, pelvic, and iliac lymphadenopathy after 4 cycles of pembrolizumab.

derived urothelial carcinoma achieved complete response on immune checkpoint inhibitor therapy and is now considering a repeat renal transplant. This case adds to the literature on a rare complication of kidney transplantation, with important features being BK viral expression in cancer cells, the indications for immunotherapy, and the consideration for redo transplant.

Many viruses have been implicated to promote oncogenesis through a variety of mechanisms not limited to tumor suppressor protein degradation, direct genome integration, and cell cycle dysregulation [15–18]. BK polyomavirus is a widespread double-stranded DNA virus that tends to pathologically manifest in immunocompromised individuals such as those who undergo organ transplantation through viral reactivation [19]. In recent years, BK polyomavirus has emerged as a source of malignant transformation in humans with improved understanding of its carcinogenic pathophysiology. The primary oncogenic driver seems to be persistent latent infection via genome integration which leads to overexpression of the viral oncoprotein and large T antigen and subsequently promotes unwarranted cellular proliferation [20–23]. Several case reports have highlighted the potential for BK viremia to predispose patients to posttransplant urothelial carcinoma through persistent infection coupled with chronic immunosuppression which serves as an ideal breeding ground for cancer development [24, 25]. A fully intact immune system is often sufficient for resuppression of BK viremia and may explain why some patients with donor-derived malignancy experience complete cancer remission upon immunosuppression discontinuation and transplantectomy alone. PD-1 plays a significant role in T cell exhaustion during chronic viral infections which can serve as one potential mechanism of efficacy for pembrolizumab as the blockade can lead to restoration of T cell function. However, the exact duration of BK viremia could not be established for our patient since she had received only one BK virus quantitative PCR which showed detectable levels several months prior to the official diagnosis of metastatic UTUC. Repeat measurement at the time of cancer diagnosis demonstrated significant elevation in the number of viral copies. PD-L1 testing performed after diagnosis was negative which makes the mechanism of favorable efficacy for pembrolizumab unclear in this case.

Standard therapy for metastatic urothelial carcinoma has historically been combination cisplatin-based chemotherapy in those who are cisplatin-eligible [26]. For those with platinum-refractory urothelial carcinoma, pembrolizumab has been an effective option with better overall survival rates as well as lower rates of adverse events when compared to standard chemotherapy regimens [27]. Pembrolizumab is an immune checkpoint inhibitor which functions by blocking the PD-1 receptor to allow a greater natural immune response against tumors [28]. Based on the findings of KEYNOTE-52, a multicenter, single-arm, phase 2 study, pembrolizumab can also serve as an effective and safe first-line therapy option in patients who are cisplatin-ineligible [29]. Many clinical trials have excluded patients with solid organ transplants who develop metastatic cancers from the use of checkpoint inhibitors due to concerns for graft rejection [30, 31]. One systematic review of 57 patients found that the use of immune checkpoint inhibitors had no significant association with graft rejection and can have clinically relevant response rates for treating metastatic cancer [30]. A recently published case series found that although immune checkpoint inhibitors can serve as a viable therapeutic option for transplant patients, prospective studies are warranted given the potential risk of allograft rejection [32]. There is currently limited data on the safety and efficacy of immune checkpoint inhibitor rechallenge after withdrawal due to complete response, but restarting immune checkpoint inhibitor therapy after progression often results in very low response rates [33, 34]. Given these studies, we could potentially provide her with another renal transplant while reinitiating pembrolizumab followed by close monitoring for both signs of graft rejection as well as signs of cancer recurrence.

There is little published experience on redo renal allotransplantation following complete remission of donor-derived malignancies. Occult metastatic disease may resurface with reinstitution of immunosuppression. Yet, most patients can safely undergo solid organ transplantation after two years of disease-free survival following treatment of most malignancies, including renal cell carcinoma. The indications for redo kidney transplant include improved quality and quantity of life compared with dialysis by eliminating scheduled dialysis sessions and minimizing cardiovascular complications [35–37]. Georgieva et al. describe 3 patients with donor-related malignancies who successfully underwent retransplantation after achieving complete remission, implying that it may be safe [7].

4. Conclusion

As the need for solid organ transplantation continues to increase, the prevalence of donor-related malignancies can be expected to also rise. More evidence is required to inform management of these uncommon malignancies that currently have high morbidity and mortality. This case includes discussion of novel etiology, investigation, treatment, surveillance, and postremission redo transplantation. With increased published experience, we may advance beyond individualized approaches to having evidence-based guidelines.

References

[1] *UNOS: transplant trends*, 2019, December 2019, https://unos.org/data/transplant-trends/.

[2] E. A. Engels, R. M. Pfeiffer, J. F. Fraumeni et al., "Spectrum of cancer risk among US solid organ transplant recipients," *JAMA*, vol. 306, no. 17, pp. 1891–1901, 2011.

[3] A. E. Grulich, M. T. van Leeuwen, M. O. Falster, and C. M. Vajdic, "Incidence of cancers in people with HIV/AIDS compared with immunosuppressed transplant recipients: a meta-analysis," *The Lancet*, vol. 370, no. 9581, pp. 59–67, 2007.

[4] R. Desai, D. Collett, C. J. Watson, P. Johnson, T. Evans, and J. Neuberger, "Cancer transmission from organ donors-unavoidable but low risk," *Transplantation*, vol. 94, no. 12, pp. 1200–1207, 2012.

[5] H. M. Kauffman, M. A. McBride, W. S. Cherikh, P. C. Spain, W. H. Marks, and A. M. Roza, "Transplant tumor registry: donor related malignancies," *Transplantation*, vol. 74, p. 358e62, 2002.

[6] M. J. Gandhi and D. M. Strong, "Donor derived malignancy following transplantation: a review," *Cell and Tissue Banking*, vol. 8, p. 267e86, 2007.

[7] L. A. Georgieva, E. M. Gielis, R. Hellemans et al., "Single-center case series of donor-related malignancies: rare cases with tremendous impact," *Transplantation Proceedings*, vol. 48, no. 8, pp. 2669–2677, 2016.

[8] T. Baudoux, K. Gastaldello, S. Rorive, A. Hamade, N. Broeders, and J. L. Nortier, "Donor cancer transmission in kidney transplantation," *Kidney International Reports*, vol. 2, no. 2, pp. 134–137, 2017.

[9] J. F. Buell, T. Gross, R. R. Alloway, J. Trofe, and E. S. Woodle, "Central nervous system tumors in donors: misdiagnosis carries a high morbidity and mortality," *Transplantation Proceedings*, vol. 37, no. 2, pp. 583-584, 2005.

[10] M. I. Bellini, J. P. Gopal, P. Hill, D. Nicol, and N. Gibbons, "Urothelial carcinoma arising from the transplanted kidney: a single-center experience and literature review," *Clinical Transplantation*, vol. 33, no. 6, article e13559, 2019.

[11] R. M. Michel Ortega, D. J. Wolff, C. A. Schandl, and H. A. Drabkin, "Urothelial carcinoma of donor origin in a kidney transplant patient," *Journal for immunotherapy of cancer*, vol. 4, no. 1, p. 63, 2016.

[12] F. J. Moloney, P. O. Kelly, E. W. Kay, P. Conlon, and G. M. Murphy, "Maintenance versus reduction of immunosuppression in renal transplant recipients with aggressive squamous cell carcinoma," *Dermatologic Surgery*, vol. 30, 4 Part 2, pp. 674–678, 2004.

[13] A. H. Waldman, J. M. McNiff, A. M. Liapakis, W. S. Asch, S. Smith-Marrone, and O. R. Colegio, "Revision of immunosuppression in a solid organ transplant recipient leads to complete remission of metastatic undifferentiated carcinoma," *JAAD Case Reports*, vol. 1, no. 6, pp. S8–S11, 2015.

[14] M. T. van Leeuwen, A. C. Webster, M. R. E. McCredie et al., "Effect of reduced immunosuppression after kidney transplant failure on risk of cancer: population based retrospective cohort study," *BMJ*, vol. 340, no. 2, p. c570, 2010.

[15] A. Bansal, M. P. Singh, and B. Rai, "Human papillomavirus-associated cancers: a growing global problem," *International Journal of Applied & Basic Medical Research*, vol. 6, no. 2, pp. 84–89, 2016.

[16] D. R. McGivern and S. M. Lemon, "Virus-specific mechanisms of carcinogenesis in hepatitis C virus associated liver cancer," *Oncogene*, vol. 30, no. 17, pp. 1969–1983, 2011.

[17] M. Tarocchi, S. Polvani, G. Marroncini, and A. Galli, "Molecular mechanism of hepatitis B virus-induced hepatocarcinogenesis," *World Journal of Gastroenterology*, vol. 20, no. 33, pp. 11630–11640, 2014.

[18] G. Niedobitek, N. Meru, and H. J. Delecluse, "Epstein-Barr virus infection and human malignancies," *International Journal of Experimental Pathology*, vol. 82, no. 3, pp. 149–170, 2001.

[19] S. M. Bennett, N. M. Broekema, and M. J. Imperiale, "BK polyomavirus: emerging pathogen," *Microbes and Infection*, vol. 14, no. 9, pp. 672–683, 2012.

[20] K. F. Harris, J. B. Christensen, E. H. Radany, and M. J. Imperiale, "Novel mechanisms of E2F induction by BK virus large-T antigen: requirement of both the pRb-binding and the J domains," *Molecular and Cellular Biology*, vol. 18, no. 3, pp. 1746–1756, 1998.

[21] D. J. Kenan, P. A. Mieczkowski, R. Burger-Calderon, H. K. Singh, and V. Nickeleit, "The oncogenic potential of BK-polyomavirus is linked to viral integration into the human genome," *The Journal of Pathology*, vol. 237, no. 3, pp. 379–389, 2015.

[22] F. Fu, W. Deng, S. Yu et al., "Occurrence and regression of BK polyomavirus associated carcinoma: a clinical and next-generation sequencing study," *Clinical Science*, vol. 132, no. 16, pp. 1753–1763, 2018.

[23] P. An, M. T. Sáenz Robles, and J. M. Pipas, "Large T antigens of polyomaviruses: amazing molecular machines," *Annual Review of Microbiology*, vol. 66, no. 1, pp. 213–236, 2012.

[24] S. P. Salvatore, P. M. Myers-Gurevitch, S. Chu, B. D. Robinson, D. Dadhania, and S. V. Seshan, "Polyoma (BK) virus associated urothelial carcinoma originating within a renal allograft five years following resolution of polyoma virus nephropathy," *Clinical Nephrology*, vol. 85, no. 3, pp. 179–183, 2016.

[25] B. A. Alexiev, P. Randhawa, E. Vazquez Martul et al., "BK virus-associated urinary bladder carcinoma in transplant recipients: report of 2 cases, review of the literature, and proposed pathogenetic model," *Human Pathology*, vol. 44, no. 5, pp. 908–917, 2013.

[26] H. von der Maase, S. W. Hansen, J. T. Roberts et al., "Gemcitabine and cisplatin versus methotrexate, vinblastine, doxorubicin, and cisplatin in advanced or metastatic bladder cancer: results of a large, randomized, multinational, multicenter, phase III study," *Journal of Clinical Oncology*, vol. 18, no. 17, pp. 3068–3077, 2000.

[27] Y. Fradet, J. Bellmunt, D. J. Vaughn et al., "Randomized phase III KEYNOTE-045 trial of pembrolizumab versus paclitaxel, docetaxel, or vinflunine in recurrent advanced urothelial cancer: results of >2 years of follow-up," *Annals of Oncology*, vol. 30, no. 6, pp. 970–976, 2019.

[28] G. Roviello, S. P. Corona, G. Nesi, and E. Mini, "Results from a meta-analysis of immune checkpoint inhibitors in first-line renal cancer patients: does PD-L1 matter?," *Therapeutic Advances in Medical Oncology*, vol. 11, 2019.

[29] A. V. Balar, D. Castellano, P. H. O'Donnell et al., "First-line pembrolizumab in cisplatin-ineligible patients with locally advanced and unresectable or metastatic urothelial cancer (KEYNOTE-052): a multicentre, single-arm, phase 2 study," *The Lancet Oncology*, vol. 18, no. 11, pp. 1483–1492, 2017.

[30] N. Abdel-Wahab, H. Safa, A. Abudayyeh et al., "Checkpoint inhibitor therapy for cancer in solid organ transplantation recipients: an institutional experience and a systematic review of the literature," *Journal for Immunotherapy of Cancer*, vol. 7, no. 1, p. 106, 2019.

[31] J. Fisher, N. Zeitouni, W. Fan, and F. H. Samie, "Immune checkpoint inhibitor therapy in solid organ transplant recipients: a patient-centered systematic review," *Journal of the American Academy of Dermatology*, vol. 82, no. 6, pp. 1490–1500, 2020.

[32] V. Kumar, A. B. Shinagare, H. G. Rennke et al., "The safety and efficacy of checkpoint inhibitors in transplant recipients: a case series and systematic review of literature," *The Oncologist*, vol. 25, no. 6, pp. 505–514, 2020.

[33] H. Watanabe, T. Kubo, K. Ninomiya et al., "The effect and safety of immune checkpoint inhibitor rechallenge in non-small cell lung cancer," *Japanese Journal of Clinical Oncology*, vol. 49, no. 8, pp. 762–765, 2019.

[34] Y. Katayama, T. Shimamoto, T. Yamada et al., "Retrospective efficacy analysis of immune checkpoint inhibitor rechallenge in patients with non-small cell lung cancer," *Journal of Clinical Medicine*, vol. 9, no. 1, 2020.

[35] T. T. Jansz, A. A. Bonenkamp, F. T. J. Boereboom, F. E. van Reekum, M. C. Verhaar, and B. C. van Jaarsveld, "Health-related quality of life compared between kidney transplantation and nocturnal hemodialysis," *PloS One*, vol. 13, no. 9, article e0204405, 2018.

[36] J. Z. Kostro, A. Hellmann, J. Kobiela et al., "Quality of life after kidney transplantation: a prospective study," *Transplantation Proceedings*, vol. 48, no. 1, pp. 50–54, 2016.

[37] M. A. Kaballo, M. Canney, P. O'Kelly, Y. Williams, C. M. O'Seaghdha, and P. J. Conlon, "A comparative analysis of survival of patients on dialysis and after kidney transplantation," *Clinical Kidney Journal*, vol. 11, no. 3, pp. 389–393, 2018.

31

Renal Metastasis of Osteosarcoma with IVC Thrombus

Prem Raj Sigdel, Diwas Gnyawali, Purushottam Parajuli, Sampanna Chudal, Durga Pandit, Bipin Guragain, Manish Man Pradhan, Sujeet Poudyal, Suman Chapagain, Bhoj Raj Luitel, Pawan Raj Chalise, and Uttam Kumar Sharma

Department of Urology and Kidney Transplant Surgery, Tribhuvan University Teaching Hospital, Institute of Medicine, Maharajgunj, Kathmandu 44600, Nepal

Correspondence should be addressed to Prem Raj Sigdel; prem.sigdel7@gmail.com

Academic Editor: Apul Goel

Renal metastasis from osteosarcoma is a rare entity, and tumour thrombus is even rarer. To date, only 15 cases of osteosarcoma with tumour thrombus have been reported in the literature. We present a case of an 18-year-old female diagnosed as having right distal femur osteosarcoma, later presenting with renal osteosarcoma with IVC thrombus.

1. Introduction

Renal metastasis from osteosarcoma is a rare entity, and tumour thrombus is even rarer. We present a case of an 18-year-old female who was diagnosed with right distal femur osteosarcoma who developed metastasis in the bilateral lungs one year later and renal metastasis after 1.5 years. Osteosarcoma with metastasis to the kidney with IVC thrombus is an aggressive tumour and has a poor prognosis. A multidisciplinary approach is required for the appropriate management.

2. Case Presentation

An eighteen-year-old female was diagnosed as having a case of right distal femur osteosarcoma 1.5 years back. The patient underwent resection of the femur with the placement of a prosthesis. Biopsy reports of the femur showed chondroblastic osteosarcoma. She received four cycles of cisplatin-based chemotherapy postoperatively. On routine CT chest after one year, nodular lesions were seen in bilateral lungs. Biopsy of these lung lesions showed metastatic osteosarcoma. She underwent right lower lobectomy and left upper lobe metastasectomy.

Six months after the lung lesions, she presented to us with complaints of vague abdominal pain. She had no haematuria or abdominal mass. She had no respiratory, urinary, or other systemic symptoms. CECT abdomen and pelvis showed right enlarged kidney with calcifications with calcified thrombus in IVC (Figures 1 and 2). CT head was done, which showed no brain metastasis.

A multidisciplinary discussion was done with provisional diagnosis of metastatic renal sarcoma with level III thrombus. She was planned for right radical nephrectomy and IVC thrombectomy. Intraoperatively, kidney mobilization and hilar dissection were done. After liver mobilization, sequential IVC clamping was done in order or infrarenal IVC, left renal vein, Pringle manoeuvre, and suprahepatic IVC. Venacavotomy and thrombus retrieval were done (Figure 3). The specimen was retrieved (Figure 4). Closure of cavotomy with sequential declamping was done. Postoperative events were uneventful.

Histopathology reports showed metastatic osteosarcoma of the kidney (Figure 5). Patients were lost to follow-up in our centre. We later knew that she developed metastatic deposits in the pelvic bones one month after surgery, but the MRI images are not available.

3. Discussion

Osteosarcoma is the most frequent malignant tumour of bones, with a peak incidence in the second decade of life

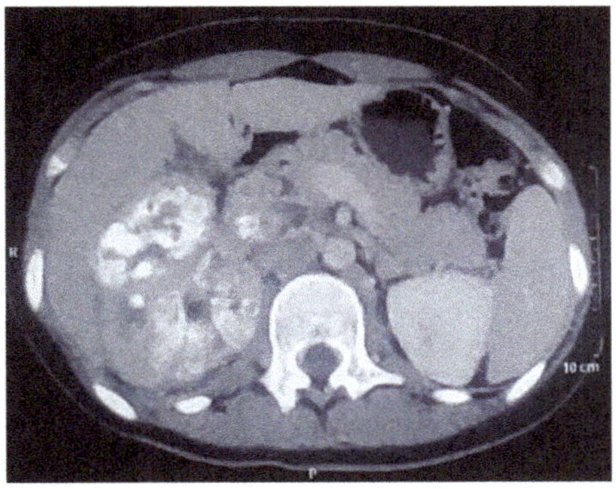

FIGURE 1: Axial CT scan showing right renal calcifications with involvement of IVC.

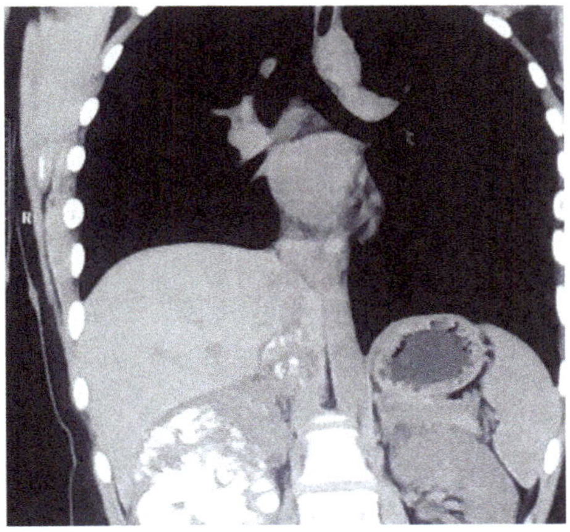

FIGURE 2: Coronal CT scan showing the involvement of IVC with the tumour thrombus.

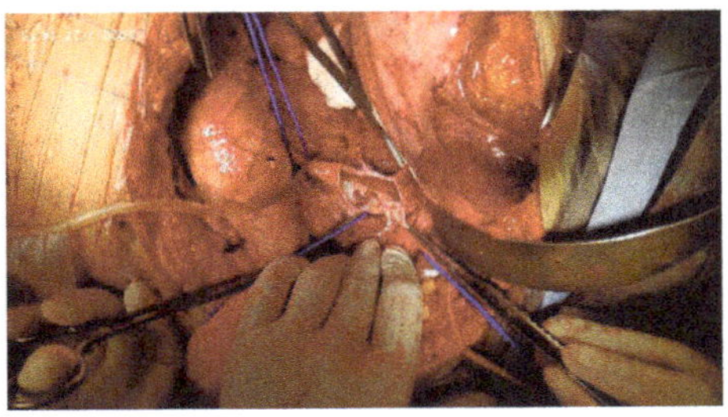

FIGURE 3: Cavotomy and removal of tumor thrombus.

[1]. The metaphyseal part of long bones is most frequently involved. The most common site of metastasis of osteosarcoma is the lung. Metastasis to soft tissues and solid organs is rare. Extrapulmonary sites are more common in treated cases because of change in the natural history of the disease by more prolonged survival of these patients and the use of multiple chemotherapy agents [2]. To date, only 15 cases of osteosarcoma with tumour thrombus have been reported in the literature [3]. The diagnosis of IVC thrombus is usually incidental. The reported incidence of renal metastasis of extrarenal neoplasms varies from 2 to 20% [4]. Metastatic osteosarcoma is usually diagnosed by imaging because of

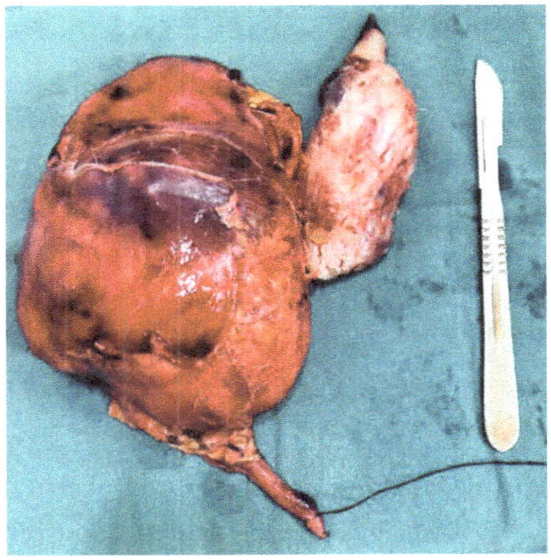

FIGURE 4: Specimen of the right kidney and IVC thrombus.

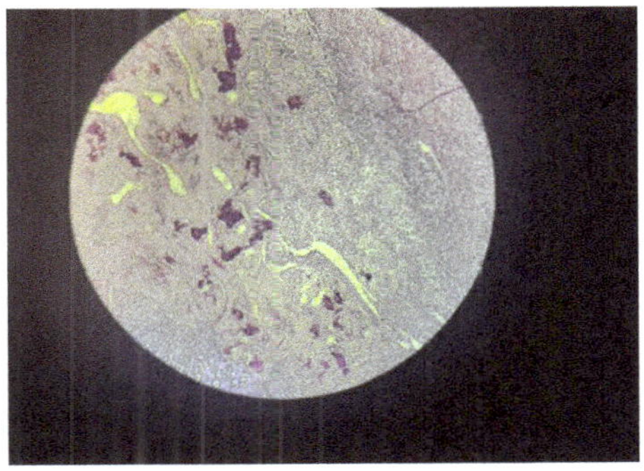

FIGURE 5: Histopathology showing renal osteosarcoma.

concern of dissemination of disease on needle biopsy [5]. Metastatic lesions usually do not have enough calcifications that can be seen in simple radiograph as compared to primary renal osteosarcoma [6]. Renal metastasis of osteosarcoma is generally detected after death as part of widespread disease; 10–12% of patient autopsies showed renal involvement [4]. Surgical resection of the intravascular/intracardiac tumour thrombus is the treatment of choice. Patients with metastatic tumour thrombus generally do not survive for more than 12 or 13 months [3].

4. Conclusion

Osteosarcoma with renal metastasis with tumour thrombus is a rare entity. Successful management of such cases relies on a careful multidisciplinary approach. Whether surgery increases the survival of these patients is still unknown and requires further investigations.

Consent

Written informed consent was taken from the patient party for the publication of this case.

Acknowledgments

I thank Dr. Benju Nepal for her assistance in the preparation of this manuscript. I thank Dr. Sabita Bishowkarma for helping to prepare pathology slides.

References

[1] Y. Akasbi, S. Arifi, K. Lahlaidi et al., "Renal metastases of a femur osteosarcoma: a case report and a review of the literature," *Case Reports in Urology*, vol. 2012, Article ID 259193, 3 pages, 2012.

[2] R. Wolf, R. F. E. Wolf, and H. J. Hoekstra, "Recurrent, multiple, calcified soft tissue metastases from osteogenic sarcoma without pulmonary involvement," *Skeletal Radiology*, vol. 28, no. 12, pp. 710–713, 1999.

[3] P. Navalkele, S. M. Jones, J. K. Jones et al., "Osteosarcoma tumor thrombus: a case report with a review of the literature," *Texas Heart Institute Journal*, vol. 40, no. 1, pp. 75–78, 2013.

[4] G. M. Jeffree, C. H. Price, and H. A. Sissons, "The metastatic patterns of osteosarcoma," *British Journal of Cancer*, vol. 32, no. 1, pp. 87–107, 1975.

[5] W. N. Raby, P. Kopplin, and S. Weitzman, "Metastatic osteosarcoma of the kidney presenting as renal hemorrhage," *Journal of Pediatric Hematology/Oncology*, vol. 18, no. 3, pp. 321-322, 1996.

[6] S. K. Lockhart, J. D. Coan, N. Jaffe, F. Eftekhari, C. David, and A. Shirkhoda, "Osteosarcoma metastatic to the kidney," *Clinical Imaging*, vol. 13, no. 2, pp. 154–156, 1989.

Page Kidney in a Child with Severe Pelviureteric Junction Obstruction

Senthil G. Kamaraj,[1] Ashita Kochunny,[2] Gopinathan Kathirvelu,[3] Praachi Singh,[4] and Naeem Samnakay[5]

[1]*Consultant Paediatric Urologist, Kanchi Kamakoti Child's Trust Hospital, 12-A, Nageswara Road, Nungambakkam, Chennai 600034, India*
[2]*Registrar in Paediatric Surgery, Kanchi Kamakoti Child's Trust Hospital, India*
[3]*Consultant Radiologist, Kanchi Kamakoti Child's Trust Hospital, India*
[4]*Registrar in Paediatrics, Kanchi Kamakoti Child's Trust Hospital, India*
[5]*Clinical Associate Professor, University of Western Australia, Paediatric Urologist, Perth Children's Hospital, 12 Hospital Ave, Nedlands, WA 6009, Australia*

Correspondence should be addressed to Senthil G. Kamaraj; dr.senthilkamaraj@gmail.com

Academic Editor: Fumitaka Koga

There are various causes of Reno Vascular Hypertension in children reported in the literature. Amongst these, Page kidney gets a rare mention. This phenomenon is a result of the accumulation of blood or urine in the perinephric or subcapsular space, resulting in compression of renal parenchyma, microvascular ischemia, alteration in the renin-angiotensin apparatus, and high renin hypertension. It has been well documented and studied in adults. Only a few cases are reported in the paediatric population. We report a rare presentation of Page kidney in a 5 year 8 months old girl. She initially presented with Dietl's crisis secondary to left Pelviureteric Junction obstruction (PUJO) causing massive hydronephrosis. She developed Page kidney phenomenon after spontaneous rupture of the pelvicalyceal system formed a tight compressive urinoma. She was managed successfully with internal JJ stenting and ultrasound-guided aspiration of the urinoma followed by elective delayed Pyeloplasty. To our knowledge, this is the first documented case of Page kidney in a child with severe PUJO.

1. Introduction

Page kidney refers to the occurrence of hypertension secondary to renal compression and is usually associated with a subcapsular or perinephric hematoma [1]. The first documented clinical case of Page kidney was reported in 1955 by Engel and Page [2]. Thereafter, many cases were reported, mainly in adults following trauma. We report a case of Page kidney in a child with PUJO, developed after spontaneous rupture of the pelvicalyceal system formed a massive subcapsular urinoma.

2. Case Report

A 5 year 8 month old presented to the emergency department with abdominal pain and non bilious vomits for 4 days. On clinical examination, there was a palpable loin mass. Ultrasound (USS) showed marked left (Figure 1) hydronephrosis with thinning of the renal cortex and severely dilated renal pelvis with an anteroposterior diameter of 6.3 cm. She was admitted to the ward for further assessment and management. EC scan, done with free draining bladder catheter, showed a differential function of 22% in the left kidney: with

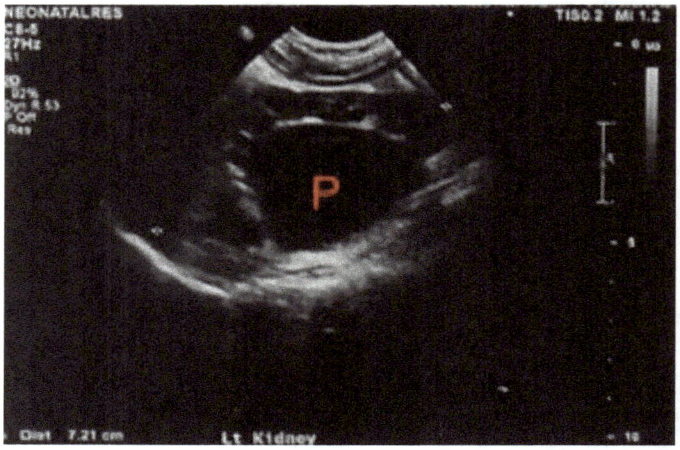

Figure 1: Ultrasound showing severe left PUJO at presentation.

an obstructive drainage pattern. The Right kidney had 78% split function and a normal drainage pattern. An early pyeloplasty during the same admission was planned.

Overnight, the girl developed seizures and elevated blood pressure of 120/78 (99th centile for age). In this acute setting, she was shifted to the Intensive care unit where she was managed with antihypertensive (Amlodipine and Prazosin) and anticonvulsant medications (Lorazepam and Levetiracetam). MRI Brain showed changes secondary to Malignant Hypertension and ruled out bleeding or infarction. With treatment, her seizures were controlled and stabilisation of blood pressure was achieved.

A repeat USS showed a large perinephric/subcapsular collection of size 18.3x10.0 cm with internal septae encompassing the left kidney. CT scan demonstrated a left PUJO associated with extravasation of contrast from the left pelvicalyceal system and dilated pelvis, forming a 13x10x6.5 cm large subcapsular collection with internal hemorrhage. This collection resulted in displacement of the left kidney and compression of left renal parenchyma—The clinical and imaging features were suggestive of Page kidney (Figure 2).

Under general anaesthetic, she underwent USS guided aspiration of the tense subcapsular collection (150 ml), followed by a Retrograde Pyelogram (RGP) and cystoscopic placement of a 3.5 F 16 cm JJ stent across the PUJO (Figures 3 and 4). She stabilised postprocedure with normalisation of blood pressure and control of seizures. Repeat USS 5 days later showed resolving perinephric collection and reduction in hydronephrosis (Figure 5). She was discharged home on antibiotic prophylaxis. The antihypertensive and antiepileptic medications were successfully tapered and ceased in the hospital prior to discharge.

Six weeks later, repeat USS showed complete resolution of the subcapsular collection and further reduction in APD of the left renal collecting system to 1.1 cm. In order to reassess the split renal function on the left, a DMSA scan was performed; Split renal function of left kidney now, with relief of acute obstruction, was 42% as compared to 22% before the stenting and drainage. She underwent a Left Anderson Hynes dismembered Pyeloplasty. The postoperative period was uneventful. JJ stent was removed 6 weeks postsurgery.

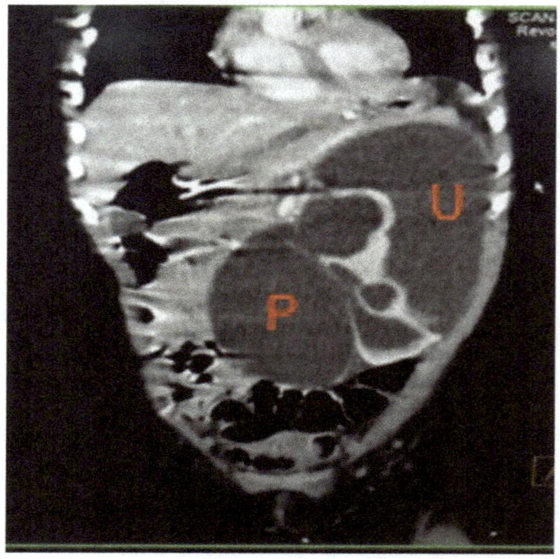

Figure 2: CT showing severe PUJO, ruptured with compressive urinoma. P: pelvis, U: compressive urinoma.

After a year of follow-up, she has been symptom-free, off medications and has minimal residual hydronephrosis on USS.

3. Discussion

The term Page kidney originated in 1939 when Dr. Irvin Page performed an experiment in which he wrapped the kidneys of dogs in cellophane [3]. He observed changes of perinephritis and the development of hypertension in these dogs. Hypertension develops due to external compression of renal parenchyma leading to microvascular ischemia and activation of Renin-Angiotension-Aldosterone System [1]. A similar response occurs when subcapsular or perinephric hematoma or encasing fibrous capsule causes induction of perinephritis and parenchymal compression [4].

Our case already had a pelvicalyceal (PCS) system under severe pressure, and after rupture of the PCS, there was in

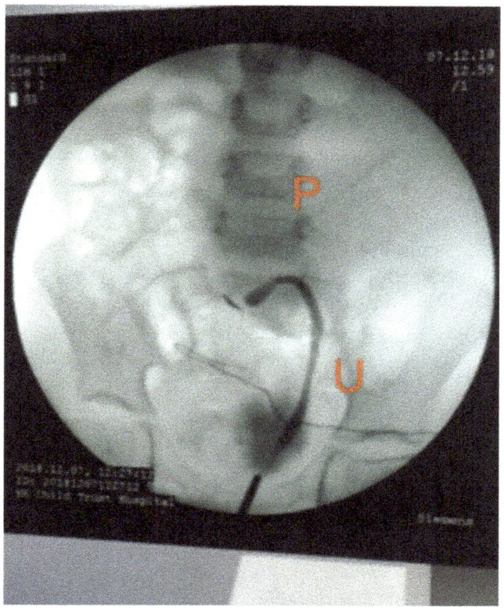

FIGURE 3: Retrograde study showing left PUJO with diluted contrast in the massive pelvis (P) and contrast in the left ureter.

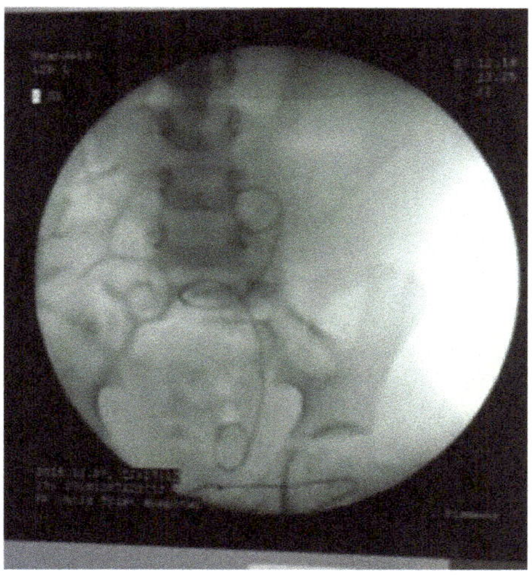

FIGURE 4: Xray KUB showing JJ stent across the left PUJ.

addition a tense external urinoma compressing the parenchyma and renal hilum further.

There have been many reports of Page kidney occurring following trauma in adults [5]. Other causes of Page kidney are tumour, arteriovenous malformation, cyst rupture, glomerulonephritis, vasculitis and native kidney biopsy, and spontaneous intrarenal haemorrhage [5, 6]. There are few reports of children with Page kidney [7]. Contrast-enhanced CT is the preferred modality to diagnose subcapsular or perinephric renal hematoma [3]. Surgical treatment is the mainstay of management including minimally invasive procedures like image-guided percutaneous aspiration of hematoma [8]. Nephrectomy may be necessary in refractory cases. Antihypertensives of choice in Page kidney induced hypertension are the Angiotensin Converting Enzyme

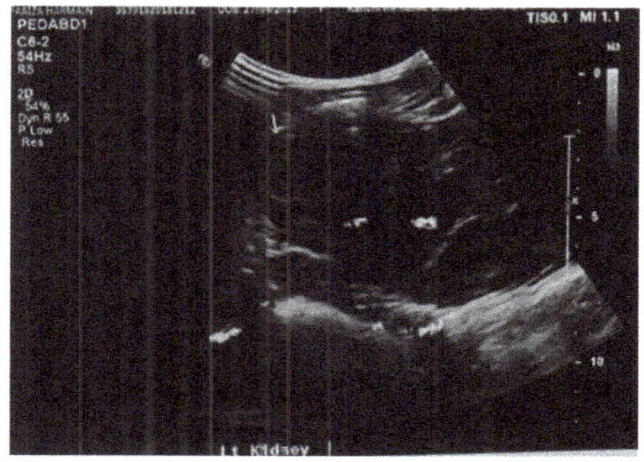

FIGURE 5: Day 5 post-JJ stenting ultrasound showing resolution of urinoma and decompression of the left kidney.

(ACE) Inhibitors [4, 6]. Generally, complete resolution of hypertension [3] follows drainage of the perirenal fluid.

Our case developed malignant hypertension after spontaneous rupture of the pelvicalyceal system, with compression of the left renal parenchyma from the resultant tense subcapsular hematoma. The hypertension settled after ultrasound-guided drainage of the subcapsular urinoma and internal drainage of the obstructed left kidney by JJ stent across the PUJO. Repeat ultrasound scan showed complete resolution of the subcapsular urinoma after 6 weeks, after which the child underwent an uneventful pyeloplasty.

Spontaneous rupture of the pelvicalyceal system is rare in PUJO. In our case, symptoms of loin pain followed by rapid development of malignant hypertension lead to the early diagnosis of Page phenomenon, resulting in prompt successful management,avoiding the morbidity of prolonged malignant hypertension. A high index of suspicion is required to diagnose Page kidney in children with suspected PUJO who develop acute or recent onset hypertension.

4. Conclusion

Page kidney is rare in children and generally posttraumatic in origin. Our case demonstrates Page kidney can occur in the setting of severe PUJO. It should be suspected early in children with suspected PUJO with acute onset hypertension.Prompt management by drainage of perinephric or subcapsular urino-hematoma, as well as internal drainage of the PUJO with JJ stenting, will help in the resolution of Page kidney hypertension and prevent further deterioration of renal function.

Acknowledgments

(1) Dr. Sairam, VK AB (Paed), AB (Paediatric Nephrology), Consultant Paediatric Nephrologist, Kanchi Kamakoti Child's Trust Hospital, Chennai and (2) Dr. Muralinath S, MD (Radio Diagnosis), Consultant Paediatric Radiologist, Kanchi Kamakoti Child's Trust Hospital.

References

[1] N. Tuong, M. Daugherty, and J. Riddell, "Acute Page kidney immediately following blunt trauma to a solitary pediatric kidney," *Canadian Urological Association Journal*, vol. 10, no. 5-6, pp. 192–E196, 2016.

[2] S.-W. Chen, Z.-J. Shen, Y.-L. Yu et al., "Subcapsular collection of glomerular filtrate: rare form of Page kidney," *Nephrology*, vol. 11, no. 4, pp. 372-373, 2006.

[3] M. Kiczek and U. Uayasankar, "Page kidney," *The Journal of Urology*, vol. 194, no. 4, pp. 1109-1110, 2015.

[4] T. R. McCune, W. J. Stone, and J. A. Breyer, "Page Kidney: Case Report and Review of the Literature," *American Journal of Kidney Diseases*, vol. 18, no. 5, pp. 593–599, 1991.

[5] C. Andrew Smyth, S. Collins, B. Thorsteinsdottir et al., "Page kidney: etiology, renal function outcomes and risk for future hypertension," *Journal of Clinical Hypertension*, vol. 14, no. 4, pp. 216–221, 2012.

[6] S. J. Dopson, S. Jayakumar, and J. C. Q. Velez, "Page Kidney as a Rare Cause of Hypertension: Case Report and Review of the Literature," *American Journal of Kidney Diseases*, vol. 54, no. 2, pp. 334–339, 2009.

[7] N. J. Vo, C. D. Hanevold, R. Edwards, F. A. Hoffer, and M. A. Koyle, "Recurrent Page kidney in a child with a congenital solitary kidney requiring capsular artery embolization," *Pediatric Radiology*, vol. 40, no. 11, pp. 1837–1840, 2010.

[8] R. Suckling, F. Uddin, J. Pilcher, I. A. MacPhee, J. B. Eastwood, and D. Banerjee, "Page kidney: successful radiological management of acute renal failure," *Nephrology, Dialysis, Transplantation*, vol. 21, no. 6, p. 1740, 2006.

33

Inflammatory Pseudotumor Formation at a Port Site after Robotic Partial Nephrectomy for Renal Cell Carcinoma

Mitsuo Ofude,[1] **Ryunosuke Nakagawa**,[1] **Satoko Urata**,[1] **Tohru Miyagi**,[1] **Takao Nakashima**,[1] **and Hiroshi Minato**[2]

[1]*Department of Urology, Ishikawa Prefectural Central Hospital, 2-1 Kuratsukihigashi, Kanazawa, Ishikawa, Japan*
[2]*Department of Diagnostic Pathology, Ishikawa Prefectural Central Hospital, 2-1 Kuratsukihigashi, Kanazawa, Ishikawa, Japan*

Correspondence should be addressed to Mitsuo Ofude; ofude_m@yahoo.co.jp

Academic Editor: Fumitaka Koga

Inflammatory pseudotumors (IPTs) are benign masses arising from nonspecific inflammatory conditions including surgical invasion. We herein report the rare case of an IPT mimicking port-site metastasis in a 69-year-old patient who underwent retroperitoneal robotic partial nephrectomy for stage T1a renal cell carcinoma. Radiological examination performed six months after the surgery revealed the presence of a mass underneath the abdominal wall which coincided with a port site. The tumor was resected by laparoscopic transperitoneal approach, and histological examination led to the diagnosis of an IPT that consists of xanthogranulomatous inflammation. We also discuss the etiology of IPT formation and features distinguishing IPTs from port-site metastasis.

1. Introduction

Inflammatory pseudotumors (IPTs) which are caused by nonspecific inflammatory conditions can develop at nearly every body site [1]. Albeit the very low frequency, several cases of patients who developed IPTs after surgery have been reported even in the era of minimally invasive surgery [2–6]. Distinguishing IPTs from local recurrence or metastasis of malignant neoplasms can be challenging. We herein present the rare case of an IPT mimicking port-site metastasis (PSM) of renal cell carcinoma (RCC) after robotic partial nephrectomy (RPN).

2. Case Presentation

A 69-year-old Japanese male with diabetes mellitus underwent right-sided retroperitoneal RPN for an incidental renal tumor (Figure 1). Five ports including a 12 mm AirSeal™ assistant port were placed in the procedure. The tumor resection was performed under warm ischemia, and the renal parenchymal defects were repaired using a continuous 2-0 V-Loc™ suture over a Surgicel™ bolster. The resected specimen was extracted using an entrapment bag. A drainage tube was left in a robotic instrument port. Port sites were closed with one stitch using 0 Vicryl™. Histological examination led to the diagnosis of grade 2, stage pT1a clear-cell RCC with negative surgical margins. No adjuvant therapy was administered.

Follow-up computed tomography (CT) scan performed six months after the surgery revealed an emerging small mass below the right side of the abdominal wall coinciding with a 12 mm AirSeal™ assistant port site (Figure 2(a)). By [^{18}F]fluorodeoxyglucose- (FDG-) positron emission tomography- (PET-) CT, the mass had a mild FDG uptake with a maximum standardized uptake value of 3.2 (Figure 2(b)). Further evaluation did not reveal elevated levels of inflammatory markers in blood. Overall, these findings were compatible with PSM of RCC.

Tumor resection was subsequently performed by laparoscopic transperitoneal approach (Figure 3). Although peeling the tumor off the abdominal wall was difficult due to strong adhesion, en bloc resection was successful. The resected specimen included a yellow mass, 25 × 20 × 13 mm in size, without foreign bodies. Histological examination revealed that the mass

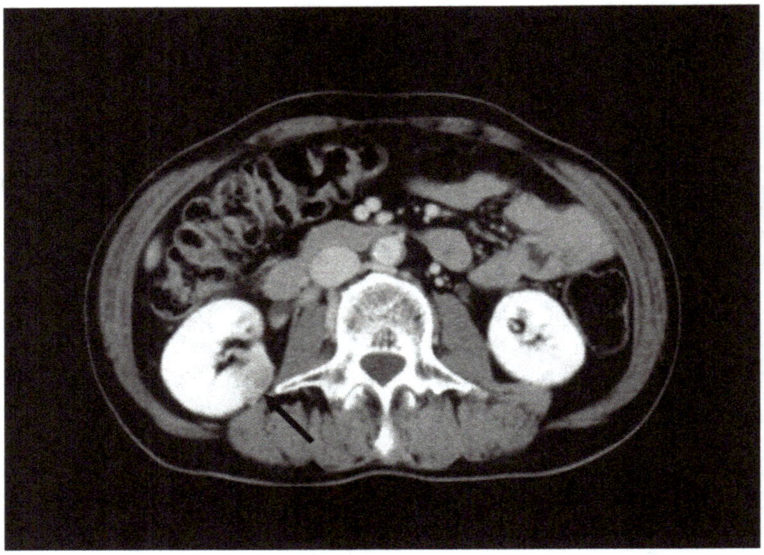

FIGURE 1: Contrast-enhanced computed tomography shows a right renal tumor (arrow) with a maximum diameter of 27 mm.

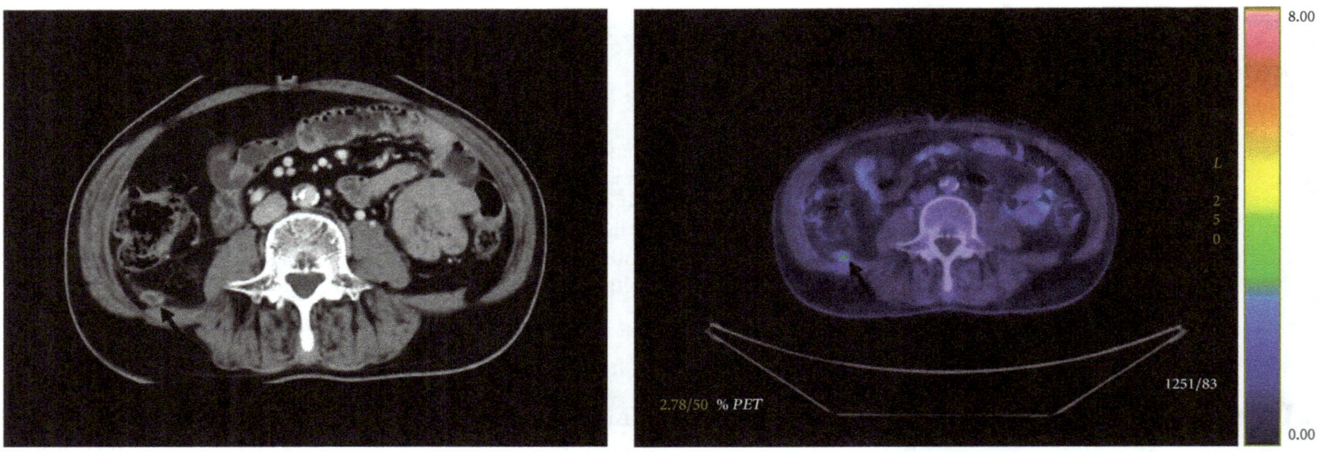

(a) (b)

FIGURE 2: Appearance of a mass underneath in right side of the abdominal wall (arrow). (a) Contrast-enhanced computed tomography. (b) [18F]fluorodeoxyglucose- (FDG-) positron emission tomography-computed tomography shows increased FDG uptake with a maximum standardized uptake value of 3.2.

was composed of aggregation of foamy histiocytes with fat necrosis (FN), lipogranulomas, fibrosis, and mild infiltration of lymphocytes and plasma cells (Figure 4). The pathological diagnosis was an IPT that consists of xanthogranulomatous inflammation. The postoperative course was uneventful, and no evidence of recurrence was observed six months after the IPT resection.

3. Discussion

IPTs are benign tumors which mimic malignant neoplasms and comprise cells associated with both acute and chronic inflammation. The pathogenesis and etiology of IPTs are unspecific; therefore, IPTs have been described under various names such as xanthogranuloma, inflammatory myofibroblastic tumor [1], and lipogranuloma [4] based on histological findings or cellulose granuloma [2], surgical granuloma [3], and Schloffer's tumor described as an immune response to foreign bodies used in surgery [5, 7] according to the antigens provoking inflammation.

Schloffer's tumor might be considered the diagnosis in the present case based on the potential etiology because it is possible that Vicryl™ suture or Surgicel™ used in RPN might have provoked a foreign body reaction. Asano et al. [5] reported four patients who developed Schloffer's tumors after colorectal surgery; absorbable sutures were used in prior surgeries in all four cases. The time interval was less than one year between the prior surgery and tumor diagnosis in three of these cases. The shared preoperative clinical findings between these cases and the present case include positive FDG-PET uptake in the absence of elevated inflammatory marker levels in peripheral blood. However, the tumor in

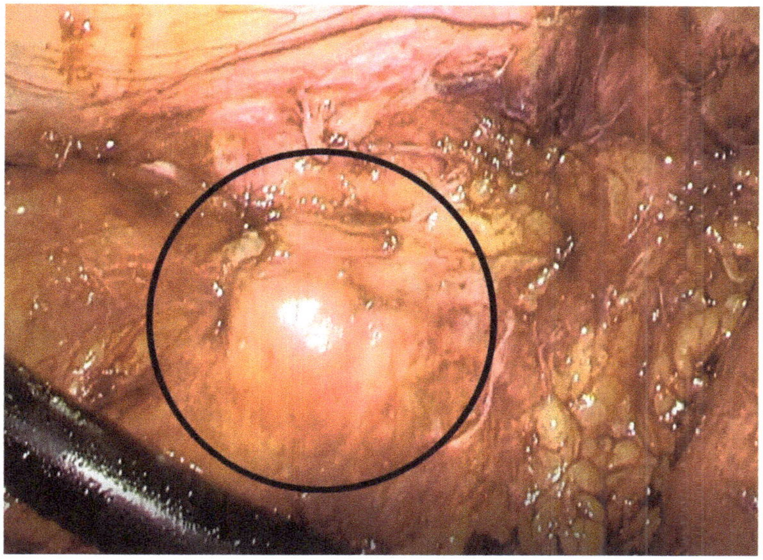

FIGURE 3: Intraoperative image reveals a mass (circle) observed in the peritoneal cavity.

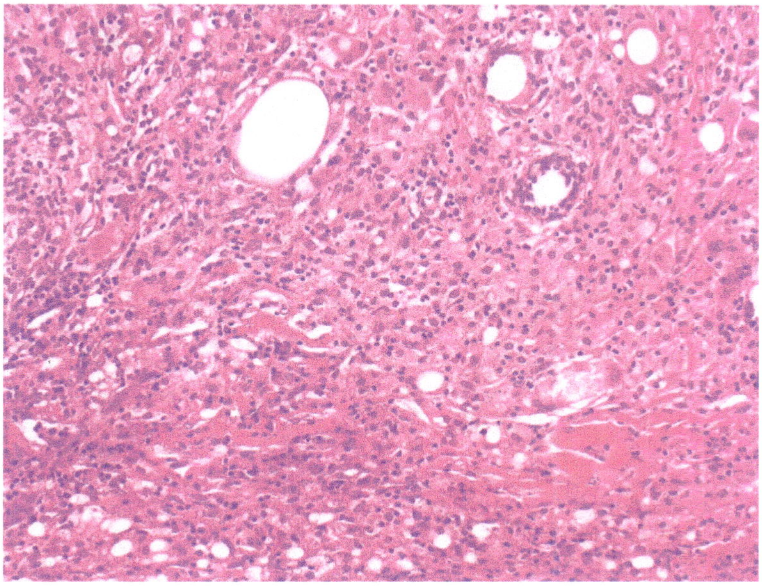

FIGURE 4: Histology of the mass at a port site showing aggregation of foamy histiocytes with lipogranulomas, mild infiltration of lymphocytes and plasma cells, and focal fibrosis.

the present case was located underneath the abdominal wall and not inside the abdominal cavity, and no tumors developed at other port sites where Vicryl™ sutures were used. These findings overall suggest that Vicryl™ sutures were not likely to have provoked a foreign body reaction.

In the present case, the Surgicel™ bolster placed on the renal parenchymal defects was nearly invisible at the IPT site. This image finding shows that the Surgicel™ bolster was normally diminished with time after surgery [8]. It is unlikely that a deviating Surgicel™ fragment provoked a foreign body reaction in the present case.

While the exact cause of IPT in the present case remains unknown, we speculate that the following two processes were more likely etiologies. The first one is chronic inflammation by microabscess formation underneath the abdominal wall, which might be partially due to diabetes mellitus. The second is the involvement of FN. Fat fragments produced in RPN might migrate to a port site and subsequently develop FN provoking chronic inflammation. Amblee and Ganesh [6] reported an interesting case of IPT formation caused by FN in right-sided upper perinephric fat after left adrenalectomy for Cushing's disease. However, the exact location of IPT seems to be unclear because tumor excision had not been performed in their case. We consider that isolated fat fragments in left adrenalectomy might lead to FN in right-sided abdominal location. We do not routinely irrigate the operative field after RPN, but careful irrigation and suction could prevent form abscess or remaining fat fragments which causes IPT formation.

The preoperative differentiation between IPT and PSM of RCC is difficult because of the rarity of both conditions, which were reported in very few case reports [2–4, 9–11]. Based on the limited information, both IPT and PSM of RCC are usually asymptomatic while retaining a small tumor burden. The diagnosis depends primarily on imaging studies; however, there are no distinguishable radiologic features of IPT, which vary according to the histological content and location [1]. Additionally, FDG-PET appears to be impractical as both conditions can display positive FDG-PET uptake [4, 5, 10].

Song et al. [11], who reported 16 cases of PSM after laparoscopic and robotic surgery for RCC, found that PSM development was associated with surgical technical approaches such as specimen morcellation before extraction, lack of entrapment bags during extraction, and tumor rupture in seven cases; the authors reported that the remaining nine cases had uniformly aggressive initial RCC of grade 3 or higher. In comparison, the risk of PSM might have been lower in the present case. However, Shimokihara et al. [10] reported a case of PSM with an initially low-risk RCC similar to the present case. Therefore, we suggest that any tumor suspicious for PSM should be resected.

Acknowledgments

We acknowledgement Enago for English language review.

References

[1] M. Patnana, A. B. Sevrukov, K. M. Elsayes, C. Viswanathan, M. Lubner, and C. O. Menias, "Inflammatory pseudotumor: the great mimicker," *AJR: American Journal of Roentgenology*, vol. 198, no. 3, pp. W217–W227, 2012.

[2] T. Tefik, O. Sanli, T. Oktar, O. B. Yucel, Y. Ozluk, and I. Kilicaslan, "Oxidized regenerated cellulose granuloma mimicking recurrent mass lesion after laparoscopic nephron sparing surgery," *International Journal of Surgery Case Reports*, vol. 3, no. 6, pp. 227–230, 2012.

[3] M. M. Agarwal, A. K. Mandal, S. Agarwal et al., "Surgicel granuloma: unusual cause of recurrent mass lesion after laparoscopic nephron-sparing surgery for renal cell carcinoma," *Urology*, vol. 76, no. 2, pp. 334-335, 2010.

[4] K. Takagi, K. Kawase, K. Minoshima, M. Yamaha, and M. Horie, "Retroperitoneal lipogranuloma mimicking recurrence of renal cell carcinoma after laparoscopic partial nephrectomy," *Urology Case Reports*, vol. 26, article 100940, 2019.

[5] E. Asano, Y. Furuichi, K. Kumamoto et al., "A case of Schloffer tumor with rapid growth and FDG-PET positivity at the port site of laparoscopic sigmoidectomy for colon cancer," *Surgical Case Reports*, vol. 5, no. 1, p. 116, 2019.

[6] A. Amblee and M. Ganesh, "Retroperitoneal fat necrosis in a patient with extensive weight loss after adrenalectomy for ACTH-independent Cushing syndrome: a case report and review of the literature," *AACE Clinical Case Reports*, vol. 2, no. 4, pp. e316–e320, 2016.

[7] F. J. Yazyi, C. M. Canullan, N. F. Baglietto et al., "Schloffer's tumor: case report and review of the literature," *International Journal of Surgery Case Reports*, vol. 5, no. 12, pp. 1234–1237, 2014.

[8] D. Pai, J. M. Willatt, M. Korobkin et al., "CT appearances following laparoscopic partial nephrectomy for renal cell carcinoma using a rolled cellulose bolster," *Cancer Imaging*, vol. 10, no. 1, pp. 161–168, 2010.

[9] J. B. Song, Y. S. Tanagho, E. H. Kim, P. H. Abbosh, G. Vemana, and R. S. Figenshau, "Camera-port site metastasis of a renal-cell carcinoma after robot-assisted partial nephrectomy," *Journal of Endourology*, vol. 27, no. 6, pp. 732–739, 2013.

[10] K. Shimokihara, T. Kawahara, D. Takamoto et al., "Port site recurrence after laparoscopic radical nephrectomy: a case report," *Journal of Medical Case Reports*, vol. 11, no. 1, p. 151, 2017.

[11] J. Song, E. Kim, J. Mobley et al., "Port site metastasis after surgery for renal cell carcinoma: harbinger of future metastasis," *The Journal of Urology*, vol. 192, no. 2, pp. 364–368, 2014.

34

Retroperitoneal Ectopic Location of an Intrauterine Device Revealed by Renal Colic: An Exceptional Case

Idriss Ziani,[1,2] **Imad Boualaoui**,[1,2] **Ahmed Ibrahimi**,[1,2] **Hachem El Sayegh**,[1,2] **Lounis Benslimane**,[1,2] **and Yassine Nouini**[1,2]

[1] *Department of Urological Surgery A, University Hospital of Rabat, Rabat, Morocco*
[2] *Faculty of Medicine-Mohammed V University RABAT, Morocco*

Correspondence should be addressed to Idriss Ziani; idrissziani20@gmail.com

Academic Editor: Apul Goel

The intrauterine device (IUD) is one of the most effective contraceptive methods. Its Pearl Index is less than 1 per 100 women. It is the most used method around the world: about 100 million users. However, its insertion can cause certain complications, such as infection, expulsion, or perforation essentially when the rules of use are poorly applied. Perforation remains exceptional but one of the most serious complications. Indeed, after a perforation, the IUD could be located in different neighboring organs. We report a new case of IUD ectopic location in the peritoneal cavity, which was diagnosed 7 years after the insertion and as part of the renal colic assessment. The surgery was performed to remove the IUD which was embedded in the peritoneum and compresses the ureter and causes dilation upstream. To our knowledge, this is the first case reported in the literature of an ectopic location in the retroperitoneal space of an intrauterine device.

1. Introduction

The intrauterine device (IUD) is one of the most effective methods of contraception. Its Pearl Index is less than 1 per 100 women [1]. It is the most widely used method around the world: about 100 million users. However, its insertion can cause some complications, such as infection, expulsion, or perforation essentially when the rules of use are poorly applied. The perforation remains exceptional but one of the most serious complications. Indeed, after a perforation, the IUD may be located in different neighboring organs. Ectopic locations at the Douglas pouch, omentum, mesentery, colon, and bladder have been described [2], often with lithiasic complications in the bladder [3].

We report a new case of IUD extralocation in the retroperitoneal cavity, which was diagnosed 7 years after the insertion and as part of the renal colic assessment. The surgery was performed to remove the IUD which was embedded in the peritoneum compressing the ureter and causing dilation upstream.

2. Patient and Observation

Mrs. A.k., 29 years old, is a primigravida by caesarean delivery with no significant pathological history and known carrier of a copper T-uterine device inserted 7 years earlier. The first control one month after insertion revealed no abnormalities. A second check 6 months after the observation by the patient of the disappearance of nylon thread and clinical examination shows an empty uterine cavity. No radiological investigation was considered at the time.

She consults for renal colic evolving since one year treated symptomatically by analgesic treatment; before the recurrence and the persistence of the symptomatology the patient consulted in our formation. The clinical examination found the patient to be in good general condition; the abdomen is supple with a slight sensitivity to palpation of the left lumbar fossa with no observation of IUD strings in the speculum examination. The vaginal examination shows a normal-sized uterus. An initial radiological assessment included an abdominal X-ray which reveals an extralocation

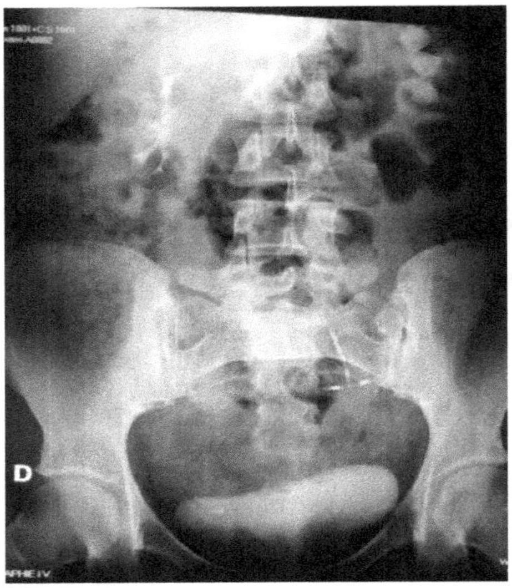

FIGURE 1: ASP while standing with an IUD at the pelvic area of the uterine.

of IUD in the left ureter path (Figure 1) and ultrasound that shows a left ureterohydronephrosis (renal pelvis at 25 mm). The abdominal CT confirms the retroperitoneal location and the left ureteral compression by the IUD (Figures 2 and 3). The diagnosis of a migratory IUD is thus retained. Given her surgical history, the patient had laparotomy for IUD removal. Surgical exploration revealed parietal adhesions that were gently released, allowing the observation of the extralocated IUD, whose vertical limb was embedded in the left ureter. The IUD was removed without difficulty after resection anastomosis of the ureter made with placement of a double J probe. No complication was noted (Figures 4 and 5).

3. Discussion

The IUD is one of the most used means for nondefinitive contraception in the world [1, 4, 5]. Like any foreign body, the IUD can have risks and complications, such as migration after uterine perforation that remains rare and infection [6]. This migration can take several directions; it is usually in the peritoneal cavity and rarely in the neighboring pelvic organs, mainly the bladder and the rectosigmoid [1, 5, 7]. Pelvic locations out of the bladder are exceptional [1, 4]. Ibghi et al. reported stenosis of the iliac vein secondary to the migration of an IUD [8]. According to our knowledge, this observation is the first case of retroperitoneal migration with ureter insertion reported in the literature.

The copper in some IUDs can trigger an inflammatory reaction leading to a contraceptive effect, but it can also be involved in the process of long-term perforation and uterine transmigration [9]. Intramyometrial migration begins with the incarceration of an IUD branch in the myometrium, and inflammatory phenomena as well as uterine contractions will allow the IUD to continue its migration [1, 6, 7]. Another study explains that the IUD is driven to abnormal sites by uterine forces. In fact, Goldstuck and Wildemeersch showed that the nature of perforation may be primary, secondary, or both. They also suggested that the forces of myometrial contractions are leading factors in IUD moving out of the uterine cavity. Moreover, they bring to light the crucial effect of force vector direction and that the summated multivectorial force determines the IUD direction [10]. Factors predisposed to this extralocation are especially a weakening of the myometrium by multiple pregnancies and caesareans, ante- or retroverted and hypoplastic uterus, and the laying of IUD too early in the postpartum period [1, 4]. The delay of this complication, which would correspond to the time between the insertion of the IUD and the appearance of the first clinical signs, can be several years (up to 36 years) [1].

Clinically, the symptomatology is variable according to the site of ectopic location and the type of IUD [10, 11]; in our case, the main symptom was renal colic because of the ureteral compression and the insertion of a branch of IUD in the ureter as well as periureteral fibrosis which was responsible for ureteral stenosis.

Thus, uterine perforation by IUD is usually asymptomatic, except when it occurs primarily at the time of the pose, resulting in violent pain, which must attract the attention of the doctor. On examination, the perforation is suspected before the disappearance of the reference thread, after ensuring that this landmark is not raised in the endocervix, and this is the case of our patient whose clinical examination shows the lack of thread in the vulva and endocervix [10–12].

The means to locate an extrauterine IUD will be ultrasound and, if unsuccessful, abdominal X-ray to look for it in the abdomen before concluding to an unknown expulsion. Computed tomography (CT) or magnetic resonance imaging will locate it precisely. When migrating, the IUD can be localized in the Douglas pouch, the broad ligament, and the omentum (45%) [13, 12]. Digestive localizations (such as the mesentery and the colon) and the bladder are less frequent [2]; no case of retroperitoneal migration has been diagnosed in the literature.

In our observation, the diagnosis was confirmed by the spiral CT with reconstruction which allows a better study of the repercussion on the upper urinary tract and specifies the exact location of the ectopic IUD.

The majority of authors believe that the removal of the device is essential given the risk of digestive and especially urological complications like the case we discussed. The removal of the migratory IUD is most often done by laparoscopy. In the literature, its success rate varies between 44 and 100% [13, 14], depending on the number of cases treated, the location of the IUD, and the experience of the operator. In our observation, we recommended a laparotomy upon seeing the patient's surgical history.

4. Conclusion

The IUD is an effective contraceptive method; its insertion is a simple medical procedure that requires minimum knowledge and experience. Perforation associated with retroperitoneal ectopic location is one of the rarest and most dangerous

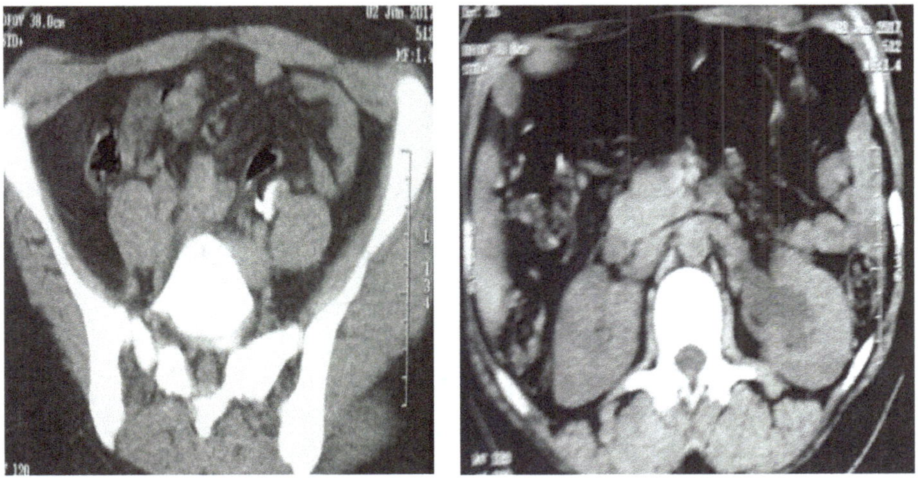

(a) (b)

Figure 2: CT image (cross section). (a) CT image showing the retroperitoneal location with left ureteral compression. (b) CT image showing left ureterohydronephrosis secondary to ureteral compression by the IUD.

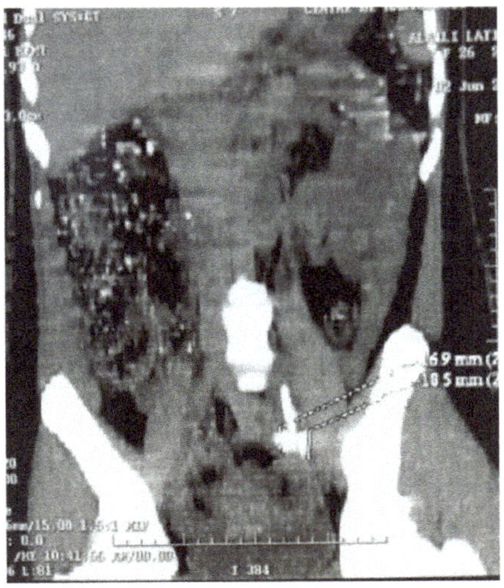

Figure 3: CT scan sagittal objective retroperitoneal localization of the IUD.

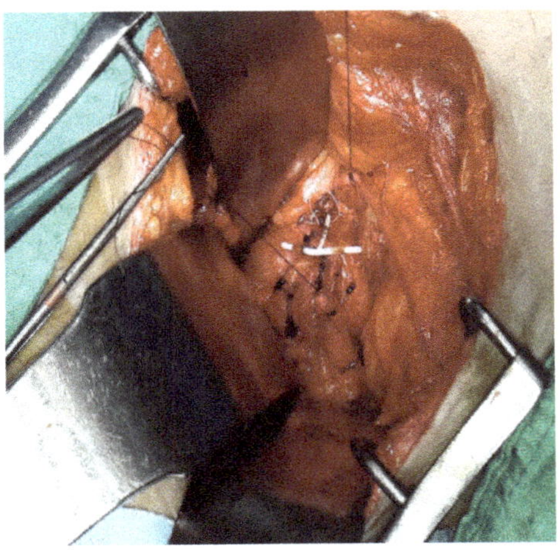

Figure 4: The IUD which vertical limb was embedded in the left ureter (intraoperative image).

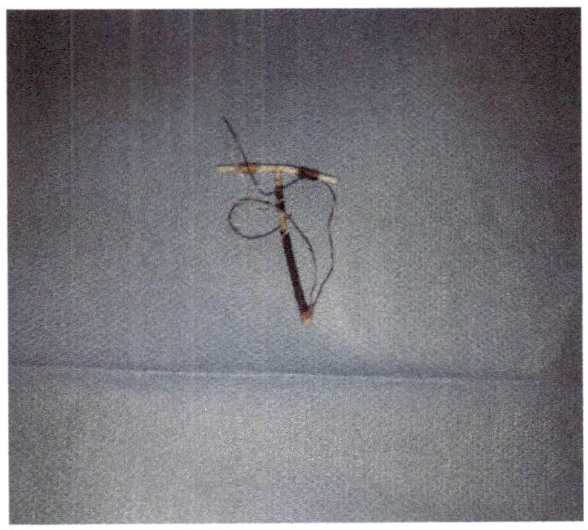

Figure 5: The IUD after surgical extraction.

complications. Laparoscopic or even laparotomic removal of the IUD is essential to avoid ureteral perforation and the repercussions on the upper urinary tract.

Abbreviations

IUD: Intrauterine device
CT: Computed tomography.

Conflicts of Interest

The authors declare that they have no conflicts of interest.

References

[1] A. Joual, B. Querfani, A. Taha et al., "Intravesical migration of an intrauterine contraceptive device complicated by stones," *Progrès en Urologie*, vol. 14, no. 3, pp. 374-375, 2004.

[2] M. Nouri, M. Fassi, A. Koutani, A. Ibn Attya, M. Hachimi, and A. Lakrissa, "Migration of an intrauterine device into the bladder. Report of a case," *Journal de Gynécologie, Obstétrique et Biologie de la Reproduction*, vol. 23, no. 2, pp. 1620–1624, 1999.

[3] M. A. Nouioui, T. Taktak, S. Mokadem, H. Mediouni, R. Khiari, and S. Ghozzi, "A mislocated intrauterine device migrating to the urinary bladder: an uncommon complication leading to stone formation," *Case Reports in Urology.*, vol. 2020, article 2091915, 4 pages, 2020.

[4] K. Bacha, M. Ben Amna, L. Ben Hassine, S. Ghaddab, and M. Ayed, "Intrauterine device migrating to the bladder," *Progrès en Urologie*, vol. 11, no. 6, pp. 1289–1291, 2001.

[5] N. Zeraïdi, "La migration intra-ovarienne d'un dispositif intra-utérin," *J. Prat.*, vol. 13, no. 3, pp. 36-37, https://scholar.google.com/scholar?cluster=7441717070383559726&hl=fr&as_sdt=2005&sciodt=0,5.

[6] D. Riethmuller, C. Gay, S. Benoit et al., "Can adbominal migration of an IUCD be responsible for uterine rupture during pregnancy? La migration abdominale d'un DIU peut-elle etre a l'origine d'une rupture uterine gravidique?," *Revue Francaise de Gynecologie et d Obstetrique*, vol. 91, no. 10, pp. 496–498, 1996.

[7] R. A. Sparks, B. G. Purrier, P. J. Watt, and M. Elstein, "Bacteriological colonisation of uterine cavity: role of tailed intrauterine contraceptive device," *British Medical Journal*, vol. 282, no. 6271, pp. 1189–1191, 1981.

[8] W. Ibghi, M. Batt, A. Bongain et al., "Iliac vein stenosis caused by intrauterine device migration," *The Journal de Gynécologie Obstétrique et Biologie de la Reproduction*, vol. 24, no. 3, pp. 273–275, 1995.

[9] B. Kassa and P. Audra, "Le sterilet migrateur: à propos d'un cas et revue de la littérature," *Contraception, Fertilité, Sexualité (1992)*, vol. 27, no. 10, pp. 696–700, 1999.

[10] N. D. Goldstuck and D. Wildemeersch, "Role of uterine forces in intrauterine device embedment, perforation, and expulsion," *International Journal of Women's Health*, vol. 6, pp. 735–744, 2014.

[11] K. Andersson, E. Ryde-Blomqvist, K. Lindell, V. Odlind, and I. Milsom, "Perforations with intrauterine devices," *Contraception*, vol. 57, no. 4, pp. 251–255, 1998.

[12] R. Brar, S. Doddi, A. Ramasamy, and P. Sinha, "A forgotten migrated intrauterine contraceptive device is not always innocent: a case report," *Case Reports in Medicine*, vol. 2010, Article ID 740642, 3 pages, 2010.

[13] A. Zouhal, N. el Amrani, F. Bensaid, H. El Fehri, and M. T. Alaoui, *Migration intra-vesicale d'un dispositif intra-uterin a propos d'un cas*, Maternité Universitaire des Orangers, Rabat, Maroc, 2001.

[14] W. S. L. de Silva, K. A. S. U. A. Kodithuwakku, G. U. E. Aponsu, R. M. M. Rathnayake, and E. Rajasegaram, "A large bladder stone caused by the intravesical migration of an intrauterine contraceptive device: a case report," *Journal of Medical Case Reports*, vol. 11, no. 1, p. 293, 2017.

35

Traumatic Blunt Force Renal Injury in a Diseased Horseshoe Kidney with Successful Embolization to Treat Active Bleeding: A Case Report and Literature Review

Chonlada Krutsri,[1] Pongsasit Singhatas,[1] Preeda Sumpritpradit,[1] Chunlaches Chaijareenont,[2] Wit Viseshsindh,[3] Tharin Thampongsa,[1] and Pattawia Choikrua[4]

[1]*Division of Trauma Surgery and Surgical Critical Care, Department of Surgery, Faculty of Medicine, Ramathibodi Hospital, Mahidol University, Bangkok, Thailand*
[2]*Department of Surgery, Faculty of Medicine, Ramathibodi Hospital, Mahidol University, Bangkok, Thailand*
[3]*Division of Urology, Department of Surgery, Faculty of Medicine, Ramathibodi Hospital, Mahidol University, Bangkok, Thailand*
[4]*Surgical Research Unit, Faculty of Medicine, Ramathibodi Hospital, Mahidol University, Bangkok, Thailand*

Correspondence should be addressed to Pongsasit Singhatas; poojeja@hotmail.com

Academic Editor: Imran Morhason-Bello

Background. Blunt force injuries in patients with preexisting kidney disease account for 19% of all kidney injuries, suggesting that diseased kidneys are more vulnerable than normal kidneys. When a horseshoe kidney (a rare anomaly: prevalence of 0.2%) is injured, treatment is challenging, especially when nonoperative management is desired. In high-grade blunt force normal kidney injury, nonoperative management has high succession rate (94.8%) with kidney-related complication (13.6%). Surgical reconstruction and preservation of a damaged horseshoe kidney is difficult because of variations in its vascular anatomy. We report successful nonoperative management of a blunt horseshoe kidney injury with active bleeding and review previous outcomes and complications. *Case Presentation.* A 57-year-old man had a head-on collision motorcycle road traffic accident. On arrival, blood pressure was 90/60 mmHg, pulse rate 140 bpm, and clear yellow urine output 200 ml. The patient was transiently responsive to fluid and blood component. Whole body computed tomography showed a high-volume retroperitoneal hematoma and multiple-lacerated lower pole of the kidney, compatible with preexisting horseshoe kidney disease with active contrast-enhanced extravasation from the accessory right renal artery. Embolization was performed Renal function, transiently impaired after embolization, normalized on day 3. An infected hematoma found on day 7 was successfully controlled with antibiotics. His recovery was uneventful. At the 6-month follow-up, his serum creatinine level had returned to normal. The average age of blunt force horseshoe kidney injury is 31.75 years and occurred more common in male (87.5%). *Conclusion.* Diseased horseshoe kidneys are prone to injury even with low-velocity impact such as a road traffic accident speed < 15 km/h. Embolization is considered the first choice for management, with its high clinical success rate leading to less need for surgical repair. Not removing a hematoma is likely to result in complications. If embolization fails to stop bleeding, life-saving surgical exploration should be mandated.

1. Introduction

Blunt force kidney damage accounts for 1%–5% of all bodily injuries. Among kidney injuries, blunt force is responsible for 93.4%, making it ninefold more common than a penetrating injury [1, 2]. Preexisting kidney disease associated with a blunt force injury comprises 19% of all kidney injuries [3]. Blunt force injury to the more vulnerable diseased kidney should raise suspicion of the diagnosis when the injury is isolated and caused by low-velocity impact [3]. The most

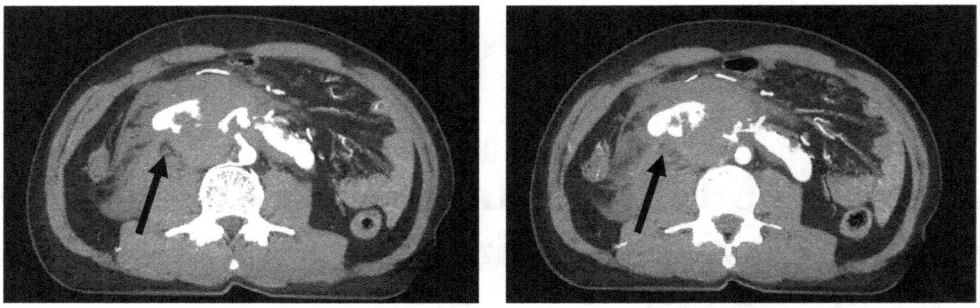

Figure 1: CT angiography in axial view, showing an active contrast extravasation from accessory right renal artery and retroperitoneal hematoma (a, b) (black arrow).

common presentation is gross hematuria, hemorrhagic shock class 2-3 based on Advanced Trauma Life Support (ATLS) principle with a retroperitoneal hematoma, and/or flank pain. Currently, a high-grade blunt force normal kidney injury can be managed nonoperatively (i.e., hemodynamic monitoring, embolization, and endovascular stent) with a high success rate of 94.8%, leading to a decreased nephrectomy rate of 5.4% [2]. A kidney-related complication (UTI, abscess, or hematuria) from nonoperative management rate is 13.6% which is not significantly different from immediate operation patients [4].

A horseshoe kidney is a rare anomaly with an overall prevalence of 0.2% with high prevalence in male to female (ratio 2 : 1) [5]. Blunt force injury to this anomalous kidney is challenging with regard to nonoperative management, especially if it is a high-grade injury with active bleeding. From the literature review of blunt force horseshoe kidney injury, the average age is 31.75 years and occurred more common in male (87.5%) [7–13].

According to the American Association for the Surgery of Trauma (AAST), the indication for surgery to treat blunt force injury of a normal kidney is the presence of unstable hemodynamics with a shattered, grade 5 kidney injury. In the presence of preexisting kidney disease, however, 57% of the indication for surgery depends on the hemodynamics and underlying parenchymal pathology, such as a tumor. For an injured diseased horseshoe kidney, surgical reconstruction and preservation of the damaged kidney is difficult because of variations in its vascular anatomy, which could lead to failed preservation of the kidney parenchyma.

We therefore report successful nonoperative management of a high-grade, actively bleeding horseshoe kidney that had been subjected to a blunt force injury. We also review the literature for outcomes and complications after various management protocols for treating horseshoe kidneys that have undergone a blunt force injury.

2. Case Report

A 57-year-old man had a head-on collision motorcycle road traffic accident to a street light pole in speed less than 40 km/h because of an acute stroke. His vitals on arrival are as follows: blood pressure 90/60 mmHg, pulse rate 140 bpm, and saturation 98%. The Advanced Trauma Life Support principle was performed, which revealed that he was transiently responsive and suffered grade 2 hemorrhagic shock. A focused assessment with sonography for trauma (FAST) was negative in all four quadrants. Physical examination found soft, no distension, no abdominal contusion, or peritonitis. A Foley catheter was inserted, which showed clear, yellow urine (200 ml).

The patient underwent whole body computed tomography (CT) scan by indication of blunt abdominal injury with hypovolemic shock grade 2, which revealed a retroperitoneal hematoma measuring 6.9 × 6.1 × 12.3 cm and multiple lacerations of the lower pole of the kidney. A CT brain (as part of whole body CT scan) shows acute ischemic stroke on MCA distribution. These findings were compatible with preexisting disease of his horseshoe kidney without a concomitant intra-abdominal organ injury or urinoma (Figures 1 and 2) There was active extravasation of contrast agent from the accessory right renal artery feeding into the lower pole of the right wing of the horseshoe kidney. This finding suggested that his transient responsiveness and grade 2 hemorrhagic shock were due to active retroperitoneal bleeding (Figures 1 and 2).

Bleeding from the accessory right renal artery was managed successfully via endovascular coil embolization (Figure 3). The patient's renal function was impaired on postembolization day 1, with the serum creatinine at 2.33 mg/dL as compared to baseline serum creatinine at 1.32 mg/dL before undergoing whole body CT scan, which recovered to 1.58 mg/dL on postembolization day 3. The patient, however, developed a low-grade fever on postembolization day 7. He then underwent CT whole abdomen, which identified an infected hematoma from a finding of multiple air-fluid level with previous hematoma. It was successfully treated with an antibiotic, without surgery. The empirical antibiotic Ceftriaxone was used based on the clinical sepsis in an immunocompetent patient of intra-abdominal infection [6]. At the 6-month follow-up, his serum creatinine level had returned to normal (1.09 mg/dL). Informed consent to publish the case was obtained from the patient.

3. Discussion

We present a patient with active bleeding from the accessory right renal artery caused by blunt injury to a horseshoe kidney with preexisting disease. Schmidlin et al. reported that

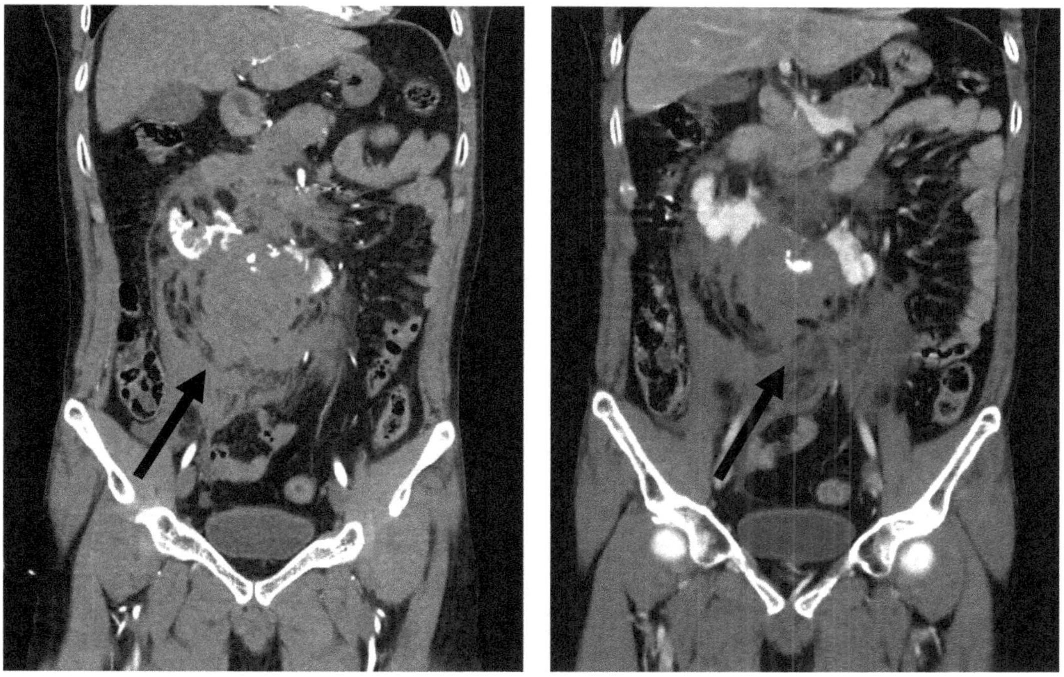

(a) (b)

FIGURE 2: CT angiography in coronal view, showing an active contrast extravasation from accessory right renal artery and retroperitoneal hematoma (a, b) (black arrow).

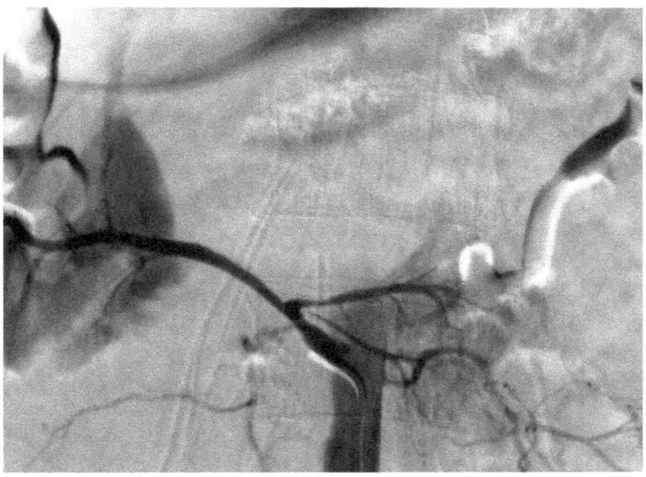

FIGURE 3: Angiogram before embolization. None of the eight patients was reported to suffer renal impairment. PR: pulse rate; BP: blood pressure; AAST: American Association for the Surgery of Trauma; PCD: percutaneous drainage.

a blunt force injury to a kidney with preexisting disease is found in 19% of all kidney injuries, suggesting that diseased kidneys are more vulnerable to violence than normal kidneys [3]. The most common presentation of a patient with blunt force injury of the kidney includes gross hematuria, frank pain, and retroperitoneal bleeding or a hematoma. We should have elevated suspicion that a preexisting kidney injury exists when the injury is due to a low-impact velocity blow with no injury of the intra-abdominal organs [3].

CT is the gold standard method for grading kidney injury and revealing preexisting kidney disease. It provides more information than intravenous pyelography and gives information of concomitant injuries that might affect the choice of a treatment modality. Currently, even high-grade blunt force injury to a normal kidney injury can be managed nonoperatively (e.g., with embolization), achieving a high success rate of 94.8% and a low rate of 5.4% requiring nephrectomy [2]. Treating an injury of a horseshoe kidney with preexisting disease nonoperatively is challenging, especially when high-grade active bleeding is present because of variations in the kidney's anatomy, vascular blood supply, and parenchyma.

The indication for surgery of the kidneys with a preexisting disease is based on the patient's hemodynamics of shock classification 3 or 4 (base on ATLS) with no response to fluid and blood component and underlying kidney pathology, keeping in mind that it is not the same as the indication for injury of a normal kidney [3]. Hence, for this reason, nonoperative management should be mandated as the gold standard for addressing blunt force injury of a normal kidney as well as for a kidney with a preexisting disease if the patient's hemodynamics are stable and/or there is transient responsiveness of hemorrhagic shock classes 2 and 3.

A horseshoe kidney is a rare anomaly with an overall prevalence of 0.2%. It is important to preserve the injured kidney's parenchyma because there is no associated risk of cancer [7]. If surgery is necessary, one must be aware that surgical reconstruction and preservation of the parenchyma in a damaged horseshoe kidney is exceedingly difficult because of variation in the vascular anatomy. Sometimes, because of the variation of the artery feeding the kidney

TABLE 1: Summary of reported treatment outcomes and complications of blunt force injuries of horseshoe kidneys.

Author (publication year)	Age (years)	Sex	PR (bpm)	BP (mmHg)	AAST (grade)	Signs and symptoms	Active extravasation of contrast medium	Management	Location of injury	Complication
Daudia (1998) [8]	25	Male	60	100/60	NA	Gross hematuria Anemia	NA	Open repair	Left lower pole	None
Legg (1998) [11]	49	Male	102	128/84	NA	Hemorrhagic shock grade 2 Anemia	Yes	Embolization	Left lower pole accessory renal artery	Retroperitoneal fluid collection
Trottier (2009) [7]	21	Male	Tachycardia (no number)	Hypotensive (no number)	4	Hemorrhagic shock grade 3	Yes	Endovascular with stent	Right polar artery arising from the common iliac artery	Compartment syndrome of the retroperitoneum
Dominguez (2010) [13]	16	Female	Stable (no number)	Stable (no number)	4	Kidney transection	No	Conservative	None	None
Molina Escudero (2011) [12]	25	Male	Stable (no number)	Stable (no number)	NA	Gross hematuria Hemorrhagic shock grade 3	Yes	Embolization	Lower branch of right renal artery	None
Paragi (2011) [9]	30	Male	Stable (no number)	Stable (no number)	NA	Expanding retroperitoneal hematoma Hypotension	NA	Open repair	Left wing of horseshoe kidney	Left subdiaphragmatic abscess
Cortese (2016) [10]	31	Male	140	80/50	4	Hemorrhagic shock grade 3	Yes	Open repair	Bilateral renal artery	None
Present case (2019)	57	Male	140	90/60	4	Hemorrhagic shock grade 2	Yes	Embolization	Lower branch of right renal artery	Infected hematoma

parenchyma, preservation of kidney parenchyma is likely to fail and nephrectomy cannot be avoided. Nonoperative management, such as embolization, is therefore preferable. A few types of nonoperative management of patients with horseshoe kidney disease who have experienced blunt force kidney damage have been proposed [7].

The present patient appears to be only the eighth reported case of blunt force injury to a horseshoe kidney and the fifth with nonoperative management. The details of our search of the English language literature on the various types of management and outcomes of blunt force-injured horseshoe kidneys are shown in Table 1 [7–13]. The average age of blunt force injury to a horseshoe kidney patients was 31.75 years, and this occurred more commonly in male patients (7/8, 87.5%). The average American Association for the Surgery of Trauma (AAST) kidney injury grade was 4. The most common presentation for this injury was gross hematuria and retroperitoneal bleeding, leading to hemorrhagic shock. Active extravasation of contrast medium, shown on CT angiography, occurred in five of the eight cases (62.5%). For the other three cases, it was not documented in two, and there was no contrast extravasation in one. Operative repair was required in three of the eight cases (37.5%).

There were three cases in which open operative repair was undertaken. In the first case, reported in 1998, the patient underwent operative repair because of hypotension and anemia [8]. In the second case, the patient was addressed surgically because of splenic rupture and an expanding retroperitoneal hematoma due to injury to a diseased horseshoe kidney [9]. During the surgery, the left-side peritoneal organs were medially rotated, revealing active bleeding from the left wing of the horseshoe kidney. The suprarenal aortic vessel was cross-clamped, and the left wing of the kidney was surgically removed [9]. The third case in which operative repair was indicated was addressed by bilateral transection of the horseshoe kidney. There had been active bleeding from the bilateral renal artery, leading to grade 3 hypovolemic shock. Embolization was not indicated because of the high risk of permanent kidney failure. Hence, medial visceral rotation was performed on both sides, after which the kidney parenchyma underwent suture repair [10].

The most common location of the injury among the eight reported patients was the lower pole (6/8 cases, 75%). This majority may be because the lower pole lies and fuses in the midline of the body, which is apt to be crushed to the lumbar spine during blunt force assault and is vulnerable to a shearing force. Embolization is the first choice of treatment of a blunt force injury to the normal kidney and, we believe, should be mandated for a diseased horseshoe kidney as well.

For management, there was a clinical success rate of 100% with embolization and endovascular stent placement. Complications occurred in three of the four (75%) patients with this treatment because the hematoma had not been removed. The complications included, respectively, an infected hematoma, retroperitoneal fluid collection, and retroperitoneal compartment syndrome even without increased bleeding [7, 11, 12]. Except for retroperitoneal compartment syndrome, these complications can be managed successfully with antibiotics and percutaneous drainage. Trottier et al. reported retroperitoneal compartment syndrome after endovascular stent placement for treating blunt force injury in a diseased horseshoe kidney [7]. Their patient had a systemic inflammatory response and renal failure secondary to the retroperitoneal compartment syndrome. The present hematoma had enlarged because of liquefaction and swelling of the retroperitoneum without increased bleeding. The clot was removed surgically, and the patient's condition dramatically improved. The retroperitoneal compartment syndrome may be caused by back bleeding from a lacerated arterial stump or parenchyma. Thus, when nonoperative management, such as embolization, is the first choice of treatment for a diseased horseshoe kidney with blunt force injury, we should be aware of that possible complication.

4. Conclusion

The number of reports of blunt force injuries in diseased horseshoe kidneys is limited because of the rare prevalence of the horseshoe kidney itself. Nevertheless, among those that are available, embolization had a high clinical success rate. Currently, nonoperative management, such as embolization, should be the first choice for management of blunt force injuries of a diseased horseshoe kidney. We should also be aware of the possibility of complications if the hematoma is not removed. If embolization fails to stop a patient's bleeding, surgical exploration should be mandated even though it is difficult because of the variation in the vascular anatomy of the horseshoe kidney.

Ethical Approval

Ethical approval has been approved by the committee of Mahidol University.

Consent

The patient consented to participate in this report.

Authors' Contributions

Chonlada Krutsri contributed to the conception and design, interpretation of data, and writing and revising of the manuscript. Pongsasit Singhatas and Preeda Sumritpradit contributed to the interpretation of data and revising of the manuscript. Chunlaches Chaijareenont contributed to the conception and design and acquisition of data. Wit Viseshsindh contributed to the acquisition of the data. Tharin Thampongsa contributed to the interpretation of data. Pattawia Choikrua contributed to the analysis and interpretation of data.

Acknowledgments

We thank Nancy Schatken, BS, MT(ASCP), from Edanz Group (https://en-author-services.edanzgroup.com/), for editing the draft of this manuscript. We also thank Miss Ticomporn Luangwattanawilai for arranging the reference list.

References

[1] S. Vozianov, M. Sabadash, and A. Shulyak, "Experience of renal artery embolization in patients with blunt kidney trauma," *Central European journal of urology*, vol. 68, no. 4, pp. 471–477, 2015.

[2] B. B. Voelzke and L. Leddy, "The epidemiology of renal trauma," *Translational Andrology and Urology*, vol. 3, no. 2, pp. 143–149, 2014.

[3] F. R. Schmidlin, C. E. Iselin, A. Naimi et al., "The higher injury risk of abnormal kidneys in blunt renal trauma," *Scandinavian Journal of Urology and Nephrology*, vol. 32, no. 6, pp. 388–392, 1998.

[4] A. M. May, O. Darwish, B. Dang et al., "Successful nonoperative management of high-grade blunt renal injuries," *Advances in Urology*, vol. 2016, Article ID 3568076, 5 pages, 2016.

[5] B. Glodny, J. Petersen, K. J. Hofmann et al., "Kidney fusion anomalies revisited: clinical and radiological analysis of 209 cases of crossed fused ectopia and horseshoe kidney," *BJU International*, vol. 103, no. 2, pp. 224–235, 2009.

[6] M. Sartelli, F. Catena, F. M. Abu-Zidan et al., "Management of intra-abdominal infections: recommendations by the WSES 2016 consensus conference," *World Journal of Emergency Surgery*, vol. 12, no. 1, 2017.

[7] V. Trottier, M. A. Lortie, E. Gouin, and F. Trottier, "Renal artery avulsion from blunt abdominal trauma in a horseshoe kidney: endovascular management and an unexpected complication," *Canadian Journal of Surgery*, vol. 52, no. 6, pp. E291–E292, 2009.

[8] A. Daudia, T. B. Hassan, and D. Ramsay, "Trauma to a horseshoe kidney," *Emergency Medicine Journal*, vol. 16, no. 6, pp. 455-456, 1999.

[9] P. R. Paragi, P. H. Go, Z. Klaassen, and M. Ingram, "Trauma to a horseshoe kidney: case report and review of the literature," *UroToday International Journal*, vol. 4, no. 4, 2011.

[10] F. Cortese, P. Fransvea, R. Marcello et al., "Challenging case of horseshoe kidney double fracture," *International Journal of Surgery Case Reports*, vol. 41, pp. 158–161, 2017.

[11] E. A. Legg, F. B. Herbert, B. Goodacre, and D. E. Neal Jr., "Super-selective arterial embolization for blunt trauma in the horseshoe kidney," *Urology*, vol. 51, no. 2, pp. 320-321, 1998.

[12] R. Molina Escudero, M. J. Cancho Gil, A. Husillos Alonso et al., "Traumatic rupture of horseshoe kidney," *Urologia Internationalis*, vol. 88, no. 1, pp. 112–114, 2012.

[13] K. Dominguez and A. P. Ekeh, "Blunt trauma causing transection of a horseshoe kidney," *The Journal of Trauma*, vol. 71, no. 2, p. 517, 2011.

36

Crisis Averted: Clinical T1b Renal Mass with Concurrent Arteriovenous Malformation and Renal Vein Thrombus

David Zekan,[1] **Kareem Wasef**,[1] **Zachary Werner**,[1] **Robert Grammer**,[2] **Cara Lombard**,[2] **Adam Luchey**,[1] **and Ali Hajiran**[1]

[1]*West Virginia University Department of Urology, 1 Medical Center Drive, Morgantown, WV 26506, USA*
[2]*West Virginia University Department of Radiology, 1 Medical Center Drive, Morgantown, WV 26505, USA*

Correspondence should be addressed to David Zekan; dszekan@hsc.wvu.edu

Academic Editor: David Duchene

Arteriovenous malformations (AVMs) secondary to renal-cell carcinoma (RCC) are well-described in the literature. Independently, renal vein and inferior vena cava tumor thrombi can be detected in locally-advanced RCC. A 67-year-old gentleman presented with a cT1b renal mass detected on workup for elevated creatinine. Multiphase CT imaging obtained for partial nephrectomy surgical-planning revealed an initially-missed renal cortical AVM. This drastically changed the plan for intervention, including use of an open approach with AVM embolization by interventional radiology prior and avoidance of a nephron-sparing approach. Final pathology confirmed the AVM and a subclinical renal vein thrombus masked by arterial flow on CT imaging, making this the first concurrent case described in the literature. Herein, we describe avoidance of catastrophic intraoperative hemorrhage by careful review of preoperative imaging and provide a literature review of imaging modalities for both renal surgical-planning and detection of tumor thrombi in RCC.

1. Introduction

In 2022, kidney cancer represents 4.1% of all adult malignancies in the United States with clear-cell renal-cell carcinoma (RCC) being the most common primary malignancy of the kidney [1]. RCC comprises 90% of primary malignant renal-neoplasms in adults and accounted for approximately 2% of all cancer deaths in 2019 [2]. It is diagnosed almost two times more in men, most commonly between the ages of 60 and 70 years [3]. With a primarily expansile growth pattern, it can spread via direct extension following breach of the renal fascia. This leads to a predilection for RCC to compress and involve hilar structures, most commonly the renal vein. Right-sided tumors are more likely to involve the vena cava due to the right renal vein's proximity and short length. RCC tumor thrombus extension can lead to involvement of the hepatic veins, supraphrenic IVC, and right atrium [4]. However, over half of RCCs are asymptomatic and diagnosed during thoracoabdominal imaging obtained for an unrelated reason. Those that do present symptomatically no longer garner the classic triad of flank pain, hematuria, and palpable abdominal mass. Instead, hematuria is most commonly the sole presenting symptom [3].

Radical and partial nephrectomy are long-established treatment modalities for suspicious renal masses. It is critical for surgeons to obtain and review dedicated high-quality cross-sectional renal imaging for presurgical planning to optimize oncologic control and minimize intraoperative complications. CT is often used over MRI due to lower cost and greater availability, and arterial- and nephrogenic-phased are recommended. At least two-phase imaging can help with pathologic subtype differentiation. Three-phase imaging is more commonly being utilized for surgical planning. Extension of RCC into the renal vein and vena cava is detected in 25% and 10% of patients, respectively, and preoperative thrombus detection is crucial for determination of surgical approach [5].

Herein, we present a rare case of a 6 cm renal mass that initially appeared to be amenable to partial nephrectomy; however, additional dedicated imaging raised concern for the presence of a cortical arteriovenous malformation (AVM), which changed the patient's surgical plan, outcome, and histologic findings.

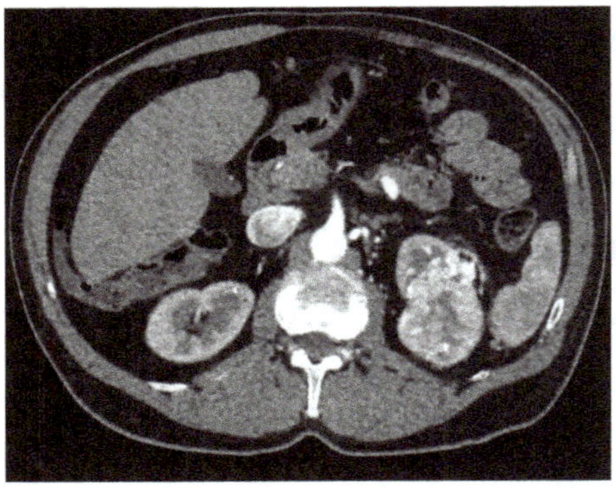

Figure 1: Axial CT scan showing posterior upper pole left enhancing renal mass concerning for malignancy.

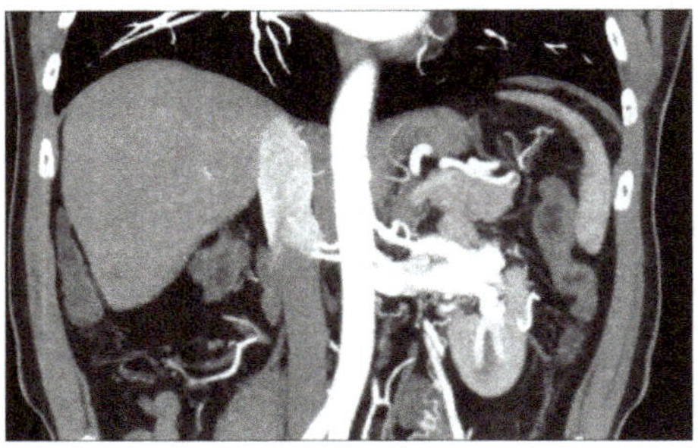

Figure 2: Coronal CT arterial phase showing two left renal arteries and early venous filling of contrast in renal vein and vena cava concerning for AVM in addition to multiple collateral vessels.

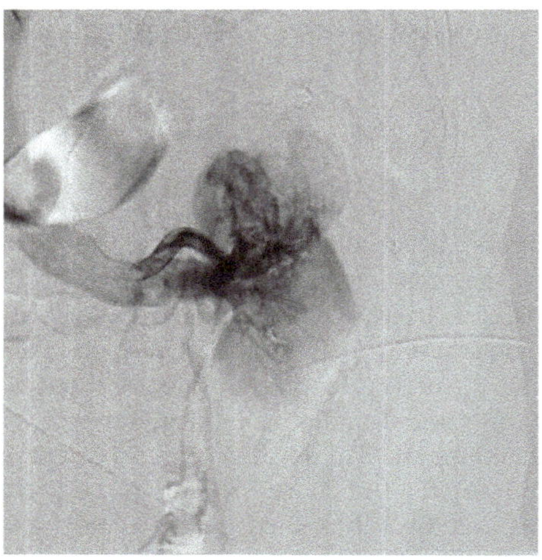

Figure 3: Selective angiography of main renal artery showing early filling of enlarged left renal vein with arterialized flow within the renal vein.

2. Case Presentation

A 67-year-old otherwise healthy male presented with a left upper pole partially endophytic T1b renal mass diagnosed incidentally on imaging during workup for elevated creatinine. He was referred to our tertiary care center for consideration for a robotic partial nephrectomy. The differential diagnosis at this point included RCC, oncocytoma, or metastatic deposit from another primary cancer. The patient presented with a CT scan of the abdomen and pelvis with and without intravenous contrast that demonstrated the tumor and, per the radiology report, no evidence of vascular invasion on portal venous phase imaging (Figure 1). Upon further review of the imaging, there appeared to be abnormal enlargement of the renal vein, prompting additional investigation with a dedicated presurgical-multiphase CT scan with an arterial phase. Subsequent findings of early venous filling and multiple engorged collateral vessels with arterialized blood flow raised concern for the presence of a cortical AVM (Figure 2). These findings proved to be critical as the presence of AVM can lead to uncontrolled intraoperative hemorrhage during renal manipulation.

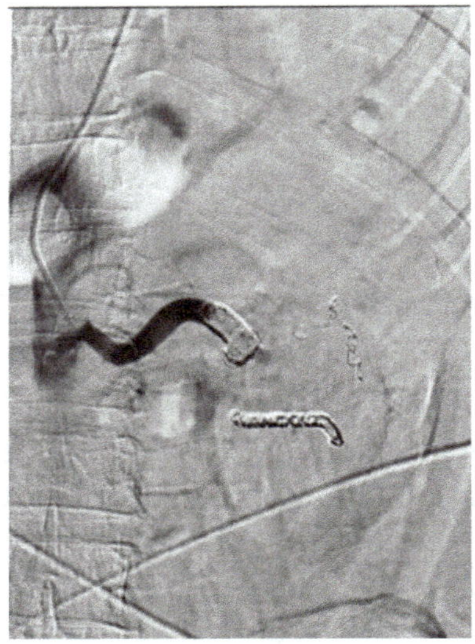

Figure 4: Status post selective coil embolization of the main renal artery at the level of the AVM with absence of early venous filling.

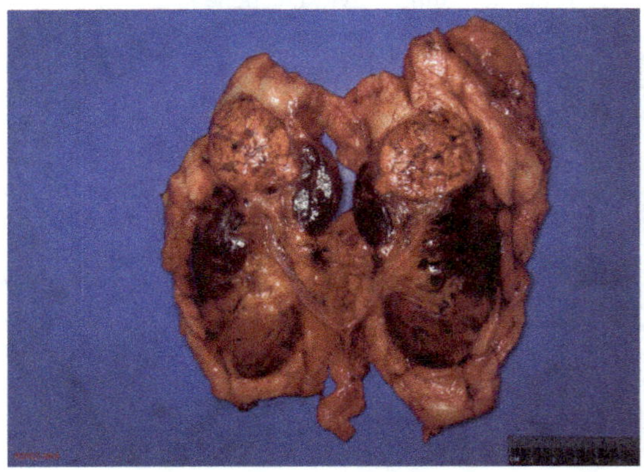

Figure 5: Gross pathology showing left kidney with upper pole renal mass, perinephric fat, and proximal ureter en bloc.

The patient subsequently underwent a selective arterial angiography with embolization by interventional radiology (Figures 3 and 4) followed by an open radical nephrectomy

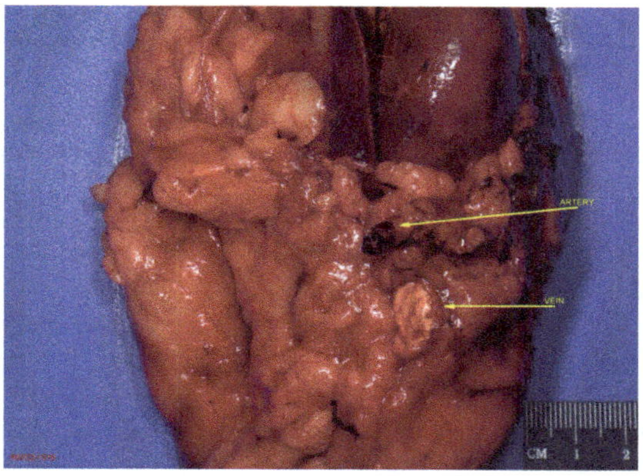

Figure 6: Gross pathology showing coil within the renal artery and tumor thrombus in the main renal vein.

within 24 hours. Intraoperatively, renal vein tumor thrombus invasion was found, which was masked by arterial flow from the AVM on imaging. The surgery was successful, and the patient recovered well without complication. Final pathology revealed clear-cell renal-cell carcinoma grade 2 with renal vein tumor thrombus, AVM within renal cortex, and tumor invasion of the renal sinus (pT3a) with negative surgical margins (Figures 5 and 6).

3. Discussion/Conclusion

AVMs arise from absence of a capillary bed resulting in aberrant shunting of blood from arterial to venous systems. Their prevalence in the general population has been approximated at 0.04% [6]. They can be congenital or acquired through trauma, biopsy, or malignancy. In the context of RCC, there have been 25 cases reported in the literature [7]. RCC can arise from VHL mutations and commonly produces high levels of angiogenic growth factor, contributing to highly vascular tumor presentations [8]. This likely contributes to their rare association with AVMs ([6, 9], and [10]). Renal AVMs can present similarly to RCC with hematuria and flank pain and can be challenging to differentiate on imaging. Indeed, there are reports of AVMs masking the presence of renal tumors on imaging [11]. Conversely, our case involved a renal mass with subsequently discovered AVM, which altered the surgical plan from partial to radical nephrectomy.

Perhaps, the largest alteration in AVM management in the past quarter century is diagnosis with contrasted CT and MRI, as opposed to direct angiography in the past [12]. Aberrant hilar vasculature or collateralization may arise following embolization. Sharma et al. described resection of a left-sided renal mass status post angioembolization characterized by multiple small arterial branches entering directly from the aorta and a large aneurysm at the junction of the renal and gonadal veins [13]. Resection of such a mass without anatomic delineation could lead to catastrophic hemorrhage. Likewise, attempted partial nephrectomy in the mass described is high risk based on both a potential for large arterial parasitic vessels when considering its relation to the renal hilum and a high pressure venous system due to aberrant arterial flow causing a potential for significant back-bleeding. One could encounter significant back-bleeding from the venous system which could compromise visualization and the ability to perform a proper partial nephrectomy without compromising oncologic control or having to convert to a radical nephrectomy. Also, arteriovenous malformations have a risk of spontaneous rupture, which could occur during renal mobilization while performing hilar dissection. In addition, in this case, flow from the arteriovenous malformation was masking a thrombus within the renal vein; so there is also a danger of proceeding with a partial nephrectomy or radical nephrectomy without preoperative angioembolization. An undiagnosed venous thrombus could contribute to a fatal embolic event and/or poor oncologic control, particularly in the setting of a high-pressure venous system. If partial nephrectomy were to be attempted in the setting of a single renal unit, preoperative anatomic delineation with a high-fidelity CT scan and intraoperative assurance of ischemia using indocyanine green as an immunofluophore would be crucial. Due to the above, an open surgical approach would be preferable, as more rapid hilar control and more reliable resection of venous thrombus in a known high-pressure system can be achieved, particularly when performed through a generous midline, hockey stick, or Makuuchi incision.

Less commonly, AVMs related to RCC can lead to appreciable systemic symptoms, such as high-output heart failure. This phenomenon was described as early as 1975, an era in which RCC was often advanced at the time of diagnosis. At that time, 30% of patients with clinically-significant fistulae presented with cardiovascular complaints, and 60% were found to have cardiovascular findings on workup, most commonly abdominal bruit (72%) [14]. AVM in the setting of a primary renal malignancy was recognized as a reversible cause of hypertension and heart failure [14]. More contemporary case reports confirm RCC as the most common source of tumor-related AVMs (22 of 30 cases in one review) [12]. An abdominal bruit, systolic murmur, and hypertension are present in over half of cases [12]. Tobe et al. described that right heart catheterization, when performed, consistently shows increased cardiac output and oxygen saturation levels, with improvement in both parameters postoperatively, indicating additional benefit gained beyond oncologic control.

Contrast-enhanced CT is the gold standard imaging modality for the detection and characterization of renal masses. Renal mass CT protocols generally consist of an unenhanced phase and three enhanced phases: corticomedullary, nephrogenic, and delayed excretory. Use of these phases is instrumental in characterizing cystic masses and can be predictive of an RCC histologic subtype. An arterial phase can provide helpful preoperative information regarding hilar anatomy, but can also highlight a potential tumor-related AVM [15]. Excretory-phase imaging highlights the tumor's relationship to the collecting system, which will also assist in surgical planning, particularly when attempting a nephron-sparing approach. Addition of three-dimensional volume rendering, multiplanar reformatting, and maximum intensity projection further clarify relationships between hilar structures and tumor and have decreased the need for diagnostic catheter angiography for the sole purpose of preoperative planning [16]. Catalano et al. describe the use of the three above phases with multidetector CT and a high-resolution protocol (one-millimeter-thick images) to correctly detect the presence and size of RCC in all studied patients. This protocol allowed for 100% diagnostic accuracy of calyceal infiltration and the presence and extent of renal vein/IVC thrombus in their cohort [17]. However, when contrasted CT scans are unavailable, clinicians should have a high suspicion for RCC when both homogenous and heterogenous renal masses are composed on noncalcific regions within 20-70 Houndsfield units (HU) [18]. Pooler et al. reviewed 193 cases of histologically-proven RCC on noncontrast CT and found that all malignancies fell within this attenuation range, defined as the "danger zone" [18]. Masses measuring less than 20 HU on noncontrast CT may still represent RCC but are generally heterogenous with irregular margins. In rare cases, particularly papillary tumors with lack of enhancement on contrasted CT, gadolinium-enhanced MRI can be beneficial in diagnosing RCC if clinical suspicion is high [19].

Herein, we present the first reported case of concurrent renal vein thrombus and AVM in the setting of clinically-localized RCC. Although Harada et al. reported a case of a 50-year-old female presenting with a 1 cm right-sided renal AVM with subsequent embolization and nephrectomy, final pathology revealed no evidence of malignancy [20]. However, this case is similar to our own in that it demonstrated the utility of multiphase CT imaging in surgical planning for preoperative planning and prevention of catastrophic tumor thrombus embolization or hemorrhage following hilar ligation or tumor resection. In our case, specifically, had a partial nephrectomy been attempted without further imaging, it could have led to uncontrolled bleeding as well as poor oncologic control due to masked renal vein tumor thrombus. AVM identification would also be crucial in this case if renal mass biopsy were proposed, as aberrant flow increases venous pressure, increasing the likelihood of significant perihilar or subcapsular hematoma and significant hemorrhage.

In summary, the rare association of RCC with AVMs is important to recognize for patient safety and surgical planning. Because of their similarity in presentation, a high index of suspicion is needed to recognize these potentially coexisting lesions. Additionally, the presence of a venous thrombus invasion masked by an AVM should be considered, along with MRI to characterize the extent of thrombus. A radical nephrectomy after embolization is a safe and definitive treatment in the case of RCC presenting with an AVM.

References

[1] R. L. Siegel, K. D. Miller, H. E. Fuchs, and A. Jemal, "Cancer statistics, 2022," *CA: a Cancer Journal for Clinicians*, vol. 72, no. 1, pp. 7–33, 2022.

[2] S. A. Padala, A. Barsouk, K. C. Thandra et al., "Epidemiology of renal cell carcinoma," *World Journal of Oncology*, vol. 11, no. 3, pp. 79–87, 2020.

[3] R. E. Gray and G. T. Harris, "Renal cell carcinoma: diagnosis and management," *American Family Physician*, vol. 99, no. 3, pp. 179–184, 2019.

[4] E. Levine, "Renal cell carcinoma: clinical aspects, imaging diagnosis, and staging," *Seminars in Roentgenology*, vol. 30, no. 2, pp. 128–148, 1995.

[5] N. R. Dunnick, "Renal cell carcinoma: staging and surveillance," *Abdominal Radiology*, vol. 41, no. 6, pp. 1079–1085, 2016.

[6] I. Fleetwood and G. Steinberg, "Arteriovenous malformations," *The Lancet*, vol. 359, no. 9309, pp. 863–873, 2002.

[7] D. Watanabe, A. Horiguchi, M. Isono et al., "Renal cell carcinoma presenting with high-output heart failure due to arteriovenous fistula," *Japanese Journal of Urology*, vol. 106, no. 1, pp. 35–39, 2015.

[8] M. M. Baldewijns, V. L. Thijssen, G. G. Van den Eynden et al., "High-grade clear cell renal cell carcinoma has a higher angiogenic activity than low-grade renal cell carcinoma based on histomorphological quantification and qRT-PCR mRNA expression profile," *British Journal of Cancer*, vol. 96, no. 12, pp. 1888–1895, 2007.

[9] S. Vasavada, S. Manion, R. Flanigan, and A. Novick, "Renal arteriovenous malformations masquerading as renal cell carcinoma," *Urology*, vol. 46, no. 5, pp. 716–721, 1995.

[10] C. Selli, C. Bartolozzi, G. Lizzadro, and D. Petacchi, "Arteriovenous fistula associated with renal cell carcinoma: demonstration by magnetic resonance imaging," *Urologic Radiology*, vol. 8, no. 1, pp. 190–193, 1986.

[11] S. Volin, P. Steinberg, and D. Mittleider, "Renal cell carcinoma initially presenting as an arteriovenous malformation: a case presentation and a review of the literature," *Case Reports in Urology*, vol. 2013, Article ID 356819, 5 pages, 2013.

[12] A. Tobe, A. Tanaka, S. Yoshida et al., "High-output heart failure caused by a tumor-related arteriovenous fistula: a case report and literature review," *Internal Medicine*, vol. 60, no. 18, pp. 2979–2984, 2021.

[13] A. P. Sharma, M. K. Gupta, G. Sharma, and R. S. Mavuduru, *Arteriovenous Malformation with a Renal Mass: A rare Association*, p. 2, 2020.

[14] M. Rodgers, A. Moss, M. Hoffman, and E. Lipchik, "Arteriovenous fistulae secondary to renal cell carcinoma. Clinical and cardiovascular manifestations: report of a case," *Circulation*, vol. 52, no. 2, pp. 345–350, 1975.

[15] A. C. Tsili, E. Andriotis, M. G. Gkeli et al., "The role of imaging in the management of renal masses," *European Journal of Radiology*, vol. 141, article 109777, 2021.

[16] A. Morshid, E. S. Duran, W. J. Choi, and C. Duran, "A concise review of the multimodality imaging features of renal cell carcinoma," *Cureus*, vol. 13, 2021.

[17] C. Catalano, F. Fraioli, A. Laghi et al., "High-resolution multidetector CT in the preoperative evaluation of patients with renal cell carcinoma," *American Journal of Roentgenology*, vol. 180, no. 5, pp. 1271–1277, 2003.

[18] B. D. Pooler, P. J. Pickhardt, S. D. O'Connor, R. J. Bruce, S. R. Patel, and S. Y. Nakada, "Renal cell carcinoma: attenuation values on unenhanced CT," *American Journal of Roentgenology*, vol. 198, no. 5, pp. 1115–1120, 2012.

[19] S. Krishna, C. A. Murray, M. D. McInnes et al., "CT imaging of solid renal masses: pitfalls and solutions," *Clinical Radiology*, vol. 72, no. 9, pp. 708–721, 2017.

[20] H. Harada, M. Togashi, T. Abe, Y. Takeyama, T. Seki, and N. Ohashi, "Renal arteriovenous malformation with thrombus in the inferior vena cava," *International Journal of Urology*, vol. 7, no. 8, pp. 310–312, 2000.

37

Successful Endoscopic Management of a Renal Fungal Ball using Flexible Ureterorenoscopy

Mahmoud Abuelnaga,[1] **Sadegh Khoshzaban,**[1] **Mahmoud Reda Badr,**[2] **and Aasem Chaudry**[1]

[1]*Department of Urology, Bedford Hospital NHS Trust, Bedford, UK*
[2]*Department of Urology, Ain Shams University Hospitals, Cairo, Egypt*

Correspondence should be addressed to Mahmoud Abuelnaga; mroshdymd@gmail.com

Academic Editor: Francesco M. Solivetti

Background. Candida as a cause for urinary tract infection in healthy individuals is unusual. The extension of fungi into the urinary collecting system rarely leads to formation of bezoars or fungus balls. This can in turn lead to hydronephrosis, obstructive uropathy and sepsis. *Case Presentation.* An eighty years old gentleman presented to A&E with confusion, severe urosepsis and acute kidney injury. CTKUB demonstrated significant right sided hydronephrosis, perinephric fat stranding and gas in collecting system. A year prior to this admission he has become known to the urology team for a fungal ball that was noted in the upper pole of the right kidney which was picked up following elective flexible ureterorenoscopy for right kidney stones. Flexible ureterorenoscopy and successful retrieval of fungal ball by basket was performed. *Conclusion.* We advocate this technique to be considered as an alternative to the current treatment offered to patients with fungal ball infections and especially so in cases were a nephrostomy is either contraindicated, unavailable, or not possible.

1. Introduction and Background

Candida as a cause for urinary tract infection in healthy individuals is unusual. The fungal species has two ways invading the urinary tract system, either via haematogenous dissemination or via the bladder and urethra referred to as antegrade and retrograde respectively [10]. Kidneys are the second major target organ following the lungs for antegrade invasion by Candida [12]. The extension of fungi into the urinary collecting system rarely leads to formation of bezoars or fungus balls. This can in turn lead to hydronephrosis, obstructive uropathy and sepsis [16].

Given the two possible routes of fungal infection in urinary tract, it can be concluded that the candida infection in the genitourinary tract maybe the cause of systemic infection or as a result of it. Following an extensive review of the cases of urinary tract infections caused by candida albicans, Fisher and associates demonstrated the following as the predisposing factors: diabetes mellitus, antibiotic administration, steroid therapy, urine flow turbulence, congenital anomalies, neurogenic bladder, indwelling catheter, and ileal conduits [9].

Fungal balls in the pelvis of kidney, also known as fungal accretions or bezoars are known to cause urinary tract obstruction. The diagnosis is often established by presence of fungi in urine culture and identification of obstructive uropathy via imaging studies such as ultrasound, intravenous pyelography and CT scan. These imaging could also identify soft tissue densities within the renal collecting system, pelvis or ureter [7].

This case report aims to demonstrate an alternative method for management of candiduria due to fungal ball in the kidney. Most reported cases in literature were managed by intravenous antifungal treatment and antifungal instillation through percutaneous nephrostomy tube [1].

2. Case Presentation

An eighty-year-old patient,who was later found to have a right sided fungal ball causing obstructive uropathy, initially presented in 2017 with renal colic. He was known to have uncontrolled type two diabetes mellitus and a history of neo-adjuvant

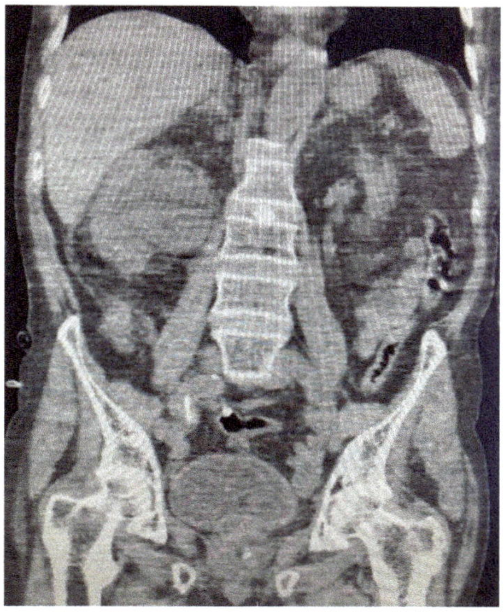

FIGURE 1: CT KUB showing significant right sided hydronephrosis along with perinephric fat stranding.

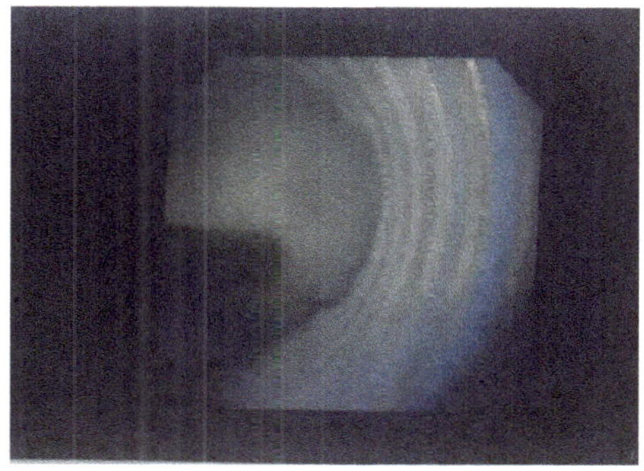

FIGURE 2: Fungal tissue inside basket within the ureteral access sheath.

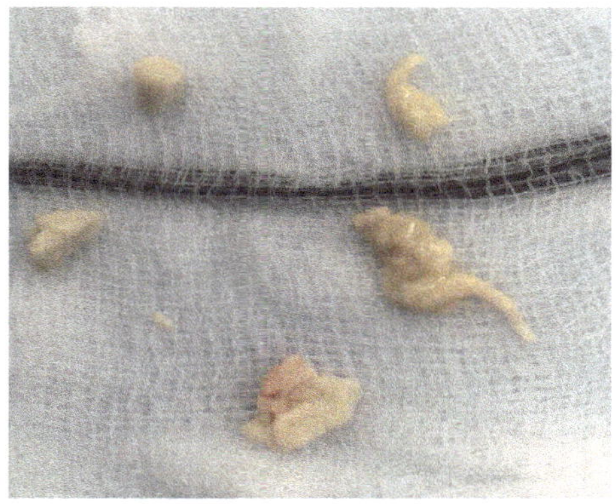

FIGURE 3: Retrieved fluffy fungal tissues by basket.

long course chemo-radiotherapy followed by low anterior resection and loop ileostomy for management of a rectal tumour.

At the time of initial presentation, he was found to have a left sided 1.2 cm mid ureter calculus for which he had a left rigid ureteroscopy and stent insertion. A follow-up ultrasound scan of his kidneys revealed bilateral small kidney stones and he subsequently had shockwave lithotripsy on the left side.

During this time the patient was admitted to the hospital under the medical team for management of diabetic ketoacidosis and it was noted that his urine culture grew candida. He came under our attention two months later when he was booked for an elective flexible ureterorenoscopy for management of his right sided kidney stones. However it was noted on URS that he had a fungal ball in the upper pole of the right kidney and therefore a JJ stent was inserted and IV antifungals were started as per microbiologists' recommendation. His creatinine at that time was 3.6 mg/dl.

One month later, he had a right flexible ureteroscopy and laser stone disintegration with partial removal of fungal ball and insertion of JJ stent. His renal function improved following the procedure (Cr 2.2 mg/dl). Since the entire fungal ball could not be removed at the time, a second-look flexible ureteroscopy was planned two weeks later while the patient was sent home with IV antifungals. Unfortunately, the patient declined the procedure following discharge and did not attend follow up clinic appointments.

Ten months later, he was admitted with severe urosepsis, confusion and acute kidney failure (Cr 4.8 mg/dl). CT KUB showed significant right sided hydronephrosis along with perinephric fat stranding and gas in the collecting system (Figure 1).

The patient underwent an urgent cystoscopy and replacement of blocked JJ stent initially following which the patient's general condition as well as renal function improved (Cr 2.2 mg/dl). During the same admission he subsequently had a right sided flexible ureteroscopy which went as follows. After the placement of ureteral access sheath, 200 mls of pure pus was drained and sent for culture. A Zero Tip Nitinol Stone Retrieval Basket was then used to remove the fluffy fungal tissues and a JJ stent was left in place (Figures 2 and 3).

The culture heavily grew candida albicans and reported as sensitive to Fluconazole. Analysis of the tissue retrieved also showed granular debris together with numerous fungal spores and hyphae which were consistent with Candida species. He was then discussed with microbiologist and specialised infectious diseases who advised long term Intravenous Fluconazole for two weeks after complete removal of fungal ball. Two weeks later, he underwent another flexible ureteroscopy and his kidney was found to be clear of fungal tissues and his stent was removed. His condition was stable, and his creatinine level settled at 1.9 mg/dl when he was discharged home.

3. Discussion

Mycosis renalis, (fungal infection of kidneys) as described by Lundquist in 1931 is a rare and serious infection which is even less common as a primary infection. Lundquist first reported on 17 patients with primary infections and demonstrated that these infections are even more serious in immunocompromised patients [11].

Common predisposing factors of fungal infections in the urinary tract are diabetes mellitus, prolonged Foley catheter, urinary tract abnormalities, prolonged antibiotic therapy, steroids, immunosuppressive therapy, malnutrition and malignancy. Formation of a fungal ball can be initiated by agglutination of a necrotic tissue nucleus (papillary necrosis), mucosus debris and foreign or stone debris. Such a fungal ball can in turn cause upper urinary tract obstruction with hydronephrosis . Most frequent pathogens seen to cause such complications are *C. albicans* and *C. tropicalis* [3, 16].

In complex fungal infections of the urinary tract, upper urinary tract imaging is essential due to high incidence of obstructive uropathy in complex fungal infections. Wainstein reviewed fifty patients who had fungal infections of the urinary tract from 1982 to 1992 and classified the fungal infections into simple infections (i.e., localised to bladder) and complex infections (i.e., those involving upper urinary tract or with systemic infections) and demonstrated that the incidence of the following were significantly higher in patients with complex infections. These, in descending order of difference in incidence, were obstructive uropathy, malnutrition, neoplasia, prolonged antibiotic use and renal failure. The high incidence of obstructive uropathy in complex infection (88%) together with the fact that fungemia being common in complex infections (81%) with a 36% mortality rate, makes upper urinary tract imaging a requirement in such patients [3].

Most of the reported cases of fungal ball in literature were managed by either long term antifungal therapy or local antifungal instillation through a nephrostomy tube [1, 12, 13, 15, 16]. Current management options for renal fungal ball include intravenous antifungal agents, percutaneous nephrostomy with instillation of antifungal agents with no consensus over the duration of instillation required. The most common antifungal agents used are fluconazole and amphotericin B due to their high urine concentration, however, amphotericin B is also nephrotoxic which complicates its use in such scenarios. Other antifungals, such as echinocandins, are not renally excreted and therefore their systemic use in such conditions is limited [4, 14].

There are very limited number of cases in the literature about endoscopic removal of fungal ball [18] and prior to the advent of endourology, open surgical procedures with pyelotomy were sometimes necessary for removal of fungal balls in the renal collecting system. The current mainstay of treatment is percutaneous nephrostomy which is used to successfully manage patients with obstructive uropathy secondary to such infections. Nephrostomy both relieves the obstruction and also provide direct access for antifungal instillation as well as percutaneous and identification and possible removal of fungal ball [2, 5].

In current practice, endoscopy and flexible ureterorenoscopy is widely available in most hospitals across UK. The use of such equipment can be helpful in management of patient in fungal ball as it can both expedite treatment and reduce length of hospital stay for such patients. This is in direct contrast with the variable and often prolonged treatment that is required with the use of current established treatment with nephrostomy and direct antifungal instillation which averages around seven days [1].

Nephrostomy service can be limited in many hospitals and is not as widely available as urological endoscopy services across UK. Furthermore, nephrostomy is contraindicated in patients with bleeding disorders and uncooperative patients. Musculoskeletal deformities, body habitus and not adequately dilated renal pelvis can also complicate nephrostomy placement [6].

5. Conclusion

Herein we demonstrated that endoscopic retrieval of renal fungal tissues using flexible ureterorenoscopy is an effective, safe and rapid intervention in dealing with an obstructing renal fungal ball. It can also significantly reduces hospital stay and toxicity associated with long-term use of either local or systemic antifungals .We advocate that it should be considered as an alternative to the current treatment offered to patients with fungal ball infections and especially so in cases were a nephrostomy is either contraindicated, unavailable, or not possible.

References

[1] O. A. Abdeljaleel, I. Alnadhari, S. Mahmoud et al., "Treatment of renal fungal ball with fluconazole instillation through a nephrostomy tube: case report and literature review," *The American Journal of Case Reports*, vol. 19, pp. 1179–1183, 2018.

[2] J. Abramowitz, J. E. Fowler, K. Talluri et al., "Percutaneous identification and removal of fungus ball from renal pelvis," *Journal of Urology*, vol. 135, no. 6, pp. 1232–1233, 1986.

[3] M. A. Wainstein, R. C. Graham, and M. I. Resnick, "Predisposing factors of systemic fungal infections of the genitourinary tract," *Journal of Urology*, vol. 154, no. 1, pp. 160–163, 1995.

[4] E. S. Ashley, R. L. Dodds, J. S. Lewis, C. Martin, and D. Andes, "Pharmacology of systemic antifungal agents," *Clinical Infectious Diseases*, vol. 43, 1, pp. S28–39, 2006.

[5] F. F. Bartone, R. S. Hurwitz, E. L. Rojas, E. Steinberg, and R. Franceschini, "The role of percutaneous nephrostomy in the management of obstructing candidiasis of the urinary tract in infants," *The Journal of Urology*, vol. 140, no. 2, pp. 338–341, 1988.

[6] BSIR, "Nephrostomy|British Society of Interventional Radiology," 2019.

[7] M. Stein, E. Laor, B. M. Tolia, and R. E. Reid, "Unusual case of renal candida fungus balls," *Urology*, vol. 41, no. 1, pp. 49–51, 1993.

[8] J. P. Burgués Gasión, J. M. Alapont Alacreu, F. Oliver Amorós, A. Benedicto Redón, F. Boronat Tormo, and J. F. Jiménez Cruz, "Pyeloureteral fungus ball in patients with urinary lithiasis. treatment with ureterorenoscopy," *Actas Urologicas Espanolas*, vol. 27, no. 1, pp. 60–64, 2003.

[9] J. F. Fisher, W. H. Chew, S. Shadomy, R. J. Duma, C. G. Mayhan, and W. C. House, "Urinary tract infections due to candida albicans," *Clinical Infectious Diseases*, vol. 4, no. 6, pp. 1107–1118, 1982.

[10] J. F. Fisher, K. Kavanagh, J. D. Sobel, C. A. Kauffman, and C. A. Newman, "Candida urinary tract infection: pathogenesis," *Clinical Infectious Diseases*, vol. 52, 6, pp. S437–S551, 2011.

[11] C. W. Lundquist, "On primary mycosis of the kidney," *British Journal of Urology*, vol. 3, no. 1, pp. 1–13, 1931.

[12] M. A. Luno and M. E. Tortoledo, "Candidiasis," G. P. Bodey and V. Fainstein, Eds., vol. 13, New York: Raven, 1985.

[13] A. Shukla, N. Shrivastava, C. A. Singh, and B. Nayak, "Percutaneous management of systemic fungal infection presenting as bilateral renal fungal ball," *Journal of Endourology Case Reports*, vol. 2, no. 1, pp. 152–54, 2016.

[14] A. N. Malani, "Failure of caspofungin for treatment of candida glabrata candiduria: case report and review of the literature," *Infectious Diseases in Clinical Practice*, vol. 18, no. 4, pp. 271–272, 2010.

[15] M. Narendrababu, S. Ramesh, B. V. Raghunath, and B. C. Gowrishankar, "Successful management of a renal fungal ball in a pretermature neonate: a case report and review of literature," *Journal of Indian Association of Pediatric Surgeons*, vol. 18, no. 3, p. 121, 2013.

[16] V. Praz, R. Burruni, F. Meid, M. Wisard, P. Jichlinski, and T. Tawadros, "Fungus ball in the urinary tract: a rare entity," *Canadian Urological Association Journal = Journal de l'Association Des Urologues Du Canada*, vol. 8, no. 1-2, pp. E118–E120, 2014.

38

Metastatic Thyroid Cancer Presenting as Renal Cortical Mass

Osamah Hasan ,[1] Matthew Houlihan,[2] Tobias S. Kohler,[2] and Courtney M. P. Hollowell[3]

[1]*Midwestern University Chicago College of Osteopathic Medicine, Downers Grove, IL, USA*
[2]*Department of Urology, Mayo Clinic, Rochester, MN, USA*
[3]*Division of Urology, Cook County Health and Hospitals System, Chicago, IL, USA*

Correspondence should be addressed to Osamah Hasan; ohasan15@midwestern.edu

Academic Editor: David Duchene

The authors present a rare case of primary diagnosis of metastatic, differentiated thyroid cancer presenting as a solitary, large renal mass. Renal cortical masses which represent metastatic primary malignancies are often small, multifocal, and in the setting of active malignancy. Surgical excision of this patient's renal mass demonstrated the unexpected diagnosis and subsequent endocrine surgical intervention.

1. Introduction

The presentation, diagnosis, and treatment of renal cortical masses, has evolved substantially over the last forty years. Historically, the standard of care has been surgical excision via partial or radical nephrectomy. Traditional therapy has evolved in the modern era due in large part to increasing incidence and earlier diagnosis of renal masses, which is due in large part to increased utilization of cross-sectional imaging in health care [1]. Management options of cT1 renal masses may include active surveillance, thermal ablation, or extirpation via partial or radical nephrectomy depending on the size and location of the tumor, as well as patient-specific factors [2]. We report a unique urologic case with a primary diagnosis of differentiated thyroid cancer after undergoing nephrectomy for a cT1bN0M0 renal mass.

2. Case Report

2.1. Patient Presentation. The patient was a 64-year-old female with a past medical history of hypertension, diabetes mellitus type 2, and hyperlipidemia referred to urology clinic for evaluation of a 5 cm left-sided renal mass that was incidentally discovered during evaluation for diarrhea and flank pain. She denied any history of gross hematuria or other urinary symptoms. She had no significant past medical history. The patient had never smoked and denied a family history of renal malignancy. On physical examination, she was found to be in no acute distress, and appeared generally well (ECOG performance status 0). There were no carotid bruits or neck masses palpated. Her chest was clear to auscultation bilaterally and her abdomen was soft, nontender, and nondistended without palpable abdominal masses or costo-vertebral angle tenderness. Laboratory evaluation including comprehensive metabolic panel, complete blood count, and urinalysis were within normal limits.

2.2. Imaging Studies. Computed tomography of the abdomen and pelvis with contrast demonstrated a 4.9 cm by 5.0 cm by 5.8 cm endophytic interpolar left renal mass (Figures 1(a) and 1(b)). Chest CT with contrast demonstrated a 12 mm right lower lobe pulmonary nodule, which was noted to have been stable on prior imaging up to eleven years previously and was interpreted as a granuloma. Finally, she was found to have a slightly enlarged thyroid gland with several small calcified nodules (Figure 2).

2.3. Surgical Management. The patient was counseled regarding options for management and underwent hand-assisted laparoscopic radical nephrectomy. The surgical procedure was uncomplicated with an estimated blood loss of 25 cc. She tolerated surgery well, and, following an uncomplicated recovery, was discharged from the hospital on postoperative day three.

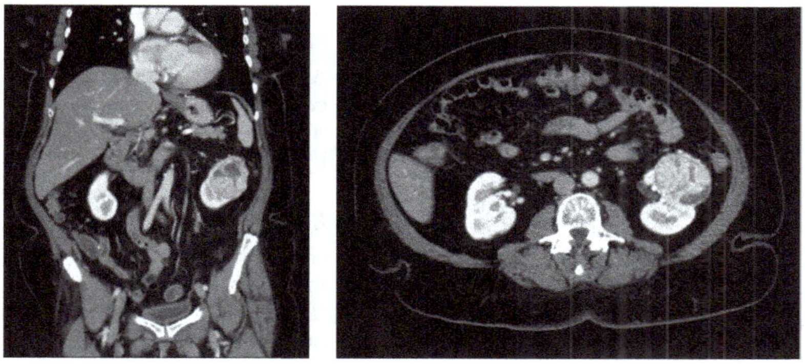

(a) (b)

FIGURE 1: CT A&P demonstrating a 4.9 cm × 5.0 cm × 5.8 cm renal mass. Coronal image (a), axial (b).

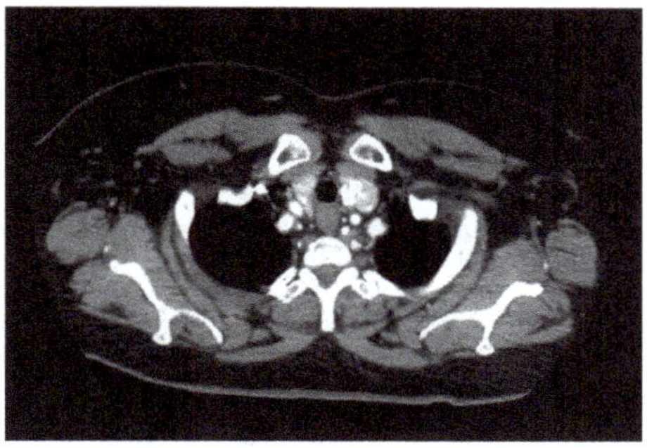

FIGURE 2: CT chest w/contrast demonstrating multinodular goiter.

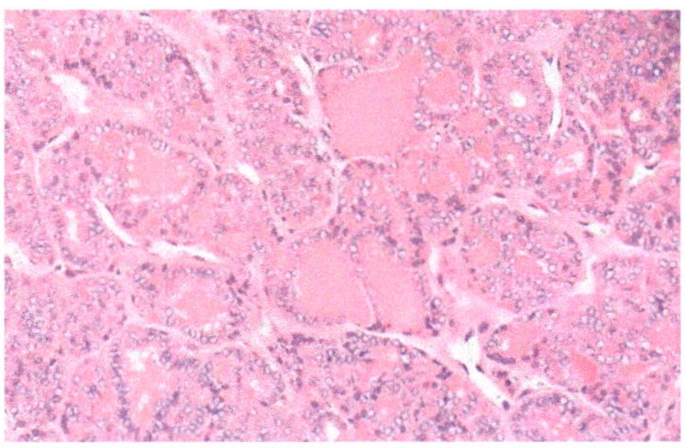

FIGURE 3: Photomicrograph showing follicular variant of papillary thyroid carcinoma (H&E stain, 100x).

2.4. Patient Outcome. Histopathology revealed a 6.5 cm mass consistent with metastatic follicular variant of papillary thyroid cancer (Figure 3). The diagnosis was confirmed with immunohistochemistry as the tumor cells were CK7 (+), TTF1 (+), and Thyroglobulin (+) but CK20 (−) and WT1 (−). The soft tissue and vascular surgical margins were negative for tumor. Given the results of the pathologic analysis and evidence of several calcified nodules within the enlarged thyroid, she was referred to endocrine surgery for further evaluation. On thyroid ultrasound, a left-sided thyroid nodule was appreciated. Her endocrine evaluation included thyroid function panel, which demonstrated an elevated thyroid-stimulating hormone (TSH) of 7.57 uIU/mL and normal T4 (0.81 ng/dL). She underwent fine-needle-aspiration of the thyroid, which showed atypia. Subsequent nuclear medicine whole body thyroid scan demonstrated no additional sites of I-131 avidity. She underwent a total thyroidectomy and radioactive iodine 3 months after. Pathology was consistent with a follicular variant of papillary thyroid carcinoma.

3. Discussion

The differential diagnosis for pathologic etiology of cT1bN0M0 renal masses is broad. Renal cortical masses may be either benign or malignant. Malignant renal cortical masses include renal cell carcinoma, metastases from other malignancies and renal medullary carcinoma [3]. Renal cell carcinoma is the most common malignant cause of renal cortical masses and can be divided into histologic subtypes including clear cell, multilocular cystic clear cell, chromophobe, papillary, collecting duct, unclassified, postneuroblastoma, and mucinous tubular and spindle cell carcinoma [4]. Clear cell renal cell carcinoma is the most common histologic subtype representing roughly 75% of malignant renal masses with papillary renal cell carcinoma representing 10–15% [4]. Patients with clear cell typically have a worse prognosis compared with other histologic subtypes [5].

Differentiated thyroid cancer consists of both papillary and follicular carcinomas. Differentiated thyroid cancer typically remains localized to the thyroid and presents with a thyroid mass. Incidence of distant metastatic disease has been studied to be less than 4% [6]. The most common sites of metastatic thyroid cancer are the cervical lymph nodes, lungs, bones, and brain [7]. It may also present with regional lymph node metastasis [8]. There are rare case reports describing metastatic thyroid cancer involving the genitourinary organs which include adrenal glands, kidneys, and penile and scrotal skin [9, 10]. Thyroid cancer is an indolent diagnosis, with overall survival greater than 85% at 20 years when localized to the thyroid gland [11]. The prognosis of well-differentiated thyroid cancer is significantly worsened by distant metastatic disease, with a 47-fold increase in risk of death [11]. Upon review of literature, 25 cases have been described involving metastatic differentiated thyroid cancer to the kidney [12]. Most cases described are in females over the age of 45 years [12]. However, diagnosis of metastatic differentiated thyroid cancer presenting as a primary renal mass has only been described in only two prior cases, per the authors' review [13, 14]. Both patients had no other evidence of metastatic disease and as such underwent uncomplicated nephrectomies with subsequent diagnosis of primary differentiated thyroid carcinoma [13, 14]. Both patients were treated post-nephrectomy with total thyroidectomies, with one patient receiving post-thyroidectomy radioactive iodine. Follow-up data was available for one patient demonstrating freedom from local or distant metastases three years following radical nephrectomy [13]. Nonrenal cell carcinoma cortical metastases from other primary tumors are typically multifocal and bilateral, discovered in the setting of other metastases, and present as small, endophytic masses [15]. Our case discussed represented a solitary lesion, 5.8 cm in greatest dimension, with primarily exophytic components without evidence of other sites of metastatic disease.

4. Conclusion

In the setting of an enlarged thyroid gland with calcified nodules during staging imaging, metastatic thyroid cancer should be included in the differential diagnosis of a localized renal mass. In such cases, baseline laboratory evaluation may include thyroid function test and preoperative consultation with endocrine surgery should be considered. Surgical excision of pT1bN0M0 renal mass via radical or partial nephrectomy in an otherwise healthy female remains the standard of care. A multidisciplinary approach to postoperative follow-up and care is essential in the setting of rare and unusual cases such as that presented here.

References

[1] J. M. Hollingsworth, D. C. Miller, S. Daignault, and B. K. Hollenbeck, "Rising incidence of small renal masses: a need to reassess treatment effect," *JNCI: Journal of the National Cancer Institute*, vol. 98, no. 18, pp. 1331–1334, 2006.

[2] R. J. Motzer, E. Jonasch, N. Agarwal et al., "Kidney cancer, version 3.2015," *Journal of the National Comprehensive Cancer Network: JNCCN*, vol. 13, no. 2, pp. 151–159, 2015.

[3] J. McKiernan, O. Yossepowitch, M. W. Kattan et al., "Partial nephrectomy for renal cortical tumors: pathologic findings and impact on outcome," *Urology*, vol. 60, no. 6, pp. 1003–1009, 2002.

[4] J. J. Patard, E. Leray, N. Rioux-Leclercq et al., "Prognostic value of histologic subtypes in renal cell carcinoma: a multicenter experience," *Journal of Clinical Oncology*, vol. 23, no. 12, pp. 2763–2771, 2005.

[5] J. C. Cheville, C. M. Lohse, H. Zincke, A. L. Weaver, and M. L. Blute, "Comparisons of outcome and prognostic features among histologic subtypes of renal cell carcinoma," *The American Journal of Surgical Pathology*, vol. 27, no. 5, pp. 612–624, 2003.

[6] A. R. Shaha, J. P. Shah, and T. R. Loree, "Differentiated thyroid cancer presenting initially with distant metastasis," *The American Journal of Surgery*, vol. 174, no. 5, pp. 474–476, 1997.

[7] E. Farina, F. Monari, G. Tallini et al., "Unusual thyroid carcinoma metastases: a case series and literature review," *Endocrine Pathology*, vol. 27, no. 1, pp. 55–64, 2016.

[8] S. V. Jagtap, D. Patil, and C. S. Gupta, "Papillary carcinoma thyroid presented with extensive local lymph nodal metastasis," *IP Archives of Cytology and Histopathology Research*, vol. 3, no. 2, pp. 113–115, 2018.

[9] M. O. Grimm, P. Spiegelhalder, H. Heep, C. D. Gerharz, H. D. Röher, and R. Ackermann, "Penile metastasis secondary to follicular thyroid carcinoma," *Scandinavian Journal of Urology and Nephrology*, vol. 38, no. 3, pp. 253–255, 2004.

[10] W. Shon, S. B. Ferguson, and N. I. Comfere, "Metastatic Hürthle cell carcinoma of the thyroid presenting as ulcerated scrotum nodules," *The American Journal of Dermatopathology*, vol. 32, no. 4, pp. 392–394, 2010.

[11] L. J. DeGroot, E. L. Kaplan, M. McCormick, and F. H. Straus, "Natural history, treatment, and course of papillary thyroid carcinoma," *The Journal of Clinical Endocrinology & Metabolism*, vol. 71, no. 2, pp. 414–424, 1990.

[12] H. J. Song, Y. L. Xue, Y. H. Xu, Z. L. Qiu, and Q. Y. Luo, "Rare metastases of differentiated thyroid carcinoma: pictorial review," *Endocrine-Related Cancer*, vol. 18, no. 5, pp. R165–R174, 2011.

[13] L. D. Graham and S. M. Roe, "Metastatic papillary thyroid carcinoma presenting as a primary renal neoplasm," *The American Surgeon*, vol. 61, no. 8, pp. 732–734, 1995.

[14] F. P. Ruggiero, E. E. Frauenhoffer, and B. C. Stack, "Papillary thyroid cancer with an initial presentation of abdominal and flank pain," *American Journal of Otolaryngology*, vol. 26, no. 2, pp. 142–145, 2005.

[15] K. Abe, T. Hasegawa, S. Onodera, Y. Oishi, and M. Suzuki, "Renal metastasis of thyroid carcinoma," *International Journal of Urology*, vol. 9, no. 11, pp. 656–658, 2002.

Unilateral Giant Hydronephrosis Secondary to Ureteropelvic Junction Obstruction in a Middle-Aged Woman

Masresha S. Dino,[1] **Seid M. Hassen**,[1] **and Tesfaye H. Tufa**[2]

[1]*Department of Surgery, Urology Unit, Addis Ababa, St. Paul's Hospital Millennium Medical College, Ethiopia*
[2]*Department of Obstetrics and Gynecology, St. Paul's Hospital Millennium Medical College, Addis Ababa, Ethiopia*

Correspondence should be addressed to Masresha S. Dino; masreshasolomon412@gmail.com

Academic Editor: Imran Morhason-Bello

Background. Giant hydronephrosis is a rare urologic problem defined as a collection of more than one liter of urine in the collecting system. The radiologic appearance may mimic benign cystic disease of the kidney. We report a case of giant hydronephrosis in a 32-year-old female who presented with progressive abdominal swelling of two-year duration, caused by ureteropelvic junction obstruction with more than nine liters of urine in the collecting system. *Conclusion.* Giant hydronephrosis is a rare differential diagnosis for cystic intra-abdominal mass in adults with progressively increasing abdominal swelling. CT and MRI are important in confirming the diagnosis by localizing the origin of the swelling. Management depends on the underlying cause and appearance of the diseased kidney.

1. Introduction

Giant hydronephrosis is defined as the presence of more than one-liter urine or 1.6% of the bodyweight of urine in the collecting system [1–3]. The development of hydronephrosis is a gradual process, and most cases are reported to have less than two liters of fluid (urine) collection [3–6]. The common presentation of these patients mimics renal stone disease. Epidemiologically, the left kidney is commonly affected. The most common underlying causes include ureteropelvic junction (UPJ) obstruction and renal stone disease. The majority of this condition will be diagnosed during childhood and infancy (congenital). If not treated early, it may cause progressive and gradual complications like hypertension, kidney rupture, renal failure, and malignant transformation because of prolonged irritation [1–5].

Urolithiasis and tumors either in the renal system or in adjacent organs can cause a compressive disease. This compression leads to obstruction of the renal collecting system leading to hydronephrosis, which gradually grows to have a cystic appearance. There are wide ranges of differential diagnoses for cystic intra-abdominal mass which resemble giant hydronephrosis, including; ovarian cysts, hepatobiliary cysts, renal cell carcinoma (RCC), retroperitoneal tumor, pseudomyxoma, splenomegaly, and ascites [6].

We present a rare case of a 32-year-old woman with long-standing abdominal pain and swelling and who was diagnosed and treated for giant hydronephrosis secondary to UPJ obstruction.

2. Case Report

A thirty-two-year-old female patient presented with progressive abdominal swelling of two-year duration. The swelling started from the left side of the abdomen and progressed to involve the whole abdomen. The swelling became prominent since one year (Figure 1), with associated dull aching left flank pain. She had no hematuria or any other urinary symptoms. On physical examination, her vital signs were within the normal range with a pulse of 83 beats per

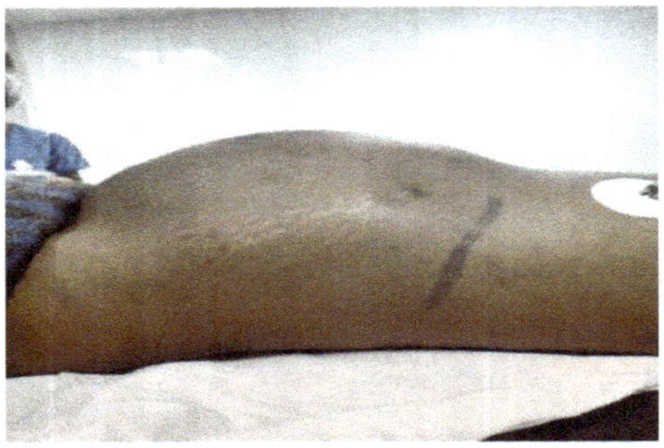

Figure 1: Abdominal examination shows a distended abdomen with cystic appearance on palpation. The marking site is left flank.

Table 1: Important laboratory investigation.

Laboratory tests	Results
Urine analysis	Non revealing
WBC	4200
Hct	41.4%
Creatinine	0.67
Urea	23.3
Potassium	4.53
Sodium	139
Chlorine	101.2

minute and blood pressure of 100/80 mmHg. On abdominal examination, she had visible abdominal swelling, which was prominent on the left side of the abdomen. The swelling was cystic with no attachment to the surrounding structure.

Laboratory findings of the patient, including urine analysis, serum electrolyte, and hematology profile, were all in the normal range (Table 1). During the initial evaluation, the ultrasound index of the left kidney showed a huge hydronephrosis passing the midline and filling almost the whole abdomen. Computerized tomography (CT) scan of the abdomen without contrast showed massive left kidney pelvicalyceal dilatation with a maximum cortical thickness of 3 mm. The dilatation spans seven vertebral lengths with the inferior border reaching the pelvis (Figure 2). The left ureter and left renal arteries are not visible, and significant mass effects on other abdominal organs were also noted.

A diagnosis of giant left hydronephrosis was made and the patient was prepared for laparotomy. The abdomen was opened with a subcostal flank incision under general anesthesia. Upon entry, 9.5 liters of urine was drained, and a left nephrectomy was performed, which was sent for histopathology. The left ureter was explored and showed severe stenosis at the level of ureteropelvic junction (Figure 3). An intra-abdominal drain was left in situ, and the abdominal wall closed in layers.

She had a smooth postoperative course following the surgery. Her postoperative hematocrit was 21.7%, for which she was transfused with one unit of crossmatched whole blood. Her postoperative serum electrolyte and renal function test were also in the normal range. The intra-abdominal drainage was removed on the 5th postoperative day, and the patient was discharged a day later with satisfactory clinical condition. Histopathologic examination of the biopsy showed a hydronephrotic kidney with no feature of malignant growth (Figure 4).

3. Discussion

Giant hydronephrosis with accumulation of more than 9 liters of fluids is an uncommon phenomenon in adults. The first reported case of giant hydronephrosis was in 1746, and etiologies include ureteric obstruction of various causes congenital or acquired, intrinsic or extrinsic, including UPJ obstruction, both renal and ureteric stone disease, and malignancy [1–3]. Patients commonly present with increasing abdominal girth and flank swelling. Other common symptoms include flank pain, hematuria, especially following trauma, and recurrent urinary tract infection. In rare circumstances, they may present with hypertension, obstructive jaundice, intestinal obstruction, respiratory distress, and contralateral hydronephrosis [3]. In our case, the patient presented with progressive abdominal swelling of two years, with associated dull aching sensation and discomfort in the flank area, which is consistent with findings in other literatures.

The first line imaging modality used was ultrasonography as a standard, and the typical finding includes hydronephrosis with a thinned out renal parenchyma. Other imaging modalities were needed to confirm the extension [5, 6]. In addition to accurately diagnosing hydronephrosis, CT and MRI are also used to exclude other causes of intra-abdominal cysts in literature [3]. We had a CT scan done without contrast which confirmed a left hydronephrosis with loss of renal parenchyma. Generally, factors that guide the management of giant hydronephrosis include the following: patient hemodynamic status, presence of functioning kidney, and associated comorbidities such as cardiac illness that can increase surgical morbidity and mortality [1–3]. Children and infants who are diagnosed with these conditions are treated with pyeloplasty which is a rare scenario in adults because of late presentation.

In a patient with a nonfunctioning kidney with loss of renal parenchyma, the recommended treatment is a simple nephrectomy because of the anticipated complication [3]. Percutaneous drainage is an alternative management option in patients with poor clinical parameters. In our case, CT scan revealed a thinned out left renal parenchyma and displaced intra-abdominal organ due to compression by the giant hydronephrosis. Considering the overall clinical picture, performing a nephrectomy was an appropriate decision. Further surgical exploration revealed a narrow left ureter confirming the diagnosis of UPJ obstruction. The patient was followed up for four months postoperatively and had a smooth postoperative course and has resumed her normal activities.

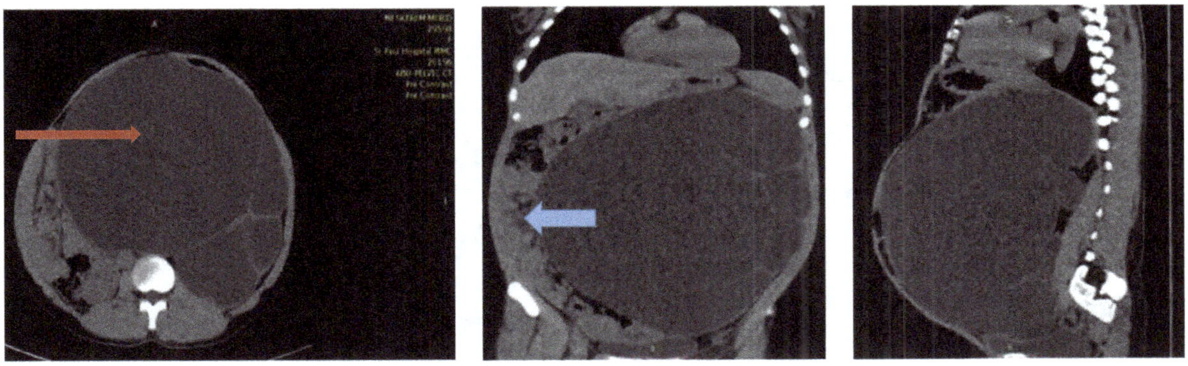

(a) (b) (c)

FIGURE 2: Noncontrast CT scan of the abdomen shows (a) axial view, (b) coronal view, and (c) sagittal view. It shows 20 cm long, 16 cm width cystic swelling (red arrow) with significant mass effect to the surrounding bowel loop (blue arrow).

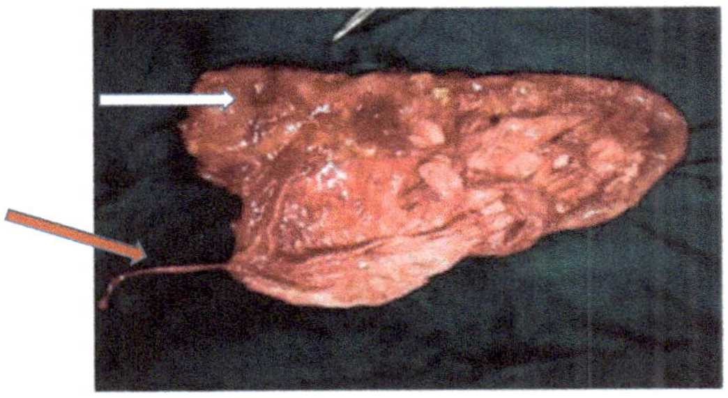

FIGURE 3: Resected sac (white arrow) with a narrowed left ureter and ureteropelvic junction (red arrow).

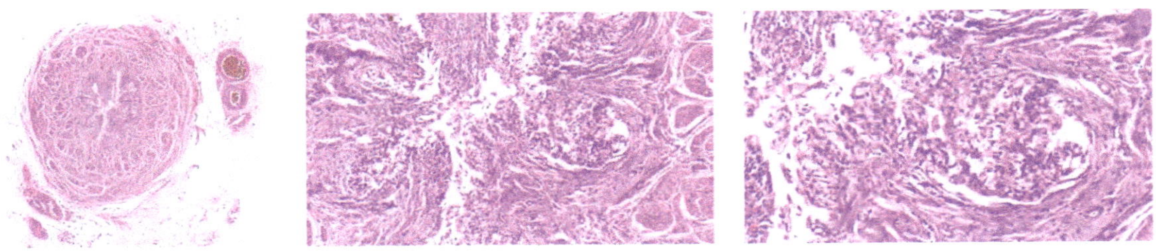

(a) (b) (c)

FIGURE 4: Histopathologic section shows an unremarkable ureteral wall with no increased wall thickness, fibrosis, or inflammation.

4. Conclusion

Giant hydronephrosis secondary to ureteropelvic junction obstruction needs to be considered in adults presenting with huge intra-abdominal cystic mass, especially if they have long-standing pain and progressive abdominal swelling. Imaging studies like CT or MRI are sufficient for diagnosing origin of the mass, but malignancy must be ruled by a histopathologic examination. Treatment of giant hydronephrosis depends on the age, underlying cause, patient clinical condition, and presence or absence of renal parenchyma.

Ethical Approval

Ethical clearance was obtained from the Institutional Research and Ethics Review Committee (IRB) of SPHMMC for the publication of the case report.

Consent

Informed and written consent was taken from the patient to publish the case report.

Authors' Contributions

MSD was involved in patient care, conceived the study, and drafted the manuscript. SMH was involved in inpatient care and critically revised the manuscript. THT is responsible for the critical revision of the manuscript and overall supervision of the manuscript. All authors have read and approved the manuscript.

Acknowledgments

We thank our patient for her consent in allowing us to share her experience. We also thank St. Paul's Hospital Millennium Medical College, Department of Surgery, Urology Unit, Addis Ababa, Ethiopia.

References

[1] Q. F. Wang, G. Zeng, L. Zhong et al., "Giant hydronephrosis due to ureteropelvic junction obstruction: a rare case report, and a review of the literature," *Molecular and Clinical Oncology.*, vol. 5, no. 1, pp. 19–22, 2016.

[2] M. F. Tazi, O. Riyach, Y. Ahallal et al., "Giant urinary bladder and bilateral giant hydronephrosis due to bladder neck obstruction: one case report and literature review," *Case Reports in Urology*, vol. 2012, 3 pages, 2012.

[3] E. Mediavilla, R. Ballestero, M. A. Correas, and J. L. Gutierrez, "About a case report of giant hydronephrosis," *Case Reports in Urology*, vol. 2013, 3 pages, 2013.

[4] C. C. Wu and G. H. Sun, "Giant hydronephrosis," *Mayo Clinic Proceedings*, vol. 84, no. 11, p. 954, 2009.

[5] Y. Golcuk, M. Ozsarac, E. Eseroglu, and M. B. Yuksel, "Giant hydronephrosis," *Western Journal of Emergency Medicine*, vol. 15, no. 4, p. 356, 2014.

[6] S. Mujagić, M. Šahinpašić, H. Huseinagić, M. Bazardžanović, and Z. Karasalihović, "Giant hydronephrosis: case report and review of literature," *Acta Medica Academica*, vol. 39, no. 1, pp. 76–79, 2010.

40

Rapidly Progressive Bladder Cancer Diagnosed because of Spontaneous Bladder Rupture

Hiroki Hagimoto,[1] Takeshi Sano,[1] Soki Kashima,[1] Takayuki Yoshino,[1] Takayuki Goto,[1] Atsuro Sawada,[1] Shusuke Akamatsu,[1] Toshinari Yamasaki,[1] Masakazu Fujimoto,[2] Yoichiro Kajita,[3] Takashi Kobayashi,[1] and Osamu Ogawa[1]

[1]*The Department of Urology, Kyoto University Hospital, Japan*
[2]*The Department of Diagnostic Pathology, Kyoto University Hospital, Japan*
[3]*Kajita Urological Clinic, Japan*

Correspondence should be addressed to Takashi Kobayashi; selecao@kuhp.kyoto-u.ac.jp

Academic Editor: Fumitaka Koga

Background. Spontaneous bladder rupture (SBR) is very rare and can be associated with advanced bladder cancer. Because of its rarity, the optimal management of bladder cancer with SBR has not been established. Herein, we report a case of SBR due to locally advanced bladder cancer, which rapidly invaded the ileum and caused peritoneal dissemination. *Case Presentation.* An 86-year-old man presented with sudden-onset lower abdominal pain and distension. The patient was diagnosed with bladder perforation and bladder tumor on contrast-enhanced computed tomography (CECT). Transurethral resection of the bladder tumor revealed an invasive urothelial carcinoma with squamous differentiation. Although radical cystectomy with lymph node dissection was planned, preoperative CECT and magnetic resonance imaging revealed enlargement of the bilateral iliac regional lymph nodes, multiple peritoneal nodules, and invasion of the bladder tumor to the ileocecum. Therefore, cystectomy and resection of ileocecum with palliative intent and bilateral cutaneous ureterostomy were performed. However, the patient's general condition rapidly worsened after surgery, and he died 74 days after the initial diagnosis. *Conclusions.* We encountered a case of SBR accompanied by bladder cancer with extremely rapid progression, which suggested the importance of short-interval repeat imaging examinations. Emergency surgery should be considered when bladder cancer is suspected in patients with SBR so as not to miss the window period of a possible cure.

1. Introduction

Spontaneous bladder rupture (SBR) is very rare and is associated with trauma, pelvic irradiation, urinary retention, chronic bladder infection, malignancy, and diverticulitis [1]. It has a mortality rate of approximately 50%, although this has declined in recent years owing to increased awareness, better imaging modalities, and better management of complications [1, 2]. Bladder cancer associated with spontaneous SBR is commonly advanced at the time of diagnosis, and the prognosis is often less than 1 year [2]. Because of its rarity, the optimal management of bladder cancer with SBR has not been established. In addition, there have been no reports showing its rapid progression using serial imaging findings. Herein, we report a case of SBR due to locally advanced bladder cancer that rapidly invaded the ileum and caused peritoneal dissemination. We performed multiple imaging to confirm the rapid growth of the tumor in a short period of time (2-4 weeks).

2. Case Presentation

An 86-year-old man was hospitalized in December 2019 with a chief complaint of sudden-onset severe lower abdominal pain. He had a medical history of appendicitis and no family history of notable medical conditions. Abdominal computed tomography (CT) revealed a thickening with calcification on the posterior wall of the bladder adjacent to the

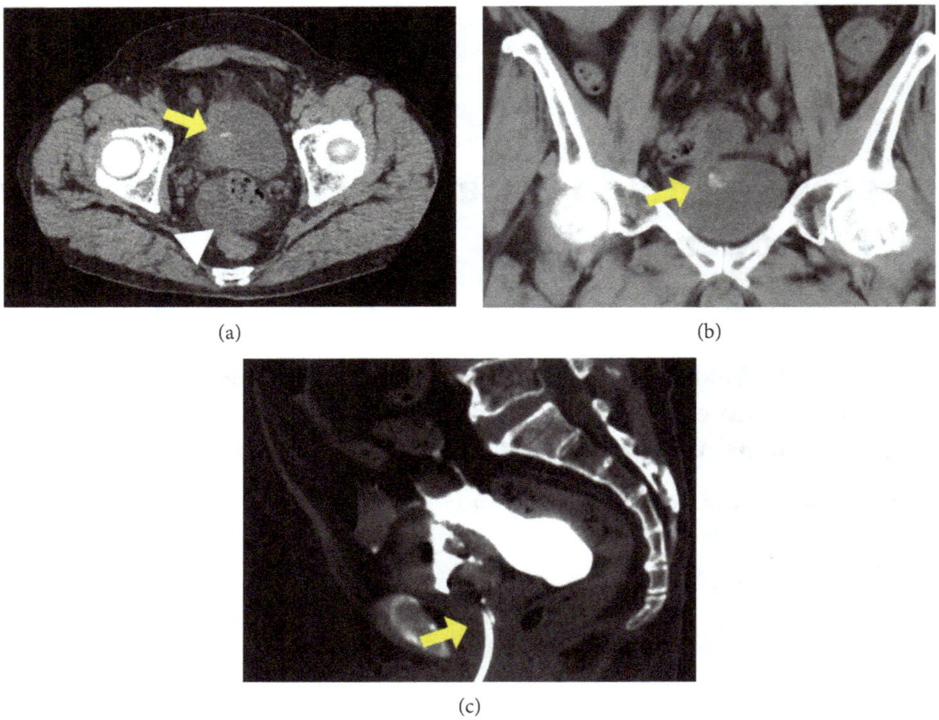

Figure 1: (a) An axial plain abdominal computed tomography (CT) scan showed bladder wall thickening with calcification (arrow) and ascites in the rectovesical pouch (white arrowhead). (b) A coronal plain abdominal CT scan showed bladder wall thickening adjacent to the ileum (arrow). (c) A sagittal CT scan after intravesical injection of contrast medium via a urethral catheter (arrow) showed leakage of contrast medium into the abdominal cavity.

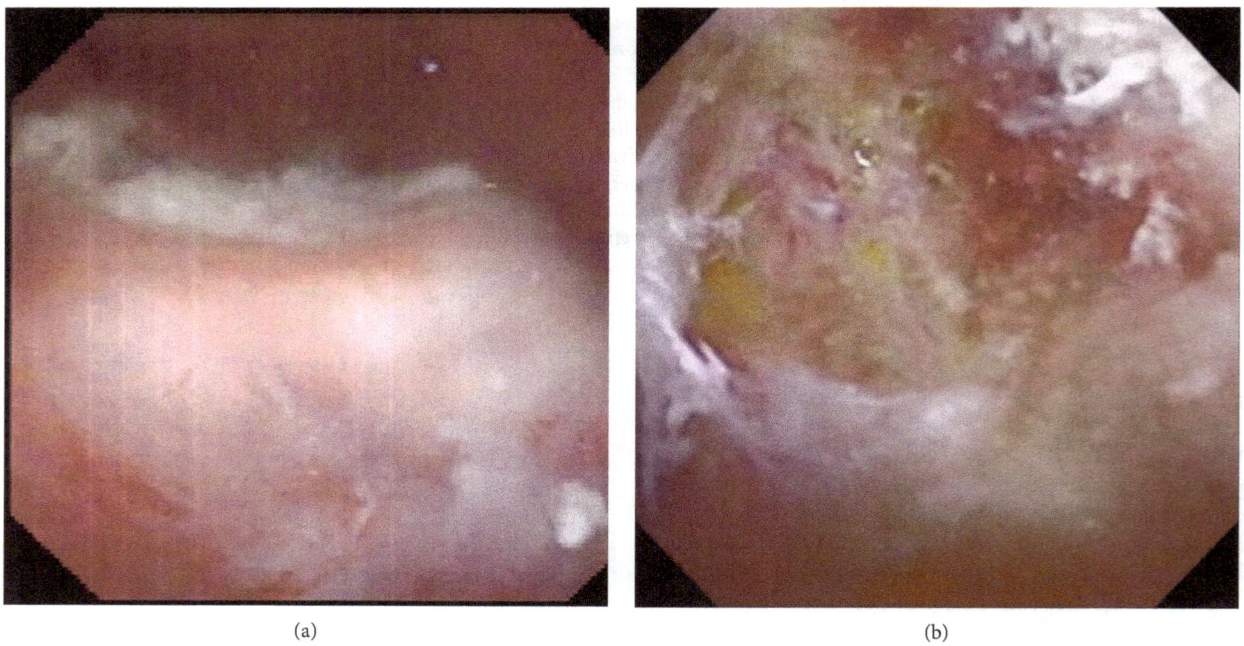

Figure 2: (a) Intravesical endoscopic imaging revealed an elevated nodule with whitish tissue and calcification on the surface. (b) Removal of the calcification exposed fat droplets on the bottom of the cavity.

ileum along with ascites in the rectovesical pouch, suggesting a spontaneous bladder perforation into the peritoneal cavity potentially associated with a bladder tumor (Figures 1(a) and 1(b)). Contrast-enhanced CT (CECT) confirmed bladder perforation in the patient (Figure 1(c)). Laboratory test results, including routine blood chemistry and complete

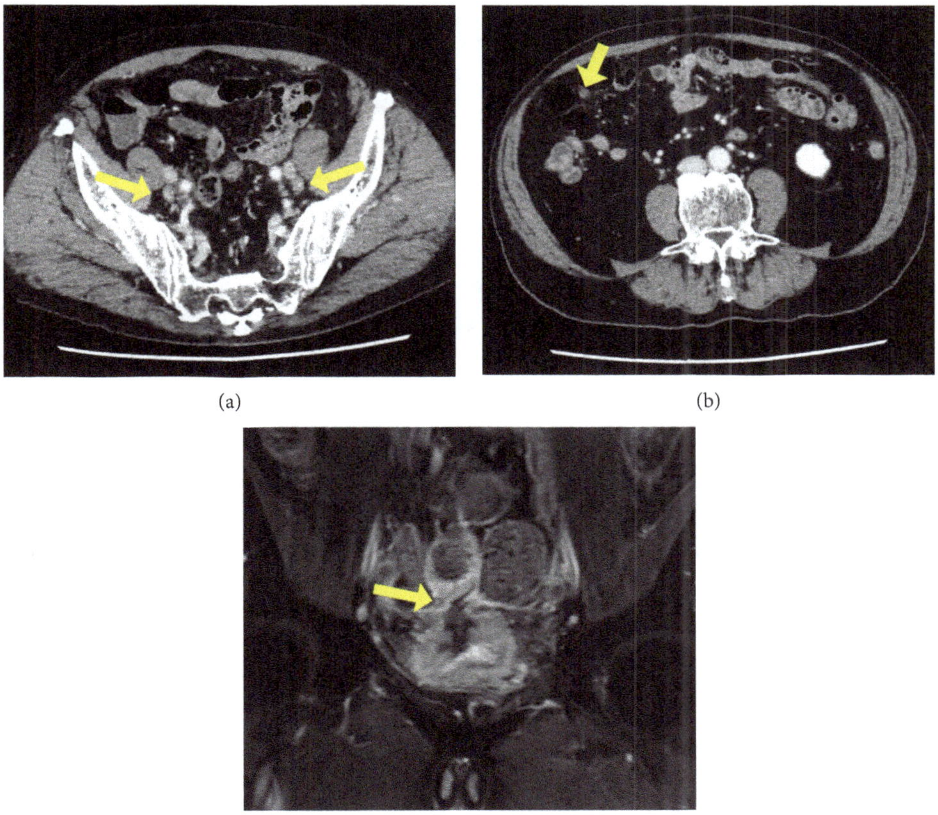

(a) (b) (c)

Figure 3: A contrast-enhanced abdominal computed tomography (CT) scan for staging showed bilateral iliac regional lymph node enlargement (a, arrow) and a small nodule in the peritoneum (b, arrow). (c) A T1-weighted TSE magnetic resonance imaging scan for preoperative local evaluation showed that the soft-tissue mass on the bladder wall extended to the small intestine (arrow), suggesting local invasion.

blood count, and tumor markers (AFP, CEA, CA19-9, and PSA) were not remarkable other than slight increases in SCC (2.0 ng/mL) and NSE (13.47 ng/mL). A urine test indicated slight microscopic hematuria and pyuria. Urine cytology was positive, suggesting high-grade urothelial carcinoma (UC). Microscopic hematuria was not observed during regular check-ups of benign prostatic hyperplasia before the onset of SBR.

Transurethral resection of the bladder tumor was performed on the 2nd day of hospitalization, and an elevated lesion with a whitish surface and calcification was observed at the posterior wall of the bladder. Removal of the calcification revealed a cavity with fat droplets at the bottom of the lesion, which was likely the perforation site (Figure 2). The pathological diagnosis of the elevated lesion was high-grade UC with squamous differentiation. Intravenous administration of fluid and antibiotics was performed for the treatment of intraperitoneal infection and impaired general condition. CT on the 11th day of hospitalization with the intent of staging showed bilateral iliac regional lymph node enlargement and scattered small nodules in the peritoneum (Figures 3(a) and 3(b)). However, it was unclear whether this was peritoneal dissemination or a secondary finding from peritonitis. Magnetic resonance imaging (MRI) performed for preoperative local evaluation on the 24th day of hospitalization showed a slight enlargement of the bilateral iliac regional lymph nodes, small peritoneal nodules suspicious for peritoneal dissemination, and a new soft-tissue mass on the bladder wall extending to the small intestine suspicious for invasion (Figure 3(c)).

Under the clinical diagnosis of cT4bN1M1b bladder cancer, open cystectomy, partial resection of the ileum, sampling of the peritoneal nodules, and bilateral cutaneous ureterostomy were performed on the 26th day of hospitalization, mainly for palliative purposes. A lower abdominal midline incision was made, and an enlarged obturator lymph node and two nodules in the greater omentum were removed for intraoperative definitive pathological diagnosis, which indicated metastatic UC. The posterior wall of the bladder strongly adhered to the ileum, suggesting infiltration of the bladder tumor, and en bloc resection of the bladder and a segment of the infiltrated ileum was performed. The specimen was a raised lesion on the posterior wall of the bladder with an irregular surface with necrotic tissue and hemorrhage (Figure 4(a)). The lesion appeared to extend to the serosa and had invaded the terminal ileum

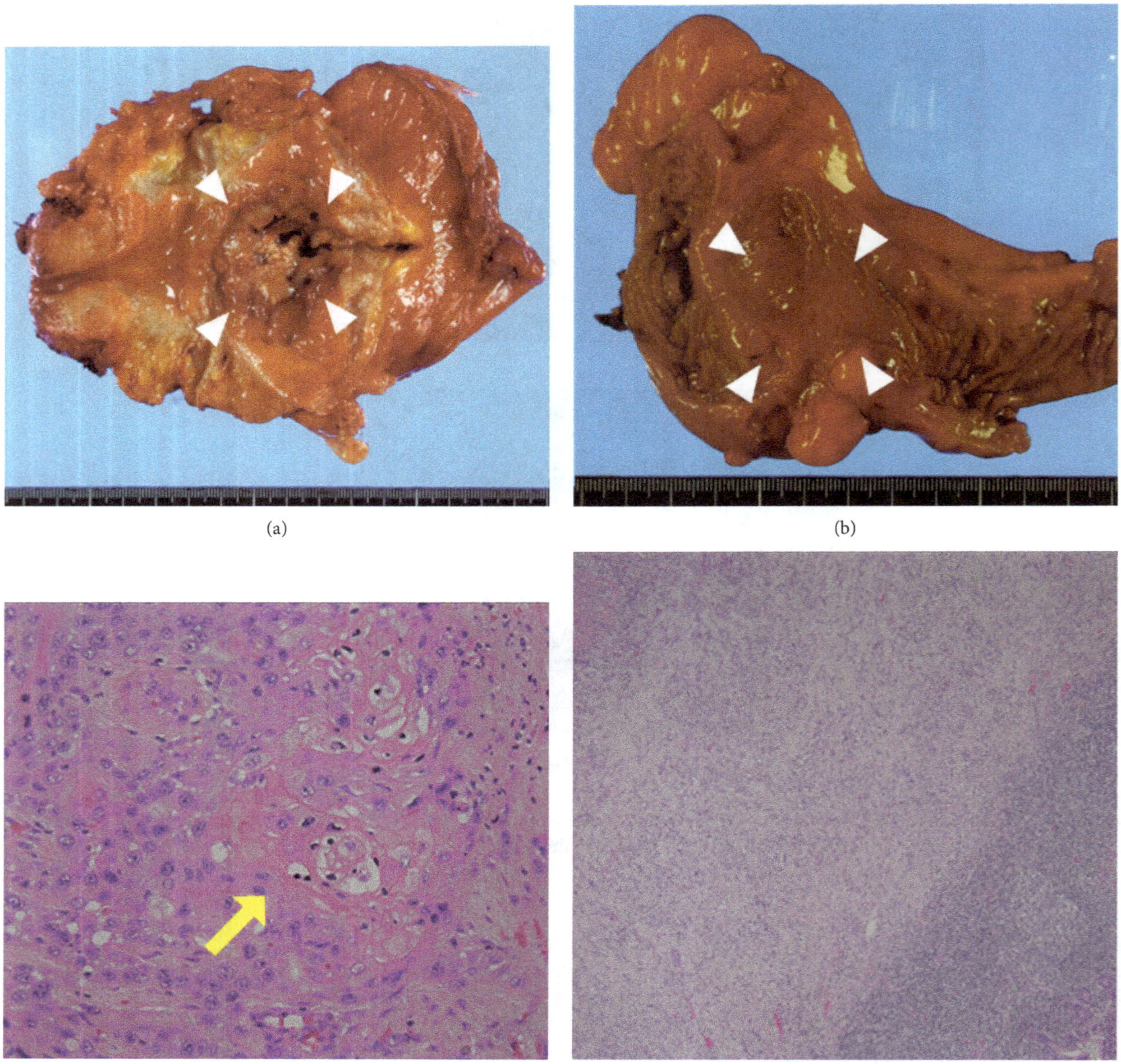

(a) (b) (c) (d)

FIGURE 4: (a) A macroscopic image of the resected bladder. The bladder tumor was a raised lesion with an irregular surface, necrotic tissue, and hemorrhage (white arrowheads). (b) A macroscopic image of the lumen of the ileum separated from the bladder. There were submucosal lesions (white arrowheads), suggesting a submucosal invasion of the bladder cancer at the terminal ileum. (c) The bladder tumor was infiltrating high-grade urothelial carcinoma with partial keratinization (arrow, hematoxylin & eosin, ×200). (d) The tumor in the terminal ileum had infiltrated the submucosal layer under the normal glandular structures (hematoxylin & eosin, ×40).

(Figure 4(b)). The pathologic diagnosis was high-grade infiltrating UC with squamous differentiation, and the pathological stage was T4bN1M1b (Figures 4(c) and 4(d)).

A CT scan on the 30th day of hospitalization showed enlargement of the left obturator lymph node and rapid growth of multiple peritoneal nodules, some of which had invaded the small intestine (Figure 5). The patient was discharged on the 58th day of hospitalization. Although systemic chemotherapy was planned, his general condition rapidly deteriorated, and he died 74 days after the initial diagnosis.

3. Discussion and Conclusions

SBR due to bladder cancer is very rare [2]. Because SBR itself is a life-threatening event and bladder cancer that causes bladder rupture is generally advanced, very few patients survive for more than a year, and most cases report a survival

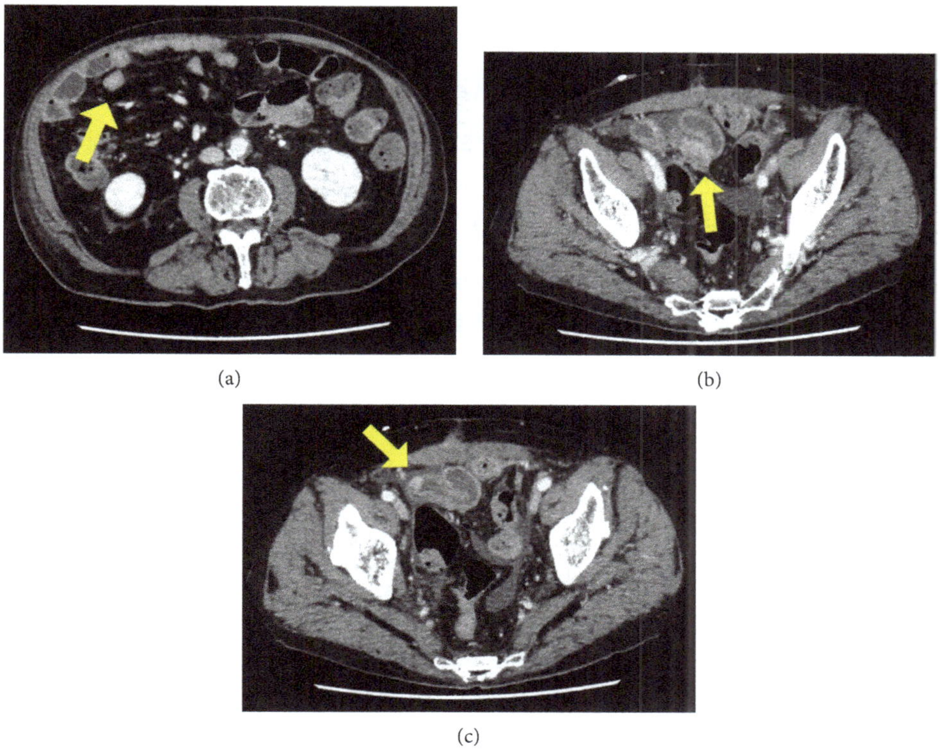

FIGURE 5: A postoperative contrast-enhanced abdominal computed tomography (CT) scan showed enlargement of one of the peritoneal nodules (a, arrow) and the invasion of nodules with edematous lumens to the small intestine (arrows) (b, c).

time after diagnosis from 10 days to several months [3, 4]. To the best of our knowledge, only 16 cases of bladder cancer with SBR have been reported between 2000 and 2022 including the present case (Table 1). All the cases revealed an SBR in the abdominal cavity, inferring that these patients had highly advanced tumors invading the peritoneum around the bladder. Four of these cases reported peritoneal dissemination at the time of diagnosis. Most patients died within a range of a few days to a few months, indicating a poor prognosis of bladder cancer in patients with SBR. Although approximately 90% of bladder cancers are UCs and only 2-5% are squamous cell carcinomas [5], squamous cell carcinomas cause half of bladder rupture cases associated with bladder tumors [3, 4]. In the present case, microscopic hematuria was not observed during regular checkups of benign prostatic hyperplasia before SBR, but mild microscopic hematuria was observed at the onset of SBR, potentially suggesting the invasive nature of the tumor to the stroma without exophytic growth and the difficulty in detecting the tumor with simple clinical testing.

Although surgical repair is generally the first choice for intraperitoneal bladder rupture [6], cystectomy is required if the cause of SBR is bladder cancer. In the present case, a CT scan at the initial diagnosis suggested the existence of bladder cancer. Hence, we performed a transurethral biopsy of the elevated lesion, which revealed high-grade UC with squamous differentiation. The tumor was localized in the bladder at the initial diagnosis. However, invasion to the ileum, lymphadenopathy, and peritoneal masses were observed on CT and MRI before cystectomy. Although bladder perforation during transurethral resection of bladder tumors is associated with an increased risk of intra-abdominal dissemination, it is very rare [7, 8]. In the present case, peritoneal masses suspicious for dissemination developed only a few weeks after the onset of bladder rupture, which suggests the extremely malignant potential of the tumor. The present case is very important because serial imaging examinations in a short period, including CT and MRI, detected the "moment" of the invasion of the bladder tumor to the ileum and revealed the speed of the development and growth of peritoneal masses in cancer-related SBR, which have not been shown previously.

Owing to the recent advancements in imaging modalities, cases in which bladder cancer is diagnosed or suspected based on imaging results before surgical repair of SBR are expected to become more common. However, there is no consensus on the next step after diagnosis. In the present case, we first performed transurethral tissue biopsy followed by cystectomy based on the pathological diagnosis. Although cystectomy was performed 23 days after the biopsy, multiple metastatic tumors were found during surgery. Based on our results, we recommend emergency laparotomy for the surgical repair of SBR. However, it may not be beneficial when the general condition of the patient is already very deteriorated. Additionally, the surgery will be only palliative and may not benefit the survival of the patient. A surgical repair

TABLE 1: Summary of reported cases of bladder cancer with spontaneous bladder rupture.

No.	Year	Author	PMID	Sex	Age	Site of rupture	Peritoneal dissemination	Treatment	Histology	Outcome
1	2001	Goel A	12230278	Male	55	Dome	None	Partial cystectomy	SCC	Alive (at least 6 months)
2	2002	Jayathillake A	12561801	Female	72	Right wall	N/A	Primary closure	SCC	Dead (10 days)
3	2002	Fujiwara A	12491613	Female	65	Dome	Yes	Radical cystectomy	Sarcomatoid carcinoma	Dead (46 days)
4	2006	Shiraishi Y	16541769	Female	71	Posterior wall	Yes	Primary closure	SCC	Dead (2 months)
5	2008	Sawazaki H	19175001	Female	90	Dome	N/A	Primary closure	SCC	Dead (2 months)
6	2009	Ahmed J	19829892	Female	47	N/A	Yes	Radical cystectomy	UC	N/A
7	2010	Lee JH	20428434	Male	75	Left wall	N/A	Palliative care	N/A	Dead (3 months)
8	2012	Stojadinović M	22511430	Male	79	Dome and posterior wall	N/A	Primary closure	Micropapillary carcinoma	Dead (12 months)
9	2013	Sallami S	24227517	Male	54	Left wall	N/A	Radical cystectomy	Sarcomatoid carcinoma	N/A
10	2015	Kivlin D	26195965	Male	72	Posterior wall	N/A	Primary closure	N/A	N/A
11	2015	Kivlin D	26195965	Male	65	Dome	N/A	Primary closure	N/A	Dead (17 days)
12	2016	Oray D	27355091	Male	56	Left wall	N/A	Palliative care	N/A	Dead (1 day)
13	2018	Al Edwan GM	29852423	Male	56	Dome	None	Radical cystectomy	SCC	Dead (7 months)
14	2020	Asano T	33102109	Female	52	Dome	N/A	Radical cystectomy	UC with squamous cell diff.	Dead (10 weeks)
15	2020	Sahnoun W	33294156	Male	63	Posterior wall	N/A	Radical cystectomy	SCC	Dead (62 days)
16	2022	Present case		Male	86	Posterior wall	Yes	Radical cystectomy	UC with squamous cell diff.	Dead (74 days)

PMID: PubMed Unique Identifier; N/A: not applicable; SCC: squamous cell carcinoma; UC: urothelial carcinoma.

should be accompanied by intraoperative pathologic examination of the bladder lesions. In case the lesion is found to be nonmalignant, a simple closure of the bladder perforation should be performed. Contrastingly, if bladder cancer is found, then the patient should undergo immediate palliative cystectomy and extensive peritoneal lavage. Considering the poor survival outcome of bladder cancer with SBR, adjuvant chemotherapy may also be considered for the survival benefit, provided the patient has a good general condition postsurgery.

In conclusion, we encountered a case of SBR accompanied by bladder cancer that showed extremely rapid progression, which suggested the importance of short-interval repeat imaging examinations, although it was localized to the bladder at the initial diagnosis. Emergency surgery should be considered when bladder cancer is suspected in a patient with SBR to avoid missing the window period of a potential cure.

Abbreviations

SBR: Spontaneous bladder rupture
CECT: Contrast-enhanced computed tomography
CT: Computed tomography
MRI: Magnetic resonance imaging
UC: Urothelial carcinoma.

Ethical Approval

The study complied with the Declaration of Helsinki guidelines and was approved by the Institutional Ethics Committee of Kyoto University Hospital.

Consent

Written informed consent was obtained from all study participants. Written informed consent was obtained from the patient's next of kin for publication of this case report and any accompanying images. A copy of the written consent is available for review by the Editor-in-Chief of this journal.

Authors' Contributions

HH and TS performed manuscript writing; HH, TS, YK, and TK performed data collection; HH, TS, SK, TY, TG, AS, SA, TY, MF, TK, and OO performed data interpretation; HH, TS, SK, TY, TG, AS, SA, TY, YK, and OO performed patient treatment; HH, TS, SK, TY, TG, AS, SA, TY, MF, YK, TK, and OO performed manuscript revision. All authors read and approved the final manuscript.

References

[1] M. M. Stojadinović, S. L. Mitrović, and D. R. Milovanović, "Micropapillary carcinoma of the bladder presented with spontaneous intraperitoneal bladder rupture," *Canadian Urological Association Journal*, vol. 6, no. 2, pp. E42–E45, 2012.

[2] D. R. Basavaraj, K. K. Zachariah, and J. G. Feggetter, "Acute abdomen–remember spontaneous perforation of the urinary bladder," *Journal of the Royal College of Surgeons of Edinburgh*, vol. 46, no. 5, pp. 316-317, 2001.

[3] J. Ahmed, I. H. Mallick, and S. M. Ahmad, "Rupture of urinary bladder: a case report and review of literature," *Cases Journal*, vol. 2, no. 1, article 7004, 2009.

[4] Y. Shiraishi, S. Moroi, H. Negoro, H. Iwamura, H. Oka, and M. Kawakita, "Squamous cell carcinoma of the bladder presenting with bladder rupture: a case report," *Hinyokika Kiyo*, vol. 52, no. 2, pp. 139–141, 2006.

[5] H. Abol-Enein, B. R. Kava, and A. J. Carmack, "Nonurothelial cancer of the bladder," *Urology*, vol. 69, no. 1, pp. 93–104, 2007.

[6] Y. Mahat, J. Y. Leong, and P. H. Chung, "A contemporary review of adult bladder trauma," *Journal of Injury and Violence Research*, vol. 11, no. 2, pp. 101–106, 2019.

[7] J. H. Kim and W. J. Yang, "Delayed spontaneous perforation of urinary bladder with intraperitoneal seeding following radical transurethral resection of invasive urothelial cancer: a case report," *BMC Research Notes*, vol. 7, no. 1, p. 167, 2014.

[8] H. C. Lim, T. L. Khong, T. A. Ong, A. C. Roslani, and C. W. Ang, "Case report: a rare case of extravesical, extraperitoneal metastasis after transurethral resection of urothelial carcinoma," *Urology Case Reports*, vol. 29, article 101017, 2020.

41

Unusual Bladder Metastasis from a Primary Gastric Carcinoma: Two Case Reports and Review of Literature

Mohamed Ali Nouioui[1] **Ahmed Saadi,**[1] **Marouene Chakroun,**[1] **Amine Oueslati,**[1] **Meriem Ksentini,**[2] **Abderrazak Bouzouita,**[1] **Amine Derouiche,**[1] **Mohamed Riadh Ben Slama,**[1] **Soumaya Rammeh,**[2] **Haroun Ayed,**[1] **and Mohamed Chebil**[1]

[1]*Department of Urology, Charles Nicolle Hospital of Tunis, University of Tunis El Manar, Tunisia*
[2]*Department of Pathology, Charles Nicolle Hospital of Tunis, University of Tunis El Manar, Tunisia*

Correspondence should be addressed to Mohamed Ali Nouioui; mednouiouimed@gmail.com

Academic Editor: Apul Goel

Primary bladder cancer is a frequent malignancy in the urology field, whereas secondary bladder neoplasms from a distant organ are extremely rare. This paper aims to report two rare cases of a secondary tumor of the urinary bladder from a primary gastric tumor and to perform a literature review of similar reported cases in order to better characterize its clinicopathological features and diagnosis in effort to shed light on this rare condition. The final diagnosis of secondary adenocarcinoma was made histologically after transurethral biopsy or resection of the bladder lesion. In one case, the bladder metastasis was a synchronous metastasis, and in the second case, it occurred under chemotherapy five months after initial diagnosis with gastric adenocarcinoma. Secondary adenocarcinoma of the bladder is extremely rare but should be considered when evaluating a bladder lesion in a patient treated for gastric cancer or presenting with gastric symptoms.

1. Introduction

Primary bladder cancer is a frequent malignancy in the urological field whereas secondary bladder tumor from distant primary foci is considered an extremely rare condition accounting for 2% from total vesical tumors [1].

Histologically, 54% of those secondary neoplasms of the bladder are adenocarcinomas of which 4.3% are originated from a primary gastric adenocarcinoma [2].

Here, we present two cases of metastatic bladder tumor from a primary gastric adenocarcinoma and a literature review of similar case reports.

2. Case Presentation

2.1. Case 1. A 72-year-old male patient with a history of smoking and no occupational exposure to urothelial carcinogens, was recently diagnosed with a poorly differentiating signet ring cell (SRC) carcinoma of the stomach based on a histological examination of endoscopic biopsy material taken from a suspicious infiltrating gastric mass.

Other than main gastric complaints, he complained of lower urinary tract storage symptoms such as frequency, nocturia, and urgency, but no haematuria was reported.

A CT scan of the abdomen and the pelvis was performed showing the malignant tumoral mass in the pylorus with peritoneal involvement and ascites associated to a diffuse thickening of the bladder wall with bilateral hydronephrosis (Figure 1).

Physical pelvic examination was normal.

Cystoscopy was performed, revealing an extensive bullous oedema of the bladder mucosa with a grape-like aspect with involvement of both the ureteric orifices initially not visualized, obscured by the lesion (Figure 2).

Transurethral biopsy of the lesion was conducted with liberation of the ureteric orifices.

Histopathological evaluation of the bladder biopsy revealed multiple signet ring cells in the lamina propria with

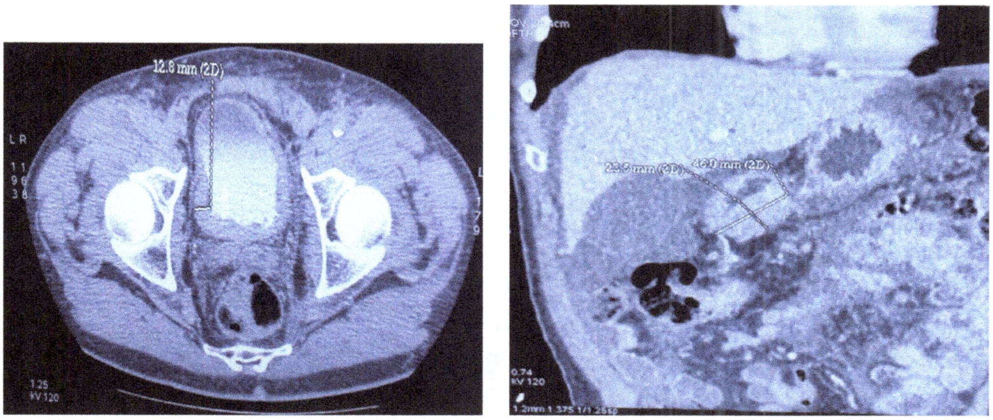

(a) (b)

Figure 1: (a) CT scan showing diffuse irregular thickening of the bladder wall. (b) CT scan showing a neoplastic gastric mass.

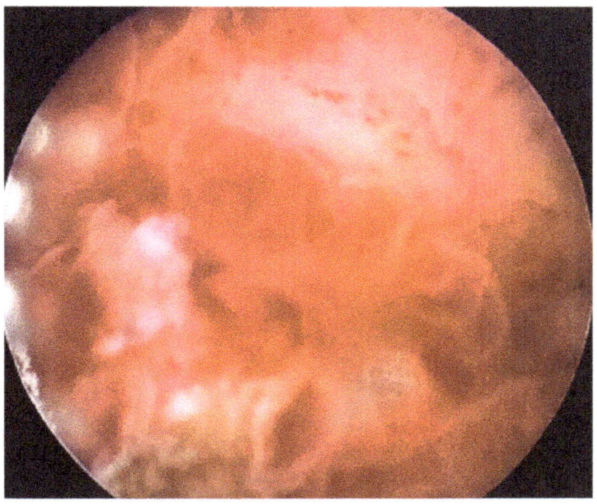

Figure 2: Macroscopic aspect of a bullous lesion of the bladder with a grape-like aspect.

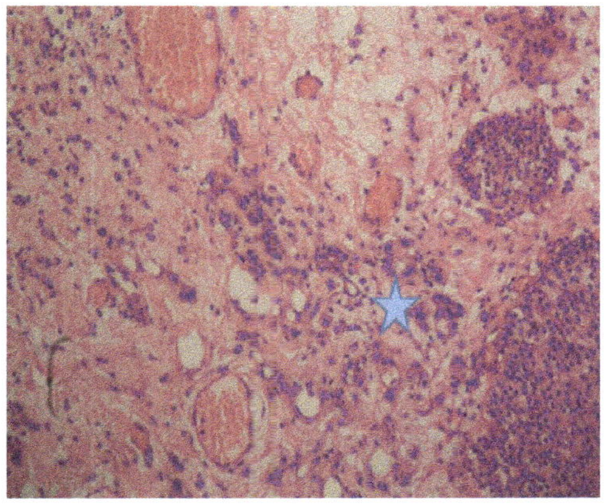

Figure 3: Infiltration of the subepithelium of the bladder with a small aggregates of neoplastic cells (H&E, ×200).

overlying transitional cell epithelium with no sign of urothelial carcinoma (Figure 3).

Based on histological findings and previous diagnosis of poorly differentiated gastric carcinoma, a diagnosis of synchronous bladder metastasis from primary gastric SRC carcinoma was made.

2.2. Case 2. A nonsmoker 36-year-old male with no occupational exposure to urothelial carcinogens, initially diagnosed five months ago with gastric signet ring cell adenocarcinoma metastatic to the bone with peritoneal involvement, initially treated with palliative chemotherapy, was referred to our urology department after he developed gross intermittent haematuria.

A CT scan of the abdomen and the pelvis detected two suspicious masses in the bladder wall, respectively, measuring 6 and 8 mm associated with homolateral hydronephrosis.

Because of our patient's history of primary gastric carcinoma, a secondary location of the bladder was suggested.

A cystoscopy showed two solid protuberant nodular lesions one in the trigone and the other in the right lateral bladder wall completely resected.

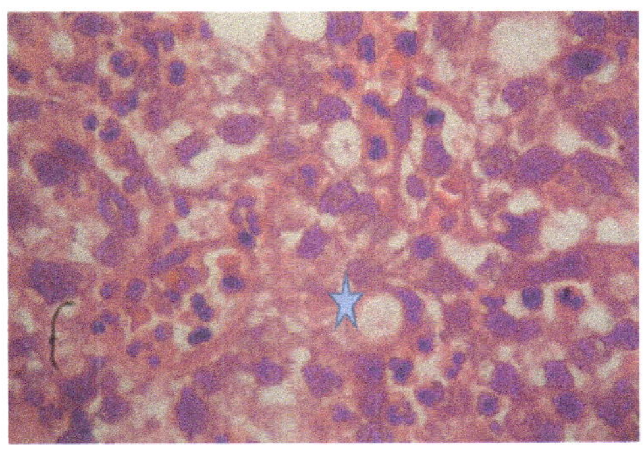

Figure 4: Signet-ring cells in the poorly differentiated adenocarcinoma (H&E, ×400).

After pathological examination of the surgical specimen, the diagnosis of metastatic poorly differentiated adenocarcinoma of the bladder from a gastric primary cancer was reached (Figure 4).

Both patients were then referred to oncology for a second-line chemotherapy.

Table 1: Review of urinary bladder metastasis from a primary gastric tumor reported in English language literature.

Author and year	Age	Gender	Primary gastric tumor stage	Clinical presentation	Haematuria	Interval between primary tumor and metastasis	Imaging findings	Presence of hydronephrosis	Other metastasis	Endoscopic findings	Management of bladder metastasis	Follow-up
Saba et al. 1997 [7]	58	M	SRC AC	Nil	Yes	7 years HC	Polypoid lesion in the bladder posterior wall	No	Retroperitoneal adenopathy	Large broad-based lesion at the posterior wall, with mucinous strands	Nil	Deceased days after diagnosis
Kim et al. 2000 [4]	60	M	AC	Sense of residual urine dysuria, non-tender supra-pubic mass	Microscopic	One year HC	Focal thickening of the bladder anterior wall	No	Nil	NR	TUR	NR
Kim et al. 2000 [4]	57	F	SRC AC	Frequency, dysuria	Microscopic	Fifteen months HC	Diffuse bladder wall thickening	No	Nil	Bullous oedema of the bladder mucosa	TUR	NR
Kim et al. 2000 [4]	42	M	SRC AC	Dysuria	Microscopic	Two years HC	Diffuse thickening of the bladder wall	No	Nil	Oedematous mucosa of the bladder with a small ulcer	Total cystectomy	NR
Antunes et al. 2004 [8]	63	F	AC	Left lumbar pain, dysuria low abdominal pain	Nil	One year and nine months	Thickened wall of the bladder	Bilateral	Ascites	Extensive vegetative lesion in the bladder	TUR	Stable condition 8 months after diagnosis
Matsuhashi et al. 2005 [9]	90	F	Tubular AC	Nausea, dysphagia	Ye	Synchronous metastasis	Thickening of the bladder wall with diverticulum enhance effect	No	Nil	Lesion in the bladder diverticulum	NIL	Deceased three months after diagnosis
Farhat et al. 2007 [10]	58	M	AC	Nil	Yes	Fifteen months HC	2 cm mass involving the trigone and the left lateral bladder wall	No	Nil	NR	TUR	NR

Table 1: Continued.

Author and year	Age	Gender	Primary gastric tumor stage	Clinical presentation	Haematuria	Interval between primary tumor and metastasis	Imaging findings	Presence of hydronephrosis	Other metastasis	Endoscopic findings	Management of bladder metastasis	Follow-up
Sharma et al. 2011 [6]	30	M	SRC AC	Weight loss	Yes	Two years HC	Localized thickening of the bladder wall	No	Nil	Multiple grape-like lesions on the dome and left bladder	TUR adjuvant chemotherapy	Alive five months after chemo
Andras et al. 2013 [11]	59	M	Tubular AC	Low abdominal pain	Nil	Ten years HC	2 × 4 cm tumor-like mass on the left posterior bladder wall	No	Nil	Mucosal hyperaemia lesion close to the ureteric orifice	TUR adjuvant chemotherapy	Colic recurrence one year after chemo
Kalra et al. 2015 [12]	60	M	SRC AC	Low urinary tract storage symptoms	Microscopic	Synchronous metastasis	Diffusely thickened bladder wall with small capacity bladder	Bilateral	Nil	Smooth wall diffusely erythematous small capacity bladder	TUR nephrostomy diversion Palliative chemotherapy	
Okutur et al. 2015 [13]	48	M	SRC AC	Abdominal pain, weight loss tenderness of hypogastric region	Yes	Synchronous metastasis	Diffuse thickening of the bladder wall	Bilateral	Peritoneum	Diffuse papillary nodular lesion	Transurethral biopsy Palliative chemotherapy	Alive 5 months after chemotherapy
Lodh et al. 2016 [14]	53	M	Tubular AC	Abdominal fullness weight loss	Yes	Synchronous metastasis	Right posterior lateral urinary bladder broad base mass	No	Nil	Protuberant mass	TUR adjuvant chemotherapy	Stable three month later
Vigliar et al. 2013 [15]	38	M	SRC AC	Abdominal pain	Yes	Seven months HC	NR	Unilateral	Ascites	NR	NIL	Deceased nine months after diagnosis
Seow-En et al. 2015 [16]	75	M	SRC AC	Frequency	Nil	Twenty years HC	Bladder wall thickening	Bilateral	Lymphadenopathy rectum	Mucosal tumor growth	Chemotherapy	Alive four months since diagnosis
Khoury et al. 2019 [17]	75	M	SRC AC	Appetite loss, lumbar pain	Nil	Two years	Diffuse thickening of bladder wall	Bilateral	NIL	Extensive vegetative lesion	NR	NR

Table 1: Continued.

Author and year	Age	Gender	Primary gastric tumor stage	Clinical presentation	Haematuria	Interval between primary tumor and metastasis	Imaging findings	Presence of hydronephrosis	Other metastasis	Endoscopic findings	Management of bladder metastasis	Follow-up
Ota et al. 1999 [18]	43	M	AC	Sense of residual urine, incontinence	Nil	Two years HC	Diffuse thickening of bladder wall	Bilateral	Nil	NR	Chemotherapy	Alive twelve months after chemotherapy

SRC: signet ring cell; AC: adenocarcinoma; TUR: transurethral resection; HC: heterochronous; NR: not reported.

3. Discussion

Bladder cancer (BC) is ranked the second most common genitourinary malignancy with an estimated 81000 new cases in the USA alone per year.

However, secondary neoplasms of the urinary bladder are rarely encountered in urology, accounting for only 2% of total vesical tumors according to the 2016 WHO classification [1].

Adenocarcinomas are the most frequent histological subtypes of such metastatic tumors [2].

Metastatic spread generally occurs by haematogenous or lymphogenous paths from distant primary foci.

Even intraperitoneal dissemination should be considered.

Bates et al. found that the most common sites of origin of cancer metastatic to the urinary bladder were the stomach yielding a figure of 4.3% of all secondary bladder neoplasms in a series of 282 cases [2].

After analysing 1000 consecutive postmortem cases of epithelial malignancies, Abrams' study yielded the same finding that gastric adenocarcinomas metastasize to the bladder more often than any other epithelial neoplasms [3].

We performed a review of PubMed for full-text peer-reviewed similar case reports published in English language since 1997.

We should point out that the majority of case reports occurred in Japan due to the high incidence of gastric adenocarcinoma there but were not included in this review due to the non-availability in English language.

15 case reports including our case report, involving 18 patients with secondary bladder tumor from primary gastric neoplasm, were included and analysed.

The features of these cases were summarised in Table 1.

The age range was 30-90, median of 60 years old.

Metastasis to the urinary bladder can be synchronous or can occur after the primary gastric tumor with an average of six years in our review.

Clinical urologic manifestations were absent in the majority of patients in whom bladder involvement was discovered postmortem [4]. However, in case one, our patient presented with lower urinary tract storage symptoms, and in case two, macroscopic haematuria was the chief complaint.

In our review, haematuria was the only consistent urinary symptom occurring in twelve of the total 18 patients.

Radiographic appearance of secondary bladder tumors may consist of focal or diffuse thickening of the bladder wall associated or not with hydronephrosis [5].

Distinction between metastatic bladder lesion and primary tumor may be hard from an imaging viewpoint which makes cystoscopy and histological examination the gold standard in making the diagnosis.

The metastatic bladder tumor can be described macroscopically as diffuse or protuberant similar to typical transitional cell carcinoma [6].

Most of the cases are protuberant in our review.

The main subsites of the secondary tumors were summarized in Table 2.

Table 2: Anatomical localization of secondary tumor deposits within the urinary bladder of the reviewed cases.

Neck	Trigone	Anterior/lateral/posterior	Fundus	Diffuse
0	3	7	0	4

Of the 12 cases for which histology subtype was available, three were tubular type adenocarcinoma, and nine were signet ring cell type, whereas in Bates et al. series, out of the 10 cases, only three were signet ring cell [2].

Without clinical history of primary malignancy elsewhere, it is often challenging to distinguish between metastatic adenocarcinoma from primary adenocarcinoma, since primary bladder adenocarcinomas have a better prognosis following cystectomy [2], making immunohistochemistry necessary in that case .

Like other metastatic tumors, secondary bladder neoplasms have a variable chemosensitivity and radiosensitivity that correlates with the primary tumor [2].

Curative intention is not possible due to the metastatic characteristic of the disease and adjuvant chemotherapy is indicated, though with unsatisfactory results [4].

4. Conclusion

Despite being a rare disease, secondary bladder neoplasm should be considered when assessing a bladder lesion whether it occurs simultaneously or years after initial diagnosis of primary cancer.

Knowledge of its clinical and radiological characteristics is important for clinicians for correct diagnosis and proper therapeutic conduct.

References

[1] P. A. Humphrey, H. Moch, A. L. Cubilla, T. M. Ulbright, and V. E. Reuter, "The 2016 WHO classification of tumours of the urinary system and male genital organs-part B: prostate and bladder tumours," *European Urology*, vol. 70, no. 1, pp. 106–119, 2016.

[2] A. W. Bates and S. I. Baithun, "Secondary neoplasms of the bladder are histological mimics of nontransitional cell primary tumours: clinicopathological and histological features of 282 cases," *Histopathology*, vol. 36, no. 1, pp. 32–40, 2000.

[3] H. L. Abrams, R. Spiro, and N. Goldstein, "Metastases in carcinoma; analysis of 1000 autopsied cases," *Cancer*, vol. 3, no. 1, pp. 74–85, 1950.

[4] H.-C. Kim, S. H. Kim, S.-I. Hwang, H. J. Lee, and J. K. Han, "Isolated bladder metastases from stomach cancer: CT demonstration," *Abdominal Imaging*, vol. 26, no. 3, pp. 333–335, 2001.

[5] V. Velcheti and R. Govindan, "Metastatic cancer involving bladder: a review," *The Canadian Journal of Urology*, vol. 14, no. 1, pp. 3443–3448, 2007.

[6] P. K. Sharma, M. K. Vijay, R. K. Das, and U. Chatterjee, "Secondary signet-ring cell adenocarcinoma of urinary bladder from a gastric primary," *Urology Annals*, vol. 3, no. 2, pp. 97–99, 2011.

[7] N. F. Saba, D. M. Hoenig, and S. I. Cohen, "Metastatic signet-ring cell adenocarcinoma to the urinary bladder," *Acta Oncologica*, vol. 36, no. 2, pp. 219-220, 1997.

[8] A. A. Antunes, T. M. Siqueira Jr., and E. Falcão, "Vesical metastasis of gastric adenocarcinoma," *International braz j urol*, vol. 30, no. 5, pp. 403–405, 2004.

[9] N. Matsuhashi, K. Yamaguchi, T. Tamura, K. Shimokawa, Y. Sugiyama, and Y. Adachi, "Adenocarcinoma in bladder diverticulum, metastatic from gastric cancer," *World Journal of Surgical Oncology*, vol. 3, no. 1, p. 55, 2005.

[10] M. H. Farhat, G. Moumneh, R. Jalloul, and Y. El Hout, "Secondary adenocarcinoma of the urinary bladder from a primary gastric cancer," *Le Journal Médical Libanais*, vol. 55, no. 3, pp. 162–164, 2007.

[11] C. András, L. Tóth, J. Pósán et al., "Occurrence of bladder metastasis 10 years after surgical removal of a primary gastric cancer: a case report and review of the literature," *Journal of Medical Case Reports*, vol. 7, no. 1, p. 204, 2013.

[12] S. Kalra, R. Manikandan, L. N. Dorairajan, and B. Badhe, "Synchronously detected secondary signet ring cell urinary bladder malignancy from the stomach masquerading as genitourinary tuberculosis," *BML Case Reports*, vol. 2015, 2015.

[13] K. Okutur, O. O. Eren, and G. Demir, "Metastasis of gastric signet-ring cell carcinoma to the urinary bladder: a case report and review of the literature," *Case Reports in Oncological Medicine*, vol. 2015, Article ID 127516, 6 pages, 2015.

[14] B. Lodh, R. Sinam, and K. Singh, "Adenocarcinoma of urinary bladder in patient with primary gastric cancer: an unusual synchronous distant metastasis," *Indian Journal of Cancer*, vol. 53, no. 1, p. 53, 2016.

[15] E. Vigliar, G. Marino, E. Matano, C. Imbimbo, D. C. Rossella, and L. Insabato, "Signet-ring-cell carcinoma of stomach metastatic to the bladder: a case report with cytological and histological correlation and literature review," *International Journal of Surgical Pathology*, vol. 21, no. 1, pp. 72–75, 2013.

[16] I. Seow-En and F. Seow-Choen, "Intestinal type gastric adenocarcinoma with unusual synchronous metastases to the colorectum and bladder," *World Journal of Clinical Cases*, vol. 3, no. 6, pp. 533–537, 2015.

[17] R. Khoury, C. Dragean, and L. Annet, "Bladder metastasis of gastric adenocarcinoma," *Journal of the Belgian Society of Radiology*, vol. 103, no. 1, p. 24, 2019.

[18] T. Ota, M. Shinohara, K. Kinoshita, T. Sakoma, M. Kitamura, and Y. Maeda, "Two cases of metastatic bladder cancers showing diffuse thickening of the bladder wall," *Japanese Journal of Clinical Oncology*, vol. 29, no. 6, pp. 314–316, 1999.

42

Solitary Renal Metastasis Arising from a Pulmonary Adenoid Cystic Carcinoma: A Case Report and Review of the Literature

Prodromos Philippou,[1,2] Anastasios Michalakis,[3] Maria Miliatou,[1,2] Christiana Poullou,[4,5] and Pavlos Constantinou[4,5]

[1]*St George's Medical School, University of Nicosia, Nicosia, Cyprus*
[2]*Apollonion Hospital, Nicosia, Cyprus*
[3]*251 Airforce Hospital, Athens, Greece*
[4]*Histopathology and Cytology Laboratory Services, Nicosia, Cyprus*
[5]*School of Medicine, European University of Cyprus, Cyprus*

Correspondence should be addressed to Prodromos Philippou; brucemed@hotmail.com

Academic Editor: Fumitaka Koga

Adenoid cystic carcinoma (ACC) is a malignancy affecting the salivary glands and rarely involving the lung. Due to its rarity, primary lung ACC remains incompletely understood. We herein report the case of a 57-year-old female patient who was initially diagnosed with primary lung ACC and was treated by lobectomy. Seven years later, an abdominal computed tomography scan performed in the context of surveillance revealed the presence of a solid lesion arising from the lower pole of the left kidney. The patient underwent left partial nephrectomy, and histopathology confirmed a completely excised metastatic ACC.

1. Introduction

Adenoid cystic carcinoma (ACC) is a rare form of malignancy that arises within secretory glands, most commonly the major and minor salivary glands of the head and neck. Other sites of origin include lacrimal glands, breast, skin, and vulva [1]. ACC tends to metastasize to the lung and, less frequently, to the brain, liver, and bones [2]. Primary salivary-type tumors including ACC account for approximately 0.1% to 0.2% of all lung cancers and are histologically indistinguishable from their salivary gland counterparts [2]. They originate from the submucosal glands of the tracheobronchial tree and usually behave as low-grade malignancies with better prognosis compared to conventional lung cancer. Due to its rarity, primary lung ACC remains incompletely understood, and its clinical behavior, optimal treatment, and long-term outcome have yet to be clarified.

Renal metastases have been described in other malignancies such as lung, breast, and gastric carcinoma. Metastatic involvement of the kidney is usually a feature of disseminated disease, while solitary renal metastases are less frequent and mimic primary renal tumors [3]. In patients harboring another malignancy, solitary renal masses may represent synchronous primary tumors of the kidney.

Herein, we report the case of a 57-year-old female patient who presented with a solitary renal metastasis of a lung ACC and was successfully managed by minimally invasive nephron-sparing surgery. We report this case to highlight its uniqueness in terms of primary site (lung) and natural history (metachronous solitary metastasis to the kidney), and we focus on relevant issues such as differential diagnosis, the role of organ-sparing metastectomy, and the need for long-term follow-up of this rare malignancy.

2. Case Presentation

A 57-year-old asymptomatic female patient was referred for a 33 × 27 mm solid lesion arising from the lower pole of the

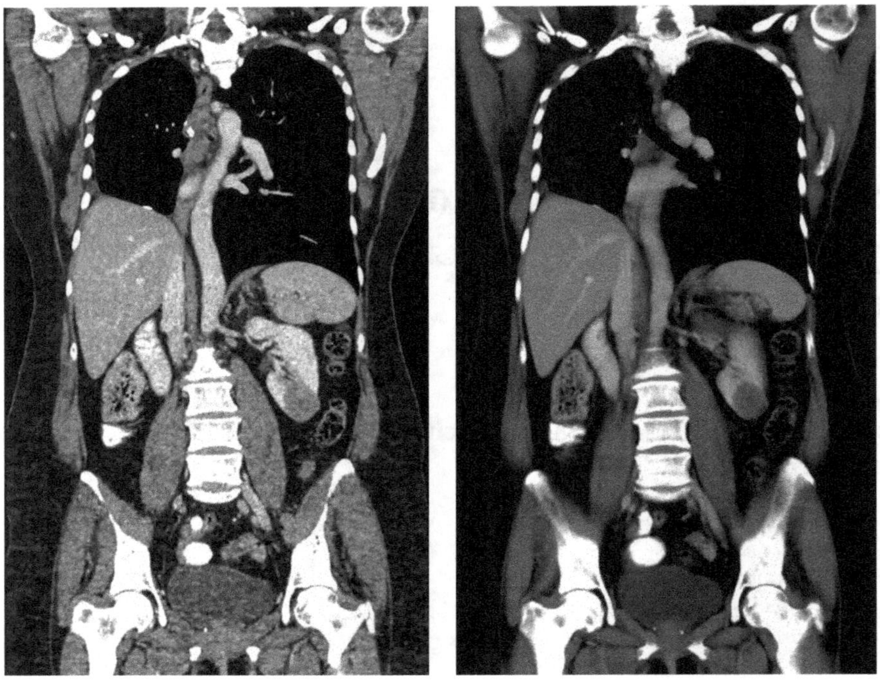

(a) (b)

FIGURE 1: Contrast-enhanced computed tomography in arterial (a) and venous (b) phases, revealing a slightly enhancing mass occupying the lower pole of the left kidney.

left kidney, which was diagnosed by computed tomography (CT) performed in the context of annual surveillance (Figure 1). She had been diagnosed with primary lung ACC seven years earlier and underwent right lower lobectomy, without any further adjuvant treatment. On precontrast CT images, the lesion appeared well-circumscribed, homogeneous, and relatively hypodense (30 +/-5 HU). It enhanced slightly in the arterial phase (45 +/-5 HU), but the enhancement was more pronounced in the venous phase (65 +/-5 HU). On 18F-fluorodeoxyglucose positron emission tomography–CT scan (Figure 2), a lump-shaped radioactive concentration shadow was observed at the lower pole of the left kidney, with a maximum standardized uptake value of 7. No other metastatic lesions were detected. Based on imaging characteristics and the patient's history, the differential diagnosis included nonclear cell renal cell carcinoma, renal metastasis, and benign renal tumors.

According to the Oncology Department's protocol for small renal masses (≤4 cm in greatest dimension) of questionable origin, percutaneous CT-guided biopsy of the renal lesion was performed, and histopathological analysis revealed a pattern compatible with ACC, similar to the primary lung tumor. Given the patient's age and the features of the tumor, nephron-sparing surgery was recommended. The patient underwent laparoscopic transperitoneal partial nephrectomy. The postoperative course was uneventful, and the patient was discharged on postoperative day two.

Gross examination of the specimen revealed a well-circumscribed, solid, and whitish tumor, measuring 37 × 39 × 35 mm. Microscopically, tumor cells were arranged in typical cribriform, tubular, and focally solid growth patterns. Neoplastic cells were small with scant cytoplasm. The stroma manifested myxoid and hyalinized features surrounded by tumor cells forming cylindrical structures (Figure 3). Immunohistochemically, neoplastic cells showed focal cytoplasmic or very weak nuclear expression of PAX8 which was considered a negative result. The strong nuclear staining of the renal tubular epithelium was used as an internal positive control. PAX8 negativity confirmed the extrarenal and extra-Müllerian origin of the tumor. The epithelial cells showed positivity for CD117 and CK7, and the myoepithelial cells showed positivity for P63, highlighting the dual cell population of the neoplasm, a typical feature of adenoid cystic carcinoma. Surgical margins were negative. These findings confirmed a completely excised metastatic ACC. Follow-up imaging at 24 months showed no evidence of recurrent disease.

3. Discussion

Historically, metastatic involvement of the kidney was considered a rare phenomenon. According to autopsy studies, the rate of renal metastases ranges from 2.4% to 7.2% [4], while detection of renal metastases in the clinical setting is less frequent [5, 6]. The most common sites of origin for tumors that metastasize to the kidney are the lung, gastrointestinal tract, breast, ovary, soft tissue, and thyroid [5]. Most patients diagnosed with renal metastases are either asymptomatic or present with nonspecific findings, such as albuminuria or microscopic hematuria [7]. In the case presented herein, the patient was diagnosed in the context of surveillance and was completely asymptomatic.

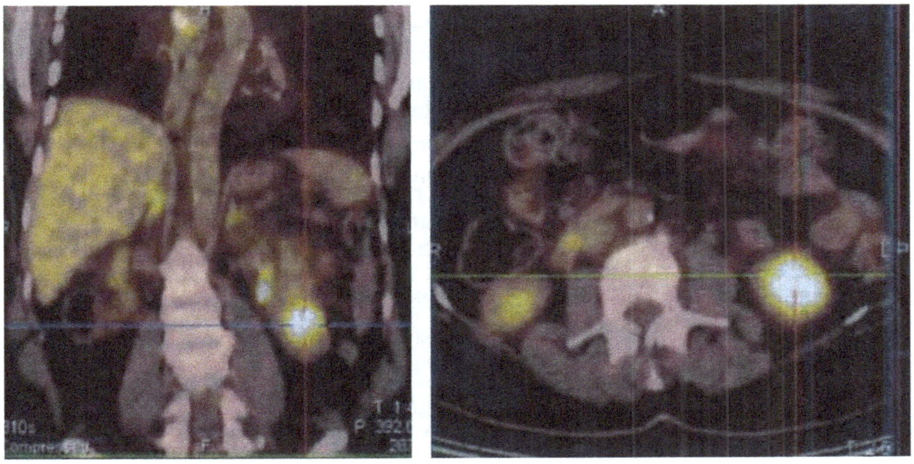

FIGURE 2: ^{18}F-Fluorodeoxyglucose positron emission tomography-computed tomography fusion scan images show a well-defined, heterogeneously low-grade fluorodeoxyglucose avid solid hypodense lesion at the lower pole of the left kidney.

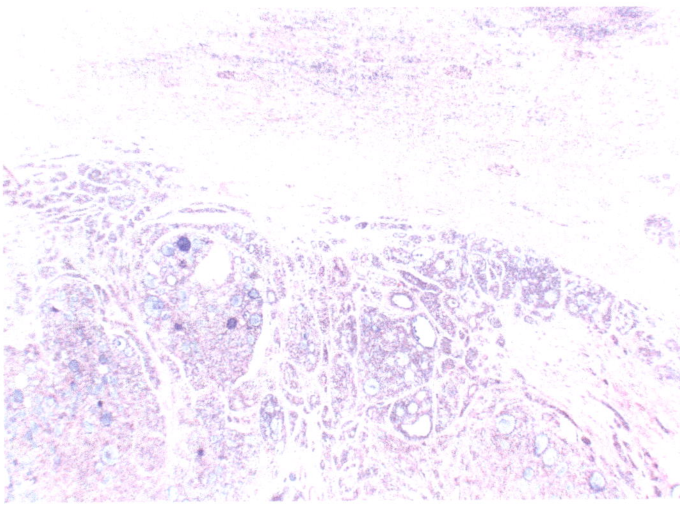

FIGURE 3: Metastatic adenoid cystic carcinoma to the kidney, showing the characteristic cribriform histological pattern of growth. Normal renal parenchyma is seen at the upper half of the image (haematoxylin-eosin stain, original magnification 40x).

Metastatic disease involving the kidney usually presents with bilateral and multiple lesions, associated with widespread dissemination of the primary tumor [8]. Solitary renal metastases, however, are uncommon [5], and most of these patients are diagnosed by routine imaging. Differentiation between a solitary renal metastasis and a primary renal tumor based on imaging can be challenging. Characteristics on CT scan suggestive of renal metastasis include endophytic growth, either isodensity or slightly lower attenuation compared to the normal renal parenchyma, hypovascularity ,and slight enhancement on contrast-enhanced images [3]. The imaging findings in this case are in accordance with these features.

In the past, the presence of a renal lesion in a patient with a history of extrarenal malignancy was considered an absolute indication for biopsy due to major treatment implications [5–9]. This approach, however, has been questioned in the context of solitary renal masses [5]. According to a previous retrospective study [8], decision-making in this setting can be based on the status of the extrarenal malignancy and the imaging characteristics of the renal lesion. The two major predictive factors for renal metastasis are evidence of clinical progression and/or other metastases from the nonrenal malignancy and lack of enhancement of the renal mass on imaging. The absence of progression of the nonrenal primary is considered a predictive factor for a renal primary over a solitary renal metastasis. In the case presented herein, the imaging characteristics of the lesion (endophytic, slightly low in attenuation, slight enhancement after intravenous contrast administration) were more typical of a metastatic lesion. The primary lesion, however, had been in remission, and no other metastatic focus was identified on imaging. The decision to perform percutaneous biopsy prior to surgical extirpation of the renal lesion in this case was based on the absence of progression of the primary tumor, even though the imaging findings were consistent with metastasis.

Table 1: Summary of primary lung ACC cases with renal metastases.

Ref no	Demographics	Treatment of primary tumor	Time interval to renal metastasis (years)	Symptoms at presentation	Metastatic tumor location/size (cm)	Management of renal tumor	Oncological outcome
[16]	47 yo male	Right pneumonectomy	23 years	Hematuria	Left kidney/9.0 cm	Radical nephrectomy	No recurrence after 12 months
[17]	79 yo male	Not done	3 years	Hematuria and right flank pain	Right kidney/4.4 cm + multiple left renal lesions	Chemotherapy	Patient died 30 months after diagnosis
[18]	50 yo male	Right lower lobectomy	7 years	Flank pain	Right kidney/9.3 cm	Radical nephrectomy (cytoreductive)	Not reported
[19]	70 yo male	Right upper lobectomy + radiotherapy	3 years	Cough, fever, weight loss	Lower and upper pole of right kidney/1.8 cm	Radical nephrectomy	No recurrence after 24 months
This case	57 yo female	Right lower lobectomy	7 years	Asymptomatic	Lower pole of left kidney/3.3 cm	Partial nephrectomy	No recurrence after 24 months

ACC is characterized by an indolent clinical course, a variable distant recurrence rate (4.1-44.7%) and a tendency for late-onset metastases [10]. The organs most frequently involved by metastatic ACC are the lungs, bones, brain, and liver [2]. On reviewing the limited cases of metastatic ACC with renal involvement, the most common primary sites are major or minor salivary glands (parotid gland, submandibular gland, palate, floor of mouth, sinonasal region), lacrimal gland, and breast [11–15]. The time interval between primary diagnosis and development of renal metastasis ranged from 3 to 14 years, with an average interval of 9.8 years, representing an indolent growth pattern and a potential for late metastases [15]. To our knowledge, only four cases of pulmonary ACC metastatic to the kidney have been described in the literature to date (Table 1) [16–19]. Two of these reports describe renal involvement in the context of widespread metastatic disease with a poor outcome [17, 18]. Surgery (with or without adjuvant radiotherapy) was the most common primary treatment modality, and the time interval between initial diagnosis of lung ACC and development of renal metastasis ranged between 3 and 23 years. All previous patients presented with symptoms indicating a renal mass (i.e., hematuria and/or flank pain), but our patient was asymptomatic and was diagnosed in the context of annual surveillance.

The prognosis of patients with distant metastases following primary lung ACC varies, but previous reports have suggested that metastases have a tendency for slow growth similar to the primary tumor [2]. In this context, complete surgical excision of metastases, if feasible, should be considered as a therapeutic option, in order to achieve control of disease and prolong survival. Given the rarity of the case presented herein, however, clear recommendations cannot be made. For metastatic ACC of the salivary glands, survival is related to the disease-free interval [20], as metastectomy for metachronous metastases (interval > 36 months) appears to achieve better disease control. While surgical excision (radical or partial nephrectomy) is considered the standard of care in patients with primary renal malignancies, there are no clear guidelines for the surgical management of renal metastases. According to the limited available data [5, 6], surgical excision of renal metastases in carefully selected patients with oligometastatic disease and good performance status achieves acceptable long-term survival rates. The role of nephron-sparing surgery in these cases is not established, since the available literature only includes case reports and nonrandomized case series. According to a large single-centre retrospective series of 151 patients, only one-third of patients were candidates for surgical excision of renal secondaries, and less than 20% of them underwent organ-sparing surgery (i.e., partial nephrectomy) [5].

Local and distant metastases of ACC are frequent due to the tumor's tendency to invade the peri-neural space [2]. Currently, there is no consensus for the treatment of metastatic ACC, as cytotoxic chemotherapy produces very low response rates (5-15%) [21, 22]. Several advances in the understanding of the pathogenesis and molecular phenotype of this malignancy have been made, and new compounds (i.e., antiangiogenic agents, tailored agents, and checkpoint inhibitors) are under investigation. Genetic analyses have shown that MYB-NFIB fusion transcripts and/or MYB overexpression are observed in the majority of ACC cases [21]. In this context, the tyrosine kinase inhibitors axitinib, dovitinib, and lenvatinib exhibited clinical activity against ACC in phase II studies [23–25]. There remains a need for further studies that incorporate molecular analysis in the management of incurable ACC, as well as the development of effective novel therapeutic approaches.

4. Conclusion

The uniqueness of the case presented herein involves metachronous solitary metastatic renal metastasis from ACC arising at an uncommon primary site, managed by organ-sparing surgery. The patient underwent laparoscopic partial nephrectomy with negative surgical margins and remained disease-free 24 months after surgery. Since late distant metastases of ACC are not uncommon, long-term follow-up is recommended.

References

[1] B. J. Resio, A. S. Chiu, J. Hoag, A. P. Dhanasopon, J. D. Blasberg, and D. J. Boffa, "Primary salivary type lung cancers in the National Cancer Database," *The Annals of Thoracic Surgery*, vol. 105, no. 6, pp. 1633–1639, 2018.

[2] J. R. Molina, M. C. Aubry, J. E. Lewis et al., "Primary salivary gland-type lung cancer: spectrum of clinical presentation, histopathologic and prognostic factors," *Cancer*, vol. 110, no. 10, pp. 2253–2259, 2007.

[3] J. E. Bailey, M. A. Roubidoux, and N. R. Dunnick, "Secondary renal neoplasms," *Abdominal Imaging*, vol. 23, no. 3, pp. 266–274, 1998.

[4] R. B. Bracken, G. Chica, D. E. Johnson, and M. Luna, "Secondary renal neoplasms: an autopsy study," *Southern Medical Journal*, vol. 72, no. 7, pp. 806-807, 1979.

[5] C. Zhou, D. L. Urbauer, B. M. Fellman et al., "Metastases to the kidney: a comprehensive analysis of 151 patients from a tertiary referral centre," *BJU International*, vol. 117, no. 5, pp. 775–782, 2016.

[6] A. Adamy, C. Von Bodman, T. Ghoneim, R. L. Favaretto, M. Bernstein, and P. Russo, "Solitary, isolated metastatic disease to the kidney: Memorial Sloan-Kettering Cancer Center experience," *BJU International*, vol. 108, no. 3, pp. 338–342, 2011.

[7] P. L. Choyke, E. M. White, R. K. Zeman, M. H. Jaffe, and L. R. Clark, "Renal metastases: clinicopathologic and radiologic correlation," *Radiology*, vol. 162, no. 2, pp. 359–363, 1987.

[8] R. F. Sánchez-Ortiz, L. T. Madsen, C. E. Bermejo et al., "A renal mass in the setting of a nonrenal malignancy: when is a renal tumor biopsy appropriate?," *Cancer*, vol. 101, no. 10, pp. 2195–2201, 2004.

[9] V. A. Sahni and S. G. Silverman, "Biopsy of renal masses: when and why," *Cancer imaging: the official publication of the International Cancer Imaging Society*, vol. 9, no. 1, pp. 44–55, 2009.

[10] D. Pandey, P. K. Garg, A. Jakhetiya et al., "Surgical experience of primary salivary gland tumors of lung: a case series," *International Journal of Surgery*, vol. 21, pp. 92–96, 2015.

[11] M. Santamaría and P. de Llano, "Adenoid cystic carcinoma metastatic to the kidney: a case report," *Acta Cytologica*, vol. 52, no. 2, pp. 215–219, 2008.

[12] S. Kala, C. Pantola, and A. Agarwal, "Metastatic adenoid cystic carcinoma of kidney masquerading as renal cell carcinoma," *Indian Journal of Pathology & Microbiology*, vol. 53, no. 4, pp. 835-836, 2010.

[13] J. Bacalja, M. Magazin, M. Ulamec, D. Rako, D. Trnski, and B. Krušlin, "Adenoid cystic carcinoma of the lacrimal gland metastatic to the kidney: case report and review of the literature," *Scottish Medical Journal*, vol. 59, no. 2, pp. e14–e17, 2014.

[14] D. S. Qiu, L. Y. Xu, and X. Y. Hu, "Imaging appearance of a singular metastatic adenoid cystic carcinoma of the right kidney: a case report and literature review," *Oncology Letters*, vol. 8, no. 6, pp. 2669–2671, 2014.

[15] L. Chen, L. Fang, Y. Zhang et al., "Adenoid cystic carcinoma of maxillary sinus metastatic to the kidney: a case report and review of the literature," *International Journal of Clinical and Experimental Pathology*, vol. 9, pp. 4061–4066, 2016.

[16] C. Ladefoged, C. Bisgaard, and J. Petri, "Solitary renal metastasis 23 years after extirpation of a bronchial adenoid cystic carcinoma," *Scandinavian Journal of Thoracic and Cardiovascular Surgery*, vol. 18, no. 3, pp. 245–248, 2009.

[17] Y. Fujii, M. Masuda, M. Hirokawa, K. Matsushita, and H. Hasegawa, "Bilateral renal metastases of lung adenoid cystic carcinoma," *Hinyokika Kiyo*, vol. 37, no. 10, pp. 1307–1311, 1991.

[18] J. Goyal, A. Sidana, M. O'Malley, and R. Rodriguez, "Large renal metastasis from rare pulmonary neoplasm," *Urology*, vol. 77, no. 5, pp. 1097-1098, 2011.

[19] N. N. Junejo, L. Almusallam, K. I. Alothman, and T. O. Al Hussain, "An unusual case report of pulmonary adenoid cystic carcinoma metastasis to the kidney. Case report and literature review," *Urology Case Reports*, vol. 27, p. 100927, 2019.

[20] L. Girelli, L. Locati, C. Galeone et al., "Lung metastasectomy in adenoid cystic cancer: is it worth it?," *Oral Oncology*, vol. 65, pp. 114–118, 2017.

[21] P. M. Dillon, S. Chakraborty, C. A. Moskaluk, P. J. Joshi, and C. Y. Thomas, "Adenoid cystic carcinoma: a review of recent advances, molecular targets, and clinical trials," *Head & Neck*, vol. 38, no. 4, pp. 620–627, 2016.

[22] G. Papaspyrou, S. Hoch, A. Rinaldo et al., "Chemotherapy and targeted therapy in adenoid cystic carcinoma of the head and neck: a review," *Head & Neck*, vol. 33, no. 6, pp. 905–911, 2011.

[23] A. L. Ho, L. Dunn, E. J. Sherman et al., "A phase II study of axitinib (AG-013736) in patients with incurable adenoid cystic carcinoma," *Annals of Oncology*, vol. 27, no. 10, pp. 1902–1908, 2016.

[24] P. M. Dillon, G. R. Petroni, B. J. Horton et al., "A phase II study of dovitinib in patients with recurrent or metastatic adenoid cystic carcinoma," *Clinical Cancer Research*, vol. 23, no. 15, pp. 4138–4145, 2017.

[25] V. Tchekmedyian, E. J. Sherman, L. Dunn et al., "Phase II study of lenvatinib in patients with progressive, recurrent or metastatic adenoid cystic carcinoma," *Journal of Clinical Oncology*, vol. 37, no. 18, pp. 1529–1537, 2019.

Primary Mature Cystic Teratoma Compressing the Prostate in a 28-Year-Old Male: A Case Report and Literature Review

Khalil Chalhoub,[1] Rawad Abou Zahr,[1] Elias Mansour,[2] Mona Aoun,[3] and Michel Jabbour[1]

[1] *University of Balamand, Saint George Hospital University Medical Center, Department of Urology, Beirut 1100 2807, Lebanon*
[2] *University of Balamand, Faculty of Medicine and Medical Sciences, Beirut 1100 2807, Lebanon*
[3] *University of Balamand, Saint George Hospital University Medical Center, Department of Pathology, Beirut 1100 2807, Lebanon*

Correspondence should be addressed to Michel Jabbour; drmjabbour@gmail.com

Academic Editor: Giorgio Carmignani

Primary mature retroperitoneal teratomas are rare tumors most commonly occurring in adult females. These tumors are usually asymptomatic since they have no attachments to specific organs. We present a rare case of a 28-year-old male with 2-month history of lower urinary tract symptoms, who was found to have a primary mature cystic teratoma abutting the prostate.

1. Introduction

Dermoid cysts or mature teratomas are neoplastic structures composed of tissues from at least two of the three germ layers (endoderm, ectoderm, and mesoderm) [1, 2]. They are most commonly located in the gonads [3]. Primary retroperitoneal neoplasms comprise only 0.1%–0.3% of all the tumors, of which the most common are metastases from gonads, and 1%–11% of those are teratomas [4, 5]. Characteristically, mature teratomas are unilocular and, in addition to cutaneous components, may contain other tissues, including hair and teeth, glandular elements, adipose tissue, cartilage, and bone as well as sebaceous material [6]. Primary retroperitoneal teratomas (RT) characteristically have no attachment to other organs such as kidneys, adrenal glands, and pancreas, with the majority being asymptomatic or discovered incidentally on routine investigations [7, 8]. Surgical excision is the diagnostic modality of choice and the mainstay of treatment [9, 10]. Prognosis is excellent after complete surgical excision with an overall five-year survival rate of nearly 100% [11]. In the literature, few cases were reported, mostly occurring in infants or young females. The most common site is sacrococcygeal area in infants and left suprarenal region in adults [12, 13]. One case of mature teratoma involving the prostate was reported in a 50-year-old male with micturition problem. The aim of this article is to present a rare case of a 28-year-old male patient with psoriasis who sought medical care after 2-month history of urinary symptoms and increased bowel movements.

2. Case Presentation

A 28-year-old male patient with psoriasis presented to our facility with two-month history of lower urinary symptoms and increased bowel movements. Physical examination and laboratory studies were unremarkable. Suprapubic ultrasonography done outside our hospital showed an enlarged prostate measuring 72mm x 76mm x 67mm and 194 cm^3 in volume. Pelvic Magnetic Resonance Imaging (MRI) showed a large mass confined to the pelvis measuring 7.2 cm in the largest diameter with predominance of cystic component without evidence of fatty content, calcification, fluid-fluid level, or suspicious enhancing nodular soft tissue thickening.

The mass was seen in the perirectal space, displacing and exerting mass effect on the seminal vesicles, prostate and abutting the bladder without clear connection with the digestive system (Figure 1).

Patient underwent a surgical resection through a suprapubic midline incision; the mass was approached from the left side after liberating and reflecting the bladder medially. Macroscopically, the mass weighs 157g and measures 7.5 x 5 x 5.5cm. It is covered by a thin membrane and is focally

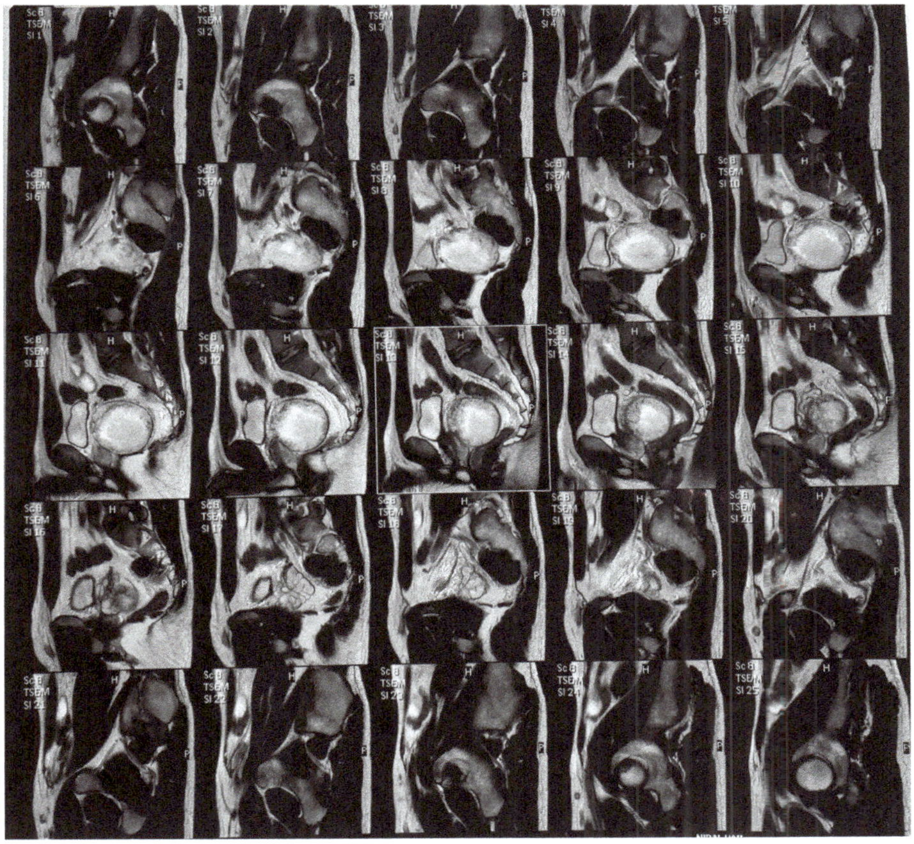

FIGURE 1: Pelvic MRI showing a large mass confined to the pelvis measuring 7.2 cm in the largest diameter with predominance of cystic component without evidence of fatty content, calcification, fluid-fluid level, or suspicious enhancing nodular soft tissue thickening.

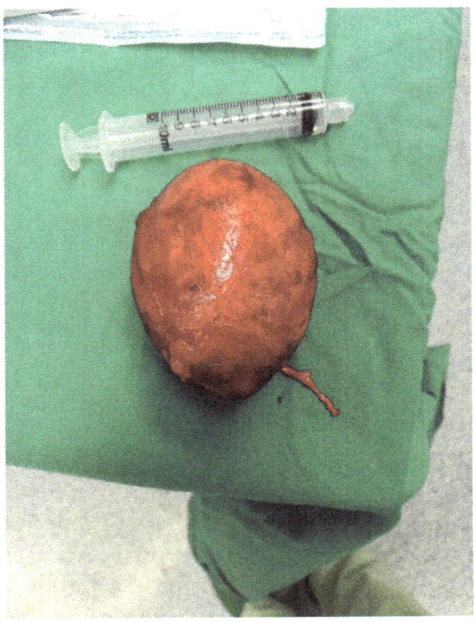

FIGURE 2: The excised mass had well-circumscribed smooth borders and rubbery consistency. It is covered by a thin and focally congested membrane. It weighs 157g and measures 7.5cm x 5.5cm x 5.5cm. Cut surface shows unilocular cystic mass filled with beige brown soft material and hair shafts.

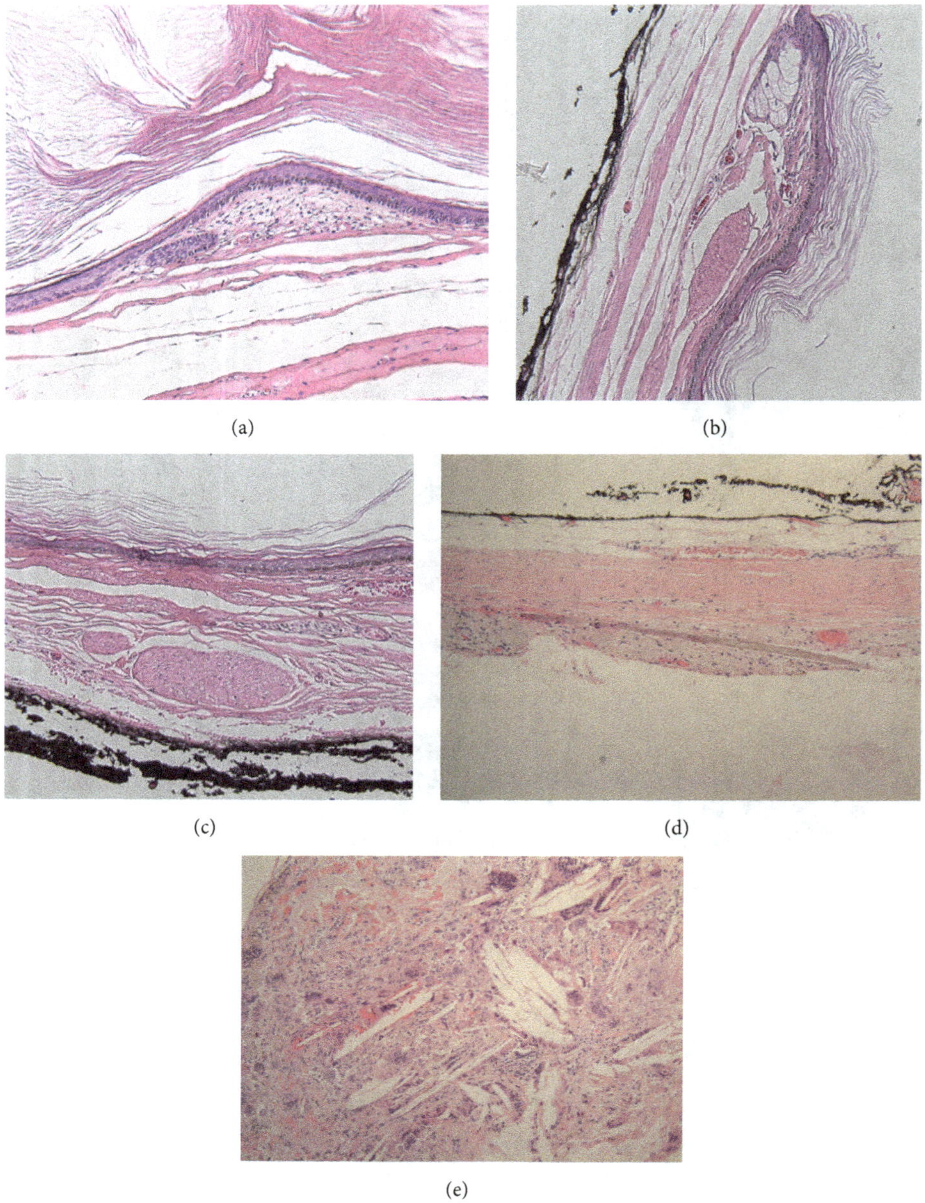

FIGURE 3: (a) & (b) Cystic cavity lined by orthokeratinized stratified squamous epithelium, with straight epithelial-connective tissue interface. Copious fibrillary keratin fills the cyst. (a) The base of a hair follicle is identified. (b) A sebaceous gland with adjacent arrector pili muscle fiber. (c) High power view of arrector pili muscle fiber. (d) A hair shaft found in the cystic wall. (e) Inflammatory reaction to keratin with multinucleated giant cells and foamy macrophages is seen. Absence of cartilage and bone in all figures.

congested (Figure 2). Cut surface shows a unilocular cystic mass filled with beige brown soft material and hair shafts.

Microscopically, the excised cystic mass is covered with a thin fibrotic wall and lined by mature squamous epithelium with few skin adnexae and hair shafts filled with fibrillary keratin. Pathology was consistent with mature cystic teratoma (Figure 3). Patient was discharged on the second postoperative day after an uneventful stay. Patient's urinary symptoms were relieved; MRI done at one year postoperatively showed no recurrence of tumor.

3. Discussion

Primary retroperitoneal teratomas constitute about 1-11% of all primary retroperitoneal tumors [14, 15]. The majority are diagnosed within the first year of life and 10-20% after 30 years of age. Adult retroperitoneal dermoid cysts commonly affect females between 15 and 40 years of age [16]. Embryologically, they originate from uncontrolled proliferation of pluripotent cells: germ cells and embryonal cells. Depending on the type of pluripotent cell, the presentation and location of teratoma may vary. Teratomas of germ cells are found in gonads (testes and ovaries). In contrast, teratomas of embryonic cell sources are always congenital and are usually found in extragonadal locations (intracranial, retroperitoneal, etc.) [17, 18]. Many theories account for the origin of the primary retroperitoneal teratomas; the most widely accepted one is that they are remnants of the Wolffian and Müllerian ducts or that they arise from pronephric or mesonephric tubules as it correlates with their midline and paramedian location [16].

Teratomas may be classified according to their location, content, epithelial lining, and degree of maturation [19]. Depending on the location, they can be gonadal or extragonadal with the former being more common. However, based on the content, teratomas can be solid, cystic, or mixed; furthermore, according to their epithelial lining, they can be divided into epidermoid, dermoid, and teratoid teratomas. Epidermoid and dermoid teratomas are lined with squamous epithelium but the latter contain dermoid elements (i.e., hair; sebaceous glands) while the teratoid type is lined by respiratory columnar epithelium and contains sebum. Besides, according to their degree of maturation, there are two types: mature and immature. Mature teratomas also called dermoid cysts are in general benign and are more common in females. The immature ones are poorly differentiated, may be benign or malignant, and are more common in males [19].

Benign teratomas are usually asymptomatic and many are discovered incidentally. Symptoms are mainly related to the mass effect of the tumor; hence they appear later as the tumor grows in the retroperitoneum and they include flank or abdominal pain, urinary symptoms as in this patient, and gastrointestinal symptoms such as constipation [16]. Physical examination may reveal abdominal mass or distention [16].

With the increased use of imaging, retroperitoneal teratomas increased in incidence. Plain radiographs may visualize calcifications but lead to nonspecific findings. Ultrasonography may be superior to radiography in delineating the cystic component but has limited specificity. Computed tomography scans and MRI are more appropriate. MRI can visualize the degree of invasion of adjacent structures as well as tumor content and may indicate if a wider resection is required [20, 21].

Complete excision of the mass is curative and is the mainstay of treatment since histological assessment is important for confirmation of the diagnosis and should be attempted since primary retroperitoneal teratomas in adults rarely infiltrate adjacent tissues [16]. In our case, histologic examination revealed all the characteristic features of dermoid cysts.

4. Conclusion

Mature (benign) retroperitoneal dermoid cysts compressing the prostate are extremely rare. Imaging should be considered when evaluating young male patients presenting with lower urinary tract symptoms. Surgical excision is the mainstay and gold standard treatment that allows symptomatic relief of the patient as well as definitive histologic diagnosis.

References

[1] R. A. Willis, Ed., *Atlas of Tumor Pathology, section III, fascicle 9*, Armed Forces, Washington, DC, USA, 1961.

[2] D. M. Yang, D. H. Jung, H. Kim et al., "Retroperitoneal cystic masses: CT, clinical, and pathologic findings and literature review," *RadioGraphics*, vol. 24, no. 5, pp. 1353–1365, 2004.

[3] H. Isaacs, "Perinatal (fetal and neonatal) germ cell tumors," *Journal of Pediatric Surgery*, vol. 39, no. 7, pp. 1003–1013, 2004.

[4] M. F. Bellin, J. J. Duron, P. Curet, E. Dion-Voirin, and J. Grellet, "Primary retroperitoneal teratoma in the adult: correlation of MRI features with CT and pathology," *Magnetic Resonance Imaging*, vol. 9, no. 2, pp. 263–266, 1991.

[5] L. T. Palumbo, K. R. Cross, A. N. Smith, and A. A. Baronas, "Primary teratomas of the lateral retroperitoneal spaces," *Surgery*, vol. 26, no. 1, pp. 149–159, 1949.

[6] H. Ye and T. M. Ulbright, "Difficult differential diagnoses in testicular pathology," *Archives of Pathology & Laboratory Medicine*, vol. 136, no. 4, pp. 435–446, 2012.

[7] J. P. K. Hui, W. H. Luk, C. W. Siu, and J. C. S. Chan, "Teratoma in the region of an adrenal gland in a 77-year-old man," *Journal of Hong Kong College of Radiologists*, vol. 7, no. 4, pp. 206–209, 2004.

[8] M. Paul, "The retro-peritoneal dermoid cysts," *ANZ Journal of Surgery*, vol. 22, no. 3, pp. 227–230, 1953.

[9] H. Liu, W. Li, W. Yang, and Y. Qi, "Giant retroperitoneal teratoma in an adult," *The American Journal of Surgery*, vol. 193, no. 6, pp. 736-737, 2007.

[10] P. Mathur, M. A. Lopez-Viego, and M. Howell, "Giant primary retroperitoneal teratoma in an adult: A case report," *Case Reports in Medicine*, vol 2010, p. 3, 2010.

[11] C. W. Pinson, S. G. ReMine, W. S. Fletcher, and J. W. Braasch, "Long-term results with primary retroperitoneal tumors," *Archives of Surgery*, vol. 124, no. 10, pp. 1168–1173, 1989.

[12] S. Bhalla, K. Masih, and R. Rana, "Teratomas of Rare Sites: a Review of Ten Cases," *Journal of the Indian Medical Association*, vol. 89, pp. 291–294, 1991.

[13] R. M. Engel, R. C. Elkins and B. D. Fletcher, "Retroperitoneal teratoma. Review of the literature and presentation of an unusual case," *Cancer*, vol. 22, no. 5, pp. 1068–1073, 1968.

[14] J. Gschwend, T. W. Burke, J. E. Woodward, and P. B. Heller, "Retroperitoneal teratoma presenting as an abdominal-pelvic mass," *Obstetrics & Gynecology*, vol. 70, no. 3, part 2, pp. 500–502, 1987.

[15] R. Lane, D. Stephens, and H. Reiman, "Primary retroperitoneal neoplasms: CT findings in 90 cases with clinical and pathologic correlation," *American Journal of Roentgenology*, vol. 152, no. 1, pp. 83–89, 1989.

[16] H. G. Gatcombe, V. Assikis, D. Kooby, and P. A. S. Johnstone, "Primary retroperitoneal teratomas : a review of the literature," *Journal of Surgical Oncology*, vol. 86, no. 2, pp. 107–113, 2004.

[17] S. Bedri, K. Erfanian, S. Schwaitzberg, and A. S. Tischler, "Mature cystic teratoma involving adrenal gland," *Endocrine Pathology*, vol. 13, no. 1, pp. 59–64, 2002.

[18] J. L. Grosfeld and D. F. Billmire, "Teratomas in infancy and childhood," *Current Problems in Cancer*, vol. 9, no. 9, pp. 1–53, 1985.

[19] A. Bhatti, H. Al-Hindi, A. Azzam, T. Amin, and A. Abu-Zaid, "Mature (Benign) cystic retroperitoneal teratoma involving the left adrenal gland in a 22-year-old male: A case report and

literature review," *Case Reports in Oncological Medicine*, vol. 2013, Article ID 610280, pp. 1–5, 2013.

[20] M. O. Cadeddu, J. Mamazza, C. M. Schlachta, P. A. Seshadri, and E. C. Poulin, "Laparoscopic Excision of Retroperitoneal Tumors," *Surgical Laparoscopy, Endoscopy & Percutaneous Techniques*, vol. 11, no. 2, pp. 144–147, 2001.

[21] A. Tiu, V. Sovani, N. Khan, and S. Hooda, "Primary retroperitoneal mature cystic teratoma (dermoid cyst) in a 51-year-old male:Case report and historical literature review," *SAGE Open Medical Case Reports*, vol. 5, 2017.

Permissions

All chapters in this book were first published by Hindawi Publishing Corporation; hereby published with permission under the Creative Commons Attribution License or equivalent. Every chapter published in this book has been scrutinized by our experts. Their significance has been extensively debated. The topics covered herein carry significant findings which will fuel the growth of the discipline. They may even be implemented as practical applications or may be referred to as a beginning point for another development.

The contributors of this book come from diverse backgrounds, making this book a truly international effort. This book will bring forth new frontiers with its revolutionizing research information and detailed analysis of the nascent developments around the world.

We would like to thank all the contributing authors for lending their expertise to make the book truly unique. They have played a crucial role in the development of this book. Without their invaluable contributions this book wouldn't have been possible. They have made vital efforts to compile up to date information on the varied aspects of this subject to make this book a valuable addition to the collection of many professionals and students.

This book was conceptualized with the vision of imparting up-to-date information and advanced data in this field. To ensure the same, a matchless editorial board was set up. Every individual on the board went through rigorous rounds of assessment to prove their worth. After which they invested a large part of their time researching and compiling the most relevant data for our readers.

The editorial board has been involved in producing this book since its inception. They have spent rigorous hours researching and exploring the diverse topics which have resulted in the successful publishing of this book. They have passed on their knowledge of decades through this book. To expedite this challenging task, the publisher supported the team at every step. A small team of assistant editors was also appointed to further simplify the editing procedure and attain best results for the readers.

Apart from the editorial board, the designing team has also invested a significant amount of their time in understanding the subject and creating the most relevant covers. They scrutinized every image to scout for the most suitable representation of the subject and create an appropriate cover for the book.

The publishing team has been an ardent support to the editorial, designing and production team. Their endless efforts to recruit the best for this project, has resulted in the accomplishment of this book. They are a veteran in the field of academics and their pool of knowledge is as vast as their experience in printing. Their expertise and guidance has proved useful at every step. Their uncompromising quality standards have made this book an exceptional effort. Their encouragement from time to time has been an inspiration for everyone.

The publisher and the editorial board hope that this book will prove to be a valuable piece of knowledge for researchers, students, practitioners and scholars across the globe.

List of Contributors

Bushra Ali Khan, Nida Saleem, Danyal Hassan, Shabaz Kiani and Muhammad Haneef
Shifa International Hospital, H-8/4, Pitras Bukhari Road, Islamabad, Pakistan

Ortwin Heißler, Maximilian Fingernagel and Claus Riedl
Department of Urology, Landesklinikum Baden-Mödling, Baden, Austria

Stephan Seklehner and Paul F. Engelhardt
Department of Urology, Landesklinikum Baden-Mödling, Baden, Austria
Paracelsus Medical University, Salzburg, Austria

Benedicta Nneoma Nnodum, Eziafa Oduah, David Albert and Mark Pettus
Berkshire Medical Center, Pittsfield, MA 01201, USA

Mahtab Poor Zamany Nejat Kermaney and Fatemeh Roodneshin
Department of Anesthesiology, Shahid Beheshti University of Medical Sciences, Tehran, Iran

Mohammad Hamidi Madani, Milad Bonakdar Hashemi and Alireza Zadmehr
Resident of Urology, Labbafinezhad Hospital, Urology Nephrology Research Center (UNRC), Shahid Beheshti University of Medical Sciences, Tehran, Iran

Mehdi Dadpour
Urology and Nephrology Research Center, Shahid Labbafinezhad Hospital, Shahid Beheshti University of Medical Sciences, Tehran, Iran

Yoichi Iwafuchi and Yuko Oyama
Department of Internal Medicine, Koseiren Sanjo General Hospital, 5-1-62 Tsukanome, Sanjo 955-0055, Japan

Tetsuo Morioka
Department of Internal Medicine, Kidney Center, Shinrakuen Hospital, 3-3-11 Shindoriminami Nishi-ku, Niigata 950-2087, Japan

Shin Goto and Ichiei Narita
Division of Clinical Nephrology and Rheumatology, Niigata University Graduate School of Medical and Dental Sciences, 1-754 Asahinachi-Dori, Niigata 951-8510, Japan

Kamal Ranabhat
Institue of Medicine, Tribhuvan University, Kathmandu, Nepal
Ministry of Health and Population, Kathmandu, Nepal

Bhuvan Saud
Department of Medical Laboratory Technology, Janamaitri Foundation Institute of Health Sciences, Lalitpur, Nepal

Saroj Adhikari
National Trauma Center, Ministry of Health and Population Kathmandu, Nepal

Suraj Bhattarai
Global Institute for Interdisciplinary Studies, Kathmandu, Nepal

Rojan Adhikari
Shahid Dharma Bhakta National Transplant Center, Bhaktapur, Nepal

Bhoj Raj Luitel and Mahesh Raj Sigdel
Institue of Medicine, Tribhuvan University, Kathmandu, Nepal

Zhiyu Qian
Division of Urology, Brigham and Women's Hospital, Harvard Medical School, USA

Emily Chou, Hanwei Zhang and Arnold I. Chin
Department of Urology, David Geffen School of Medicine at UCLA, USA

Jing Yang and HuiHui Ye
Department of Pathology, David Geffen School of Medicine at UCLA, USA

Sandy T. Liu
Department of Medicine, Division of Hematology and Oncology, David Geffen School of Medicine at UCLA, USA

Panagiotis I. Georgianos, Vasilios Vaios, Eleni Leontaridou, Athanasios Sioulis, Elias V. Balaskas and Pantelis E. Zebekakis
Section of Nephrology and Hypertension, 1st Department of Medicine, AHEPA Hospital, Aristotle University of Thessaloniki, Thessaloniki, Greece

Georgia Karayannopoulou and Triantafyllia Koletsa
Department of Pathology, Aristotle University of Thessaloniki, Thessaloniki, Greece

Hugo Otaola-Arca
Clínica Alemana, Santiago, Chile
School of Medicine, Clínica Alemana-Universidad del Desarollo, Santiago, Chile

Patricio Vargas, Daniel Hasson, Marcelo Orvieto and Hugo Bermúdez
Clínica Alemana, Santiago, Chile

Carmen Niño-Taravilla
Clinica INDISA, Santiago, Chile

Amanda Smart and Michael Wynne
Department of Urology, George Washington University Hospital, Washington, DC, USA

Ezra Baraban
Department of Pathology, Johns Hopkins University School of Medicine, Baltimore, MD, USA

Yasser Ged
Department of Oncology, Johns Hopkins University School of Medicine, Baltimore, MD, USA

Armine Smith
The James Buchanan Brady Urologic Institute and Department of Urology, Johns Hopkins University School of Medicine, Baltimore, MD, USA

Imad Boualaoui, Idriss Ziani, Ahmed Ibrahimi, Hachem El Sayegh and Yassine Nouini
Department of Urology A, Mohammed V University in Rabat, Ibn Sina University Hospital, Rabat, Morocco

Salma Marrakchi
Department of Radiology, Mohammed V University in Rabat, Ibn Sina University Hospital, Rabat, Morocco

Mohammed Raiss
Surgical Department "C", Mohammed V University in Rabat, Ibn Sina University Hospital, Rabat, Morocco

Fouad Zouidia
Department of Anatomopathology and Cytology, Mohammed V University in Rabat, Ibn Sina University Hospital, Rabat, Morocco

Julien Sarkis, Elie Hanna and Elie Nemr
Department of Urology, Hôtel-Dieu de France, Beirut, Lebanon

Fady Haddad
Department of Internal Medicine, Hôtel-Dieu de France, Beirut, Lebanon

Sarah Nasr
Department of Pathology, Hôtel-Dieu de France, Beirut, Lebanon

Ahmad Mroueh
Department of Nephrology, Hôtel-Dieu de France, Beirut, Lebanon

Takao Natsuyama, Masato Uetani, Shigeyuki Ohta and Shin-ichi Hisasue
Department of Urology, Chiba-Nishi General Hospital, 270-2251 Chiba, Japan

Yozo Mitsui
Department of Urology, Chiba-Nishi General Hospital, 270-2251 Chiba, Japan
Department of Urology, Toho University Faculty of Medicine, 143-8540 Tokyo, Japan

Taro Ikeda, Noboru Hara and Tsutomu Nishiyama
Department of Urology, Uonuma Institute of Community Medicine, Niigata University Medical and Dental Hospital, Minamiuonuma, Niigata, Japan

Kazunori Matsumoto
Department of Radiation Engineering, Uonuma Institute of Community Medicine, Niigata University Medical and Dental Hospital, Minamiuonuma, Niigata, Japan

Go Hasegawa
Department of Pathology, Uonuma Institute of Community Medicine, Niigata University Medical and Dental Hospital, Minamiuonuma, Niigata, Japan

Yohei Ikeda
Department of Diagnostic Radiology, Uonuma Institute of Community Medicine, Niigata University Medical and Dental Hospital, Minamiuonuma, Niigata, Japan

Facundo Davaro and Lindsay Lombardo
Division of Urology, Department of Surgery, Saint Louis University, 3635 Vista Ave, 3rd Floor Desloge Towers, St. Louis, MO 63110, USA

Elizabeth Davaro and Amna Qureshi
Department of Pathology, Saint Louis University, 3635 Vista Ave, 4th Floor Desloge Towers, St. Louis, MO 63110, USA

Fadhel Yusuf, Amr Elmekresh, Senthil Kumar and Fariborz Bagheri
Department of Urology, Dubai Hospital, Dubai, UAE

Sumi Dey and Sabrina L. Noyes
Spectrum Health, Department of Urology, Grand Rapids, MI, USA

Ghayas Uddin
Spectrum Health, Department of Pathology, MI, USA

Brian R. Lane
Michigan State University College of Human Medicine, Grand Rapids, MI, USA

David G. Jackson
Department of Surgery, University of Miami Miller School of Medicine, USA

Phillipe Abreu
Multi-Organ Transplant Program, University of Toronto, Canada

Manuel Anthony Moutinho and Antonio Marttos
Ryder Trauma Center, Jackson Memorial Hospital, University of Miami Miller School of Medicine, USA

George W. Burke III and Gaetano Ciancio
Miami Transplant Institute, Jackson Memorial Hospital, University of Miami Miller School of Medicine, USA

Nicholas Namias
Ryder Trauma Center, Jackson Memorial Hospital, University of Miami Miller School of Medicine, USA
Miami Transplant Institute, Jackson Memorial Hospital, University of Miami Miller School of Medicine, USA

Bela Tallai, Tawiz Gul Gulistan, Maged Nasser Aa B. Alrayashi, Hatem Mostari Kamkoum, Mohamed Ali A. Ebrahim, Mohamed Abdelkarim Ali Abdelkarim and Morshed Ali Salah
Urology Division of Surgery Department, Hazm Mebaireek General Hospital, Hamad Medical Corporation, Industrial Area Street No. 33, Doha, Qatar

Salah Abdulhabeb Abdulwali Al Mughalles
Clinical Imaging Department, Hazm Mebaireek General Hospital, Hamad Medical Corporation, Industrial Area Street No. 33, Doha, Qatar

Amal Fekkar, Kaoutar Znati, Fouad Zouaidia, Hafsa Elouazzani, Zakia Bernoussi and Ahmed Jahid
Department of Pathology, Ibn Sina University Hospital Center, Rabat, Morocco

Abhishek Bhat, Bruno Nahar, Vivek Venkatramani and Indraneel Banerjee
Department of Urology, University of Miami Miller School of Medicine, Miami, FL, USA

Oleksandr N. Kryvenko
Department of Urology, University of Miami Miller School of Medicine, Miami, FL, USA
Department of Pathology and Laboratory Medicine, University of Miami Miller School of Medicine, Miami, FL, USA
Sylvester Comprehensive Cancer Center, University of Miami Miller School of Medicine, Miami, FL, USA

Dipen J. Parekh
Sylvester Comprehensive Cancer Center, University of Miami Miller School of Medicine, Miami, FL, USA

Zeynep G. Gul, Christine W. Liaw, Avinash Reddy and Reza Mehrazin
Department of Urology, Icahn School of Medicine at Mount Sinai, New York, NY, USA

Yuichi Machida and Junji Uchida
Department of Urology, Osaka Metropolitan University Graduate School of Medicine, 1-4-3 Asahi-machi, Abeno-ku, Osaka 545-8585, Japan

Hiroki Yoshiuchi, Yuko Kitano, Yoshikazu Kuroki and Masato Kamizuru
Department of Urology, Yao Municipal Hospital, 1-3-1, Ryuge-cho, Yao-City, Osaka 581-0069, Japan

Hamza Dergamoun, Abdelilah El Alaoui, Imad Boualaoui, Hachem Sayegh, Lounis Benslimane and Yassine Nouini
Department of Urology A, Ibn Sina Hospital, Mohammed V University, Rabat, Morocco

Honoka Fuse, Masaya Ito, Kosuke Takemura, Madoka Kataoka and Fumitaka Koga
Department of Urology, Tokyo Metropolitan Cancer and Infectious Diseases Center Komagome Hospital, Tokyo, Japan

Shuzo Ikuta
Department of Radiology, Tokyo Metropolitan Cancer and Infectious Diseases Center Komagome Hospital, Tokyo, Japan

Toru Motoi
Department of Pathology, Tokyo Metropolitan Cancer and Infectious Diseases Center Komagome Hospital, Tokyo, Japan

Tomotake Okuma
Department of Musculoskeletal Oncology, Tokyo Metropolitan Cancer and Infectious Diseases Center Komagome Hospital, Tokyo, Japan

Serozsha Goonewardena, Umesh Jayarajah, Sanka Nalinda Kuruppu and Manoj Hilary Fernando
Department of Urology, National Hospital of Sri Lanka, Colombo, Sri Lanka

Fayez T. Hammad
College of Medicine and Health Sciences, United Arab Emirates University and Mediclinic Al Ain, Al Ain, UAE

Constantinos D. Georgakopoulos, Athina Pallikari, Panagiotis Plotas and Olga E. Makri
Department of Ophthalmology, Medical School, University of Patras, Rio, 265 04 Patras, Greece

Supun De Silva and Lalani De Silva
Postgraduate Institute of Medicine, University of Colombo, Sri Lanka

Susantha De Silva
Urology Unit 02, National Hospital of Sri Lanka, Colombo, Sri Lanka

Priyani Amarathunga
Department of Pathology, Faculty of Medicine, University of Colombo, Sri Lanka

Ryan S. Chiang
Department of Medicine, Stanford University Medical Center, Stanford, CA, USA

Ashton A. Connor and Aparna S. Rege
Division of Abdominal Transplant Surgery, Department of Surgery, Duke University School of Medicine, Durham, NC, USA

Brant A. Inman
Division of Urology, Department of Surgery, Duke University School of Medicine, Durham, NC, USA

Wen-Chi Foo, David N. Howell and John F. Madden
Department of Pathology, Duke University School of Medicine, Durham, NC, USA

Matthew J. Ellis
Divisions of Nephrology and Abdominal Transplant, Departments of Medicine and Surgery, Duke University School of Medicine, Durham, NC, USA

Michael R. Harrison
Division of Medical Oncology, Department of Medicine, Duke University School of Medicine, Durham, NC, USA

Prem Raj Sigdel, Diwas Gnyawali, Purushottam Parajuli, Sampanna Chudal, Durga Pandit, Bipin Guragain, Manish Man Pradhan, Sujeet Poudyal, Suman Chapagain, Bhoj Raj Luitel, Pawan Raj Chalise and Uttam Kumar Sharma
Department of Urology and Kidney Transplant Surgery, Tribhuvan University Teaching Hospital, Institute of Medicine, Maharajgunj, Kathmandu 44600, Nepal

Senthil G. Kamaraj
Consultant Paediatric Urologist, Kanchi Kamakoti Child's Trust Hospital, 12-A, Nageswara Road, Nungambakkam, Chennai 600034, India

Ashita Kochunny
Registrar in Paediatric Surgery, Kanchi Kamakoti Child's Trust Hospital, India

Gopinathan Kathirvelu
Consultant Radiologist, Kanchi Kamakoti Child's Trust Hospital, India

Praachi Singh
Registrar in Paediatrics, Kanchi Kamakoti Child's Trust Hospital, India

Naeem Samnakay
Clinical Associate Professor, University of Western Australia, Paediatric Urologist, Perth Children's Hospital, 12 Hospital Ave, Nedlands, WA 6009, Australia

Mitsuo Ofude, Ryunosuke Nakagawa, Satoko Urata, Tohru Miyagi and Takao Nakashima
Department of Urology, Ishikawa Prefectural Central Hospital, 2-1 Kuratsukihigashi, Kanazawa, Ishikawa, Japan

Hiroshi Minato
Department of Diagnostic Pathology, Ishikawa Prefectural Central Hospital, 2-1 Kuratsukihigashi, Kanazawa, Ishikawa, Japan

Idriss Ziani, Imad Boualaoui, Ahmed Ibrahimi, Hachem El Sayegh, Lounis Benslimane and Yassine Nouini
Department of Urological Surgery A, University Hospital of Rabat, Rabat, Morocco
Faculty of Medicine-Mohammed V University RABAT, Morocco

Chonlada Krutsri, Pongsasit Singhatas, Preeda Sumpritpradit and Tharin Thampongsa
Division of Trauma Surgery and Surgical Critical Care, Department of Surgery, Faculty of Medicine, Ramathibodi Hospital, Mahidol University, Bangkok, Thailand

Chunlaches Chaijareenont
Department of Surgery, Faculty of Medicine, Ramathibodi Hospital, Mahidol University, Bangkok, Thailand

Wit Viseshsindh
Division of Urology, Department of Surgery, Faculty of Medicine, Ramathibodi Hospital, Mahidol University, Bangkok, Thailand

Pattawia Choikrua
Surgical Research Unit, Faculty of Medicine, Ramathibodi Hospital, Mahidol University, Bangkok, Thailand

David Zekan, Kareem Wasef, Zachary Werner, Adam Luchey and Ali Hajiran
West Virginia University Department of Urology, 1 Medical Center Drive, Morgantown, WV 26506, USA

Robert Grammer and Cara Lombard
West Virginia University Department of Radiology, 1 Medical Center Drive, Morgantown, WV 26506, USA

Mahmoud Abuelnaga, Sadegh Khoshzaban and Aasem Chaudry
Department of Urology, Bedford Hospital NHS Trust, Bedford, UK

Mahmoud Reda Badr
Department of Urology, Ain Shams University Hospitals, Cairo, Egypt

Osamah Hasan
Midwestern University Chicago College of Osteopathic Medicine, Downers Grove, IL, USA

Matthew Houlihan and Tobias S. Kohler
Department of Urology, Mayo Clinic, Rochester, MN, USA

Courtney M. P. Hollowell
Division of Urology, Cook County Health and Hospitals System, Chicago, IL, USA

Masresha S. Dino and Seid M. Hassen
Department of Surgery, Urology Unit, Addis Ababa, St. Paul's Hospital Millennium Medical College, Ethiopia

Tesfaye H. Tufa
Department of Obstetrics and Gynecology, St. Paul's Hospital Millennium Medical College, Addis Ababa, Ethiopia

Hiroki Hagimoto, Takeshi Sano, Soki Kashima, Takayuki Yoshino, Takayuki Goto, Atsuro Sawada, Shusuke Akamatsu, Toshinari Yamasaki, Takashi Kobayashi and Osamu Ogawa
The Department of Urology, Kyoto University Hospital, Japan

Masakazu Fujimoto
The Department of Diagnostic Pathology, Kyoto University Hospital, Japan

Yoichiro Kajita
Kajita Urological Clinic, Japan

Mohamed Ali Nouioui, Ahmed Saadi, Marouene Chakroun, Amine Oueslati, Abderrazak Bouzouita, Amine Derouiche, Mohamed Riadh Ben Slama, Haroun Ayed and Mohamed Chebil
Department of Urology, Charles Nicolle Hospital of Tunis, University of Tunis El Manar, Tunisia

Meriem Ksentini and Soumaya Rammeh
Department of Pathology, Charles Nicolle Hospital of Tunis, University of Tunis El Manar, Tunisia

Prodromos Philippou and Maria Miliatou
St George's Medical School, University of Nicosia, Nicosia, Cyprus
Apollonion Hospital, Nicosia, Cyprus

Anastasios Michalakis
251 Airforce Hospital, Athens, Greece

Christiana Poullou and Pavlos Constantinou
Histopathology and Cytology Laboratory Services, Nicosia, Cyprus
School of Medicine, European University of Cyprus, Cyprus

Khalil Chalhoub, Rawad Abou Zahr and Michel Jabbour
University of Balamand, Saint George Hospital University Medical Center, Department of Urology, Beirut 1100 2807, Lebanon

Elias Mansour
University of Balamand, Faculty of Medicine and Medical Sciences, Beirut 1100 2807, Lebanon

Mona Aoun
University of Balamand, Saint George Hospital University Medical Center, Department of Pathology, Beirut 1100 2807, Lebanon

Index